IE

The White Labyrinth

A Foreign Policy Research Institute Book

This book is part of a series of works sponsored by the
Foreign Policy Research Institute in Philadelphia.
Founded in 1955, the Institute is an independent, nonprofit
organization devoted to research on issues affecting
the interest of the United States.

THE WHITE LABYRINTH

Cocaine and Political Power

Rensselaer W. Lee III

Transaction Publishers
New Brunswick (U.S.A.) and London (U.K.)

Second printing 1990
Copyright (c) 1989 by Transaction Publishers,
New Brunswick, New Jersey 08903

Library of Congress Catalog Number: 88-36845
ISBN: 0-88738-285-1
Printed in the United States of America

Library of Congress Cataloging-in-Publication Data
Lee, Rensselaer W. (Rensselaer Wright) III, 1937
    The white labyrinth : cocaine trafficking and political power in the
Andean Countries / Rensselaer W. Lee, III.
        p. cm.
    "A Foreign Policy Research Institute book."
    Bibliography: p.
    Includes index.
    ISBN 0-88738-285-1
    1. Cocaine industry—Andes Region. 2. Corruption (in politics)—
Andes   Region. 3. Andes   Region—Politics   and   govern-
ment. 4. Narcotics, Control of—United States. I. Title
HV5840.A5L44   1989
363.4'5'098—dc19   88-36845
                                                           CIP

Contents

Figures and Tables

Figures and Tables

Acknowledgments

This volume presents the results of a study of the South American cocaine industry as it has evolved in the 1980s. Research for the study emphasized a survey of Spanish-language materials, but also drew extensively from U.S. journalistic sources, U.S. government reports (including internal cables and memoranda), transcripts of Congressional hearings, and the writings of other scholars who have examined the narcotics trafficking problem.

Research for the study also relied on several field trips to Colombia, Bolivia, and Peru between February 1986 and October 1988. The author is grateful for information and insights provided by South American government officials, especially representatives of the following organizations:

- The Ministry of Interior in Peru
- Peru's National Coca Enterprise (ENACO)
- The Project for Coca Reduction in the Upper Huallaga (CORAH)
- The Special Project for the Upper Huallaga (PEAH)
- The Peruvian Directorate of Anti-Drug Police (DIPOD)
- The Peruvian National Senate
- The Ministries of Finance and Interior in Bolivia
- The Bolivian Sub-Secretariat for Social Defense
- The Bolivian Sub-Secretariat for Alternative Development and Substitution of Coca
- The Secretariat for Development of the Bolivian Tropics
- The Ministry of Justice in Colombia
- The Colombian National Anti-Narcotics Command (CONAN)
- Colombia's Banco de la República
- Colombia's Institute for the Development of Renewable Resources (INDERENA).

The author also interviewed Colombian, Bolivian, and Peruvian business-men, writers, academics, and other private citizens who are knowledgeable about different aspects of the cocaine trade.

The author owes special thanks to the overseas representatives of the State Department's Bureau of International Narcotics Matters (INM), the U.S. Drug Enforcement Agency (DEA), and the U.S. Agency for International Development (AID). These officials provided an understanding of the complex organization and operations of the international cocaine traffic and furnished invaluable background information on U.S. antinarcotics programs in the Andean countries. These officials are to be commended for their exceptional courage, ingenuity, and tenacity in waging what is obviously an uphill battle against the cocaine trade. Officials of the political, economic, and press sections of U.S. embassies in these countries also contributed in important ways to the research for this study. The extensive files of newspaper clippings maintained by the press sections in Bogotá and La Paz constituted perhaps the most important single resource used in the project.

The H. John Heinz Fund of the Pittsburgh Foundation supplied financial support for the book. The Foreign Policy Research Institute (FPRI) in Philadelphia, Pennsylvania, served as the institutional sponsor for the project. The views expressed in the study are those of the author and should not be ascribed to the Pittsburgh Foundation, FPRI, or any other institution.

The author wishes to express his appreciation to Marcie Walsh, Nan Nida, Paul Haber, and Dan Zeiger, who assisted with the research. A special debt of gratitude is owed to Sallie Chafer, without whose editorial, production, and logistical support this book would never have come into being.

Preface

In recent years, the abuse and control of illicit narcotics have come to pervade U.S. relations with the Third World. The drug issue is a source of conflict and mutual recrimination between North and South. The main consumer countries are rich and industrialized; the main drug-producing countries are poor and predominantly agricultural. The drug trade generates an annual transfer of billions of dollars from North to South and has gained a powerful economic foothold in some Third World countries. Producing countries and consuming countries blame each other for the accelerating drug traffic and advocate, respectively, demand-side and supply-side solutions. U.S. programs to control drug cultivation and production overseas often engender nationalist resentment. Moreover, political elites in some Third World countries view antidrug crusades as imposing significant economic and social costs and as creating new and formidable political challenges.

The cocaine traffic in the Western Hemisphere constitutes a particularly severe manifestation of the North-South conflict over drugs. U.S. concerns over cocaine are fairly clear-cut. Although U.S. imports of heroin and marijuana remained roughly stable from 1977 to 1987, imports of cocaine apparently increased five- to ten-fold during that time. Traffickers are "literally just throwing it at our shores," in the words of the U.S. Commissioner of Customs.[1] Abuse of cocaine and its derivative "crack"— a highly toxic and addictive substance—has become a fairly serious U.S. public health problem. According to data from the Drug Abuse Warning Network, cocaine overdoses were the main cause of 46,331 hospital emergency cases and 1,696 deaths in 1987; in contrast, in 1980, the corresponding figures were, respectively, 4,154 and 250. "Cocaine wars" among rival gangs of dealers have raised the murder rate and lowered the quality of life in Washington, New York, Miami, and other U.S. cities.

xiii

The United States expends considerable diplomatic energy on pressing Colombia, Bolivia, and Peru—the major countries producing cocaine—to curb illicit drug cultivation and refining. The United States also provides funding, technical assistance, and personnel for narcotics control programs in the three countries; such arrangements total about $50–$60 million annually. In addition, since 1983, the U.S. Congress has increasingly linked foreign aid to performance in narcotics control. Countries that do not take adequate steps to control illicit drug production, trafficking, and money laundering can lose certain specified economic and military assistance and trade preferences, such as sugar quotas or Caribbean Initiative benefits.

Supply-side approaches, however, have obviously failed to stem the flow of cocaine into U.S. markets. Latin American governments lack the resources to counter the traffic: There is no correspondence between the resources available to cocaine traffickers and the resources available to combat them. Perhaps more important, however, governments and important constituencies in the main producing countries do not give the war against cocaine their unconditional support. This is true even though the cocaine traffic in many respects damages the source countries—rampant corruption, rising numbers of drug addicts, escalating levels of violence, declining moral standards, and a deteriorating national image are among the more obvious consequences. The reasons for this Latin American reticence are complex and are detailed in the following chapters. Several points, however, deserve mention at the outset.

First, moving against the cocaine traffic entails serious economic and political costs. Narco-dollars have represented a relatively important source of foreign exchange for Andean countries, as traditional sources—foreign investment, bank loans, and earnings from Andean exports such as oil, gas, copper, and fishmeal—have contracted. The cocaine industry is an important source of jobs and income in regions characterized by desperate poverty and widespread unemployment. An estimated 500,000 to one million people are employed directly in the upstream and downstream phases of the industry—cultivation, initial processing, refining, and smuggling. Coca farmers receive less than one percent of the final street value of their crop—that is, the equivalent value of refined cocaine sold to consumers in industrialized countries—yet, they typically earn several times the income they would receive from growing alternative crops such as cacao, oranges, and coffee. All along the cocaine production-logistics chain, people receive substantially higher wages than they would in the licit economy.

Second, the cocaine industry as a whole has accumulated significant political clout. Coca farmers are numerous and well organized; in Bolivia, national labor and campesino organizations provide direct political support to farmers. Cocaine traffickers play the role of power brokers and are a major source of funding for political campaigns. Traffickers also have penetrated and corrupted nearly every important national institution: police forces, military establishments, legislatures, key government ministries, the judiciary, the church, and the news media. Some cocaine traffickers exhibit a rudimentary sense of social responsibility—a critically important development that enabled them to build a popular following by sponsoring public works and welfare projects that benefit the urban and rural poor.

Third, the war on cocaine is not especially popular in South America—it is perceived as a program imposed on South America by the United States. Certain U.S.-initiated measures—such as extradition, the spraying of illicit crops, U.S. military intervention against cocaine laboratories, and economic sanctions against cocaine-exporting countries—have provoked considerable anti-Yankee sentiment. Furthermore, most Latin American leaders see the supply-side approach to drug control as fundamentally flawed: In the Latin American view, demand, not supply, drives the international drug traffic. Says Peru's Alan García: "I have always thought of drug trafficking as the final stage of capitalist consumerism. The problem does not lie in the fact that a poor town produces coca leaves in the Peruvian jungle. The basic problem lies in the world's big consumer markets consisting of the richest societies."[2]

This is not to say that the drug war in South America is totally useless. It at least limits the inroads that traffickers can make into the political system. Today, it is significantly harder than it was in the early 1980s for cocaine dealers to run for political office, to form "nationalist" political parties, and to occupy cabinet-level positions. Yet, limiting the more outrageous political manifestations of the cocaine trade is not the same as curbing exports of cocaine from South America. On this count, U.S. programs and those of the Andean countries themselves have largely failed.

This book was not written as a polemic against supply-side approaches to drug control. However, the research and interviews conducted by the author and subsequent analyses lead inevitably to several conclusions that advocates of supply-side programs will find discouraging. First, the cocaine trade has altered irrevocably the economic and political landscape of the Andean countries. Cocaine traffickers constitute an interest group with extensive resources and political connections, just like the coffee barons in Colombia or the mining elites in Peru and Bolivia. Indeed, studies of these countries' development patterns, decisionmaking processes, and relations with other countries are no longer possible without reference to coca and cocaine.

Second, the drug war in South American source countries presents difficult if not unmanageable problems for both South American governments and the U.S. government. The drug war requires that Andean countries address a host of obstacles, such as national economic dependence on drugs, powerful narcotics lobbies, indifferent or hostile publics, weak political structures, and porous systems of criminal justice. In addition, other compelling U.S. interests in the region—such as promoting economic stability, preserving democracy, or preventing the emergence of Marxist regimes—are not necessarily compatible with aggressive drug control programs.

Third, even with significant U.S. help, Andean governments will make little progress in controlling cocaine production. Eradication campaigns, occasional large drug busts, and a few major arrests (like the highly publicized arrests of Carlos Lehder in Colombia and Roberto Suarez in Bolivia) will continue in the Andean countries. Nonetheless, the basic structure of the cocaine industry—its agricultural base, manufacturing infrastructure, leadership, smuggling networks, and so on—will remain more or less intact. The corollary: Victory in the war against cocaine cannot be won in the jungles, shanty towns, and trafficking capitals of South American countries; only when Americans decide that they will no longer be the drug lords' customers will the industry collapse.

Notes

1. Joel Brinkley, "Experts See U.S. Cocaine Problem as Continuing Despite Anti-Drug Raids," *The New York Times,* August 23, 1986, p. 26.
2. "President García Grants Interview to TV Latina," Panama City Panavision, July 5, 1987.

Introduction

Policy Issues

U.S. foreign policy toward Latin America during the 1980s can genuinely be characterized as drug diplomacy. Once an issue far out of the diplomatic mainstream, narcotics control has become a vital component of U.S. relations with countries such as Bolivia, Peru, Colombia, Mexico, Jamaica, and Panama. Controlling drug production and exports officially carries the highest U.S. diplomatic priority in Colombia and one of the top two or three such priorities in Bolivia and Peru. The United States allocates economic aid accordingly: Narcotics-related assistance rose from 30 percent of all U.S. aid to Colombia in fiscal year 1984 (FY 1984) to more than 90 percent in FY 1988.[1] Moreover, Congress now ties foreign aid to measurements of recipient countries' drug control efforts. For instance, in 1986 and 1987, the United States withheld $17.4 million in aid from Bolivia, primarily because coca crop-eradication targets were not met.[2]

Drug diplomacy, however, is largely a region-specific tool: The United States never seriously threatened to cut off economic and military aid to Pakistan (the world's largest heroin producer) or to stop supplying Stinger missiles to the Afghan freedom fighters (who cultivate opium extensively). The United States can pressure Latin America more intensely about drug policies in part because the region does not abut the major communist powers. A more important reason is that Latin America supplies most of the marijuana, about 40 percent of the heroin, and all of the cocaine entering U.S. markets.[3] Cocaine represents the biggest concern—the war against cocaine now consumes the bulk of the federal government's drug-fighting resources. Public and Congressional outrage over the U.S. cocaine epidemic—there are an estimated six million regular users of the toxic and highly addictive drug—has prompted Congress to expand its role in foreign

1

policymaking and has altered, perhaps irrevocably, the shape of American diplomacy in the Western Hemisphere. Replying to criticism that the United States was scapegoating the region, a member of the House Committee on Foreign Affairs staff notes, "We have focused more on Latin America, because cocaine has been more of an issue."[4]

This study profiles the South American cocaine industry, describing the industry's economic dimensions, its search for power and legitimacy, its place on the political spectrum, and the challenges that it poses to U.S. policy. The industry is a powerful antagonist—largely because it has cultivated extensive ties with the existing power structures in the Andean countries. Several conclusions are highlighted below.

- Although an inefficient engine of economic growth, the cocaine industry serves as an important source of jobs, income, and foreign exchange. The industry compensates for the failings of formal economies, especially in Peru and Bolivia.
- Powerful and politically articulate constituencies have developed around the cocaine industry in both its upstream (agricultural) and downstream (processing and distribution) phases. Coca farmers are blocking eradication programs in Peru and Bolivia, and cocaine syndicates are using their massive financial and logistical resources to undermine criminal justice systems and to buy a share of political power.
- In its higher value-added stages, the cocaine industry has little in common with the revolutionary left. Marxist insurgents have gained a foothold among the coca-growing peasantry, but large trafficking organizations remain generally hostile to guerrillas and to the left. Indeed, informal anticommunist alliances have developed among cocaine dealers, right-wing military officers, and large landowners, especially in Colombia.
- Andean governments cannot muster the resources, strategic reach, and political clout to confront the cocaine industry. Furthermore, governments do not view the industry as a serious threat to their own survival. In Colombia and Peru, left-wing guerrillas are the principal enemy, and the war against drugs conflicts in part with counterinsurgency efforts. Andean leaders also fear that a successful crackdown on drugs would destabilize the economy and breed new and lethal political challenges.

Three policy implications follow from the above conclusions. First, U.S. interests in cutting the supply of cocaine are not necessarily compatible with the interests of the producer nations. Second, U.S. drug diplomacy as currently practiced probably will exacerbate tensions in U.S.-Latin American relations. Third, the marginal impact of expanding supply-side programs is likely to be low. U.S. narcotics assistance programs are admittedly poorly funded—the $50–$60 million that the United States spends annually in Colombia, Peru, and Bolivia compares rather unfavorably with the $5–$6 billion that South American cocaine dealers earn each year. However, political, economic, and law enforcement conditions do not warrant massive infusions of U.S. aid, which probably would be wasted. (Moreover, given current U.S. budget deficits, Congress would be unlikely to allocate the additional funds.) The solution, if there is one, lies not in the Andean jungles but in the United States: The six million people who now consume cocaine must be persuaded to change their habits and preferences.

Economic Pressures

Each year, South American drug traffickers earn an estimated $5 billion to $6 billion by selling cocaine in international markets.[5] Most of this money stays abroad, stashed in offshore tax havens such as Panama and the Cayman Islands or invested in foreign real estate, securities, and businesses. (The Medellín syndicates alone reputedly have at least $10 billion worth of fixed and liquid assets in North America, Europe, and Asia.) Some drug earnings are spent on imported inputs for the cocaine industry—for example, chemicals, raw materials, aircraft, microwave ovens, and weapons. However, as much as $2 billion returns annually to the principal cocaine-producing countries—Colombia, Bolivia, and Peru. Measured in repatriated dollars, cocaine exports equal an estimated 10–20 percent ($500 million to $1 billion) of Colombia's legal 1987 exports, 25–30 percent ($600 million to $700 million) of Peru's, and 50–100 percent ($250 million to $450 million) of Bolivia's.[6]

Although theoretically dedicated to combatting the drug traffic, Andean governments have not discouraged the inflow of narco-dollars. As an official at Colombia's Banco de la República remarked in an April 1986 interview, "Why should we drive all this money into the black market and into foreign banks?" In Colombia, tax amnesties were declared at the beginning of the last four presidential administrations—those of Lopez-Michelsen, Turbay, Betancur, and Barco. In Peru and Bolivia, traffickers who repatriate dollars are by government decree protected from tax penalties and to some extent from criminal investigation. In Peru, the government overvalued the local currency (the INTI) and set high INTI interest rates for depositers, apparently trying to attract additional cocaine dollars and to keep them in Peru. Peruvian banking officials make no secret of their view that cocaine dollars partially substitute for the foreign investment and bank loans that traditionally have spearheaded Peru's economic growth.[7] Such traditional sources, of course, have virtually dried up in recent years, largely in response to Peru's nationalistic economic policies.

Large infusions of dollars from any source are important to poor countries such as Colombia, Bolivia, and Peru. Drug dollars stabilize the currency, help finance needed exports, stimulate some industries, and create pockets of prosperity. Some benefits accrue to specific localities. For example, in 1975, the city of Medellín (the administrative center of most of Colombia's drug trade) accounted for 10 percent of the new building permits issued in Colombia. By 1986, Medellín's share had risen to 23 percent. Between September 1979 and September 1986, the ratio of bank deposits in Medellín to total national bank deposits rose by 29 percent.[8] Yet, the cocaine industry conveys an overwhelming impression of conspicuous waste. The drug earnings are not converted efficiently into national economic growth. Some proportion of cocaine traffickers' earnings is recycled directly into buying factors of production (chemicals, raw materials, equipment, labor), building clandestine airstrips, and arranging transportation. Creating a secure climate for business operations consumes perhaps 10–20 percent of all operating funds. These funds underwrite the purchase of weapons and private security forces, information networks, bribes to law enforcement officials, contributions to political campaigns, and "war taxes" paid to guerrilla groups.

Conspicuous consumption constitutes another hallmark of the cocaine industry in both upstream and downstream phases. The coca boom has brought modern consumer life styles to remote jungle towns. However, because governments have no power to tax the coca trade, these towns lack the most elementary public services—paved streets, drinking water, sanitation systems, and decent schools. In South American cities such as Medellín, Colombia, and Santa Cruz, Bolivia, cocaine capos flaunt ostentatious life styles, buying luxury high-rise apartment buildings, Mercedes Benzes and BMWs, helicopters, and antiques.[9] Much of this consumer spending leaves or never enters the economies of cocaine-exporting countries.

At the same time, some drug money does contribute to economic growth, but in an unbalanced fashion. Most investments are made in agriculture and services rather than in traditional extraction and manufacturing industries and infrastructure projects. For example, the Rodríguez Orejuela and Santa Cruz families assembled an extensive business empire in Cali that includes—or did include until recently—banks, construction companies, pharmaceutical companies, sports clubs, private security companies, automobile dealerships, 28 radio stations, and two higher educational institutions. Several Medellín-based traffickers—Gonzalo Rodríguez Gacha, Pablo Escobar, and the Ochoa clan—own cattle ranches, dairy farms, and horse ranches. Escobar and his wife have 96 registered pieces of property in the city of Medellín alone, including 16 residences in Medellín's El Poblado district. Nearly all of these homes are outfitted with heliports. In Bolivia, where the cocaine mafia is largely coterminous with the rural elite, traffickers plow their drug profits into expanding herds, cross-breeding cattle, or improving cotton and sugar cane yields. Characteristic investments by major drug capos also include executive air transport services (which may or may not be used for drug trafficking), restaurants, and resort hotels (especially hotels on Colombia's Caribbean coast and on San Andres Island).[10]

Drug traffickers in South America, Jamaica, and Honduras also invest some of their profits on social welfare activities, earning themselves a significant popular following. Pablo Escobar, for example, built 450 to 500 two-bedroom cement-block houses in a Medellín slum now renamed the "Barrio Pablo Escobar." Escobar also financed many other Medellín projects—sewer repair, educational facilities, clinics, and sports plazas. In addition, he reputedly donated a church to the town of Doradal in the Middle Magdalena Valley, about 180 kilometers (km) from Medellín. Carlos Lehder organized and funded a major earthquake relief effort in the city of Popayan and also built a housing project for the poor in his native Armenia. Gonzalo Rodríguez Gacha donated an outdoor basketball court to his home town of Pacho (in Cundinamarca) and repaired the facade of Pacho's town hall. In Bolivia, the "King of Cocaine," Roberto Suarez, paved streets, restored churches, and donated sewing machines to poor women in his Beni home town of Santa Ana de Yacuma. Moreover, Suarez reportedly provided college scholarships for needy students in the Beni region.[11]

The relation between drug dollars and economic growth is by no means clear. Most narco-dollars probably are banked or invested abroad, and traffickers' domestic spending priorities certainly do not coincide with those of national economic planners. Core economic activities such as mining, manufacturing, and commercial transport seem to be short-changed. Some scholars argue that coca cultivation diverts land and labor from traditional agriculture and thus reduces food production, although food production elsewhere in the country may increase in response.[12] Because of its status as a renegade industry, the cocaine sector probably will not catalyze the economic take-off of the Andean countries. However, the industry does generate important economic effects, briefly noted below.

First, even apparently unproductive expenditures create numerous economic linkages—multiplier effects—that stimulate the economy. For example, traffickers' demand for luxury housing boosts the business of building contractors and, indirectly, domestic producers of construction materials such as cement, bricks, and glass. (This pattern has been especially pronounced in Colombia.) Local industrialists may have built new manufacturing capacity to accommodate the cocaine industry's demand for farm equipment, simple chemicals, filters, centrifuges, and other tools of the trade. Many banks, law firms, and accounting firms apparently specialize in goods and services for cocaine syndicates. In short, the cocaine trade creates reciprocal patterns of economic activity elsewhere in the economy, and these interactions over time can facilitate economic growth in Colombia, Bolivia, and Peru.

Second, the cocaine industry, especially in Peru and Bolivia, serves as an important economic safety valve, providing income, jobs, and foreign exchange when the formal economy falters. For example, according to the Bolivian government's "Triennial Program for the Battle Against Drug Trafficking" document, the official unemployment rate more than tripled from 1980 to 1986 (from 5.7 percent to 20 percent), but so did the number of families reportedly growing coca. During 1986, more than 20,000 Bolivian miners lost their jobs, and as many as 5,000 may have sought work in the coca fields. As Bolivian President Victor Paz Estenssoro noted, cocaine "has gained an importance in our economy in direct proportion to the shrinking of the formal economy."[13] Cocaine exports can compensate for the loss of foreign exchange from traditional sources. For example, from 1983 to 1987, Bolivia's licit exports shrank by 38 percent and Peru's by 15 percent, primarily because world prices for traditional Andean commodities—oil, natural gas, and tin—declined precipitously over the same period.[14] Cocaine export income also replaces international loans to Peru and Bolivia, which are no longer creditworthy in the eyes of commercial bankers. (In fact, Peru receives few if any international loans from any source.)

Third, the cocaine industry directly employs hundreds of thousands of people in the Andean region. Approximately 500,000 to 600,000 people, largely in Peru and Bolivia, cultivate and harvest coca leaves. Tens of thousands more work in the downstream phases: macerating coca leaves, building maceration pits, buying and selling leaves or paste, refining and smuggling cocaine, building clandestine airstrips, and smuggling precursor chemicals (i.e., chemicals used to convert coca into cocaine). An estimated 350,000 Bolivians, more than 5 percent of that country's total population, work directly in one phase or another of the trafficking cycle.[15] Such activity is not necessarily a full-time occupation; in Bolivia, for example, some farmers cultivate coca in the Chapare during the summer months and farm their traditional plots in the Upper Cochabamba Valley during the winter. Nonetheless, coca cultivation may constitute the margin between subsistence and a decent standard of living. Furthermore, the multiplier effects of the industry generate substantial indirect employment—many people make a living by selling goods and services to coca growers and cocaine traffickers.

Obviously, the cocaine industry has an extensive foothold in the Andean economies. If the industry shut down tomorrow, economic and political chaos would reign in Bolivia and Peru and possibly in Colombia as well. At the same time, the industry has spawned powerful and politically articulate constituencies. Farmers defend their right to cultivate coca, and cocaine dealers employ comprehensive protection strategies—a range of subtle and not-so-subtle influences over criminal justice systems.

The Politics of Cocaine

The Coca Lobby

The cocaine industry also has amassed significant political clout in the Andean countries because of the industry's large popular base in the upstream phases and its enormous financial and logistical capabilities in the downstream phases. Farmers who cultivate illicit coca—the most visible cocaine constituency—are highly organized, sometimes well-armed, and capable of exerting tremendous pressure on governments.

In Peru's Upper Huallaga Valley, where more than 90 percent of farm income stems from coca cultivation, coca farmers are represented by provincial and district self-defense fronts (FEDIPs). FEDIPs are heavily influenced by the political left (the Izquierda Unida) and also receive support from the Sendero Luminoso (Shining Path) and Tupac Amaru guerrilla movements.[16] FEDIPs lobby for the legalization of coca cultivation and challenge government eradication teams with strikes, roadblocks, and other forms of mass violence. Because of coca growers' opposition and security problems, a U.S.-Peruvian eradication project in the Valley ground to a virtual halt in 1987. That year, only 355 hectares were destroyed, compared to 2,575 in 1986 and 4,830 in 1985.[17] In 1988, the total increased to 5,130 hectares, primarily because eradication teams cut down coca bushes instead of uprooting them. The trouble with cutting down plants is that they grow back and can be in full production again in 18 months. Unless Peru can proceed with an aerial spraying program—and to date there is no demonstrably safe and effective herbicide against coca—control of coca cultivation in the Upper Huallaga is most likely a lost cause.

In Bolivia, the dynamics look even worse: An estimated 70,000 coca-growing families (organized in 10 regional federations in the Yungas and the Chapare) receive direct political support from national mass member-ship organizations—the 1.3-million-member Bolivian Workers Congress and its main affiliate, the Confederation of Bolivian Peasant Workers. In a country of only 6.4 million people, such support constitutes a significant deterrent to narcotics control programs.[18] U.S.-Bolivian attempts to pres-sure coca farmers by destroying crops or by regulating the sale of coca leaves trigger organized resistance on a national scale. The Bolivian coca lobby has the power to shut down parts of Bolivia's fragile transportation system. For example, coca farmers and their worker-peasant allies have sealed off Cochabamba, Bolivia's third largest city, four times since 1983 to protest several anti-coca policies of the Bolivian government. Bolivia did eradicate slightly more than 1,000 hectares of coca in 1987, but only by undertaking a complex process of bargaining with federations and individual syndicates and by paying peasants $2,000 for each hectare eradicated.[19] Involuntary eradication on any significant scale is probably a political impossibility in Bolivia.

Trafficking Syndicates

The criminal syndicates that refine, smuggle, and distribute cocaine are equally important in the political scheme of things and overwhelmingly important in Colombia. The South American cocaine trade displays vary-ing degrees of concentration. For example, five loosely organized syndi-cates headquartered in Medellín and Cali control an estimated 70–80 percent of the cocaine exported from Colombia and about 60–70 percent of all cocaine sold in the United States.[20] Bolivia's cocaine trade is controlled by some 12-to 25 families; most of them run cattle ranches or commercial farms in the Beni, Cochabamba, and Santa Cruz regions.[21] In Peru, on the other hand, the industry is highly fragmented and disorgan-ized and, to a large extent, dominated by Colombian traffickers.

Colombia is clearly the linchpin—the *país clave*—of the South American cocaine industry. The Medellín-Cali syndicates procure raw materials in Peru and Bolivia, manufacture refined cocaine in Colombia, ship cocaine in large loads of 300 kilograms (kilos) or more to the United States, and wholesale the cocaine in smaller lots within the United States. The big Colombian syndicates do not form a cartel in the sense of being able to maintain prices (cocaine wholesale prices in the United States dropped from $55,000 per kilo in 1980 to $15,000 in mid-1988). These syndicates probably do not control more than 70 percent of the total world trade in cocaine; competition comes from Colombian independents and from those Bolivian and Peruvian refiners who can market their product in the United States. There is bad blood between the Medellín and Cali groups, stemming from Medellín's attempts to poach on Cali's sales territory in New York City. Yet, there is considerable business collaboration within each group: Traffickers cooperate on insuring cocaine shipments, engage in joint ventures, exchange loads, and jointly plan assassinations. Moreover, cocaine barons share a common political agenda that includes blocking the extradition of drug traffickers, immobilizing the criminal justice system, and selectively persecuting the Colombian left.

The 20–30 percent of the Colombian trade not controlled by syndicates is distributed among scattered small processors and refiners who often have links to Revolutionary Armed Forces of Colombia (FARC) guerrillas. In fact, the FARC may possess its own cocaine processing capability in some regions. The small producers cannot access the cocaine mafia's distribution capabilities; they rely heavily on mules (hired couriers) to smuggle cocaine into the United States.[22]

The top tier of the Colombian cocaine elite comprises approximately 100 people, many on the U.S. government's list of "extraditables." At the apex of the trafficking pyramid are seven men: five Medellín-based capos— Jorge Ochoa Vazquez and his brothers Fabio and Juan David, Pablo Escobar Gaviria, and José Gonzalo Rodríguez Gacha from the town of Pacho in Cundinamarca—and two Cali drug lords, Gilberto Rodríguez Orejuela and José Santa Cruz Londoño.[23] Pablo Escobar, Jorge Ochoa, and Gonzalo Rodríguez are reputedly three of the world's richest men: They made *Forbes* Magazine's July 1988 list of 125 non-U.S. billionaires.[24] By the end of the mid-1980s, the Medellín and Cali organizations together probably grossed $3 billion to $4 billion annually from international cocaine sales, primarily in the U.S. market—and 70 percent or more of that figure is profit.

The Mafia and the Political System

The cocaine industry has been called a "clear and present danger to the survival of democratic institutions" and a "first-order geopolitical threat."[25] Such characterizations, however, are not entirely accurate. Unlike guerrillas, whose objective is seizing power, traffickers are not ultimately interested in destroying a social order that nurtures them. Just like mafia organizations elsewhere, the Colombian mafia basically seeks to prosper commercially without being disturbed. However, when an industry as large as the cocaine industry searches for protection, corruption is spawned on a massive and unprecedented scale. Cocaine traffickers have bought into the political system and can successfully manipulate key institutions—the political parties, press, police, military, and judiciary. Traffickers maintain de facto control of major cities such as Medellín and of entire regions, such as parts of the departments of Antioquia, Meta, and Cordoba in Colombia and much of the Beni region in Bolivia. Moreover, traffickers do not hesitate to use violence against government officials and other public figures to promote limited political objectives, such as deactivating the U.S.-Colombian extradition treaty.

The cocaine mafia's complex protection strategy in Colombia and other countries operates on many levels. First, and most basic, the mafia makes large outlays for weapons and guard forces to protect laboratories, clandestine airfields, drug shipments, and key personnel. Drug traffickers are generally better armed than national police forces and use better communications equipment and faster aircraft. Second, traffickers attempt to neutralize the effectiveness of law enforcement institutions by paying police or military officers to look the other way—that is, to overlook cocaine refineries or drug smuggling operations. Traffickers also maintain an elaborate network of informants that provides advance warning of the timing and location of raids and checkpoints. When traffickers are caught in the net, they pay police to release them. For example, Pablo Escobar, Colombia's biggest cocaine dealer, was arrested by accident in November 1986 at a police checkpoint in southern Antioquia and was released after paying a bribe of $250,000 to $375,000.[26]

The Colombian mafia also cultivates a strategic intelligence capability. The Ochoa family, for example, reportedly supports informants in the Ministry of Justice and the Ministry of Foreign Affairs.[27] Some U.S. narcotics experts in Bogotá believe that the Medellín syndicates have infiltrated the U.S. embassy and that they read some of the embassy's cable traffic. The cocaine mafia may well be privy to secret U.S.-Colombian deliberations on drugs and to plans for major new antidrug initiatives.

The mafia also influences the judicial system. Judges trying drug trafficking cases in Colombia are offered the proverbial choice of "*plomo o plata*" (lead or silver)—death if they convict, a bribe if they set aside the charges. Not surprisingly, few judges opt to convict. In the past 2 years, criminal court judges released from jail or dropped charges against four major cocaine dealers: Gilberto Rodríguez Orejuela, José Santa Cruz Londoño, Evaristo Porras, and Jorge Luis Ochoa. (The U.S. government has offered $500,000 for the latter's arrest and conviction.) Ochoa was released twice within 16 months, and corrupt judges apparently played a role on both occasions. Indeed, the Colombian criminal justice system has almost ceased to function in drug trafficking cases. Recently in Medellín, police arrested a middle-ranking trafficking chief implicated in the murder of Guillermo Cano (the editor of the Bogotá daily *El Espectador*). After several days in jail, he was released, because no Medellín judge was willing to try the case.[28]

Protection to the Colombian mafia is protection writ large, encompassing influence over public opinion and the political process itself. Mafia-owned publications such as Carlos Lehder's *Quindío Libre* and the Escobar family's *Medellín Cívico* carry out an unremitting campaign against the U.S.-Colombian extradition treaty, portraying it as "a monstrous legal absurdity" and "the ultimate surrender of sovereignty."[29] Moreover, these publications depict drug dealers as progressive and public-spirited citizens. (*Medellín Cívico* praises Escobar's "great human and social sensitivity" and his dedication to "redeeming the forgotten people of Antioquia.")[30] Mafia-controlled columnists in more "respectable" publications convey these same messages. In addition, as already noted, major drug capos build a popular following by sponsoring a vast array of public works and social services. These narco-welfare projects reach communities that governments cannot reach; for instance, Escobar reportedly has built more public housing in Medellín than the government. Although the cost of such projects represents a tiny fraction of total cocaine-industry resources, the political impact—the winning of hearts and minds—is incalculable.

Cocaine traffickers in Colombia and many other Latin American countries play the role of power brokers. In Colombia, where political campaigns are not funded from the state treasury, drug money serves, in fact, as an important underpinning of the entire democratic process. Traffickers contribute indiscriminately to campaigns, often through front organizations, and frequently hedge their bets. For instance, Pablo Escobar (affiliated with the Liberal Party) gave money to both candidates in the 1982 Colombian presidential campaign. Moreover, drug capos prepare their own slates of candidates for political office and several times have run for office themselves. Escobar was elected in 1982 as an alternate deputy for Jairo Ortega's seat in the Colombian House of Representatives, and Carlos Lehder ran unsuccessfully (from hiding) for the Colombian Senate in the March 1986 election. Such high-profile activities stem more from personal ambition than from a desire for protection: Indeed, they are bad for business. Escobar's election, for example, made him the target of intense public scrutiny, and some old drug trafficking charges against him were reactivated. A kind of dual morality operates here: Traditional politicians, although glad to accept money from the drug mafia, are highly offended at the thought of serving with them in the Colombian Congress.

Finally, the cocaine mafia tries to dictate the national rules of the game on narcotics control. The mafia's number-one political objective is persuading the Colombian government to scuttle the U.S.-Colombian extradition treaty. Here, violence rather than bribery constitutes the mafia's favored political weapon. In the past several years, mafia henchmen murdered several prominent Colombian supporters of extradition: two newspaper editors, a Colombian Supreme Court justice, a Medellín Superior Court judge, and most recently a Colombian Attorney General. Mafia violence and threats have paralyzed the Colombian criminal justice system and effectively blocked extraditions—understandably, no one wants to assume responsibility for implementing the treaty.

Cocaine Traffickers and Guerrillas

The connection between the cocaine industry and Marxist guerrilla groups in Colombia and Peru represents a continuing source of much speculation and controversy in Washington. Both countries must contend with sizable left-wing guerrilla movements. Insurgents and drug dealers sometimes share the same territories, thriving in areas without strong central government control and without a naturally integrated economic structure. The question is: Do drug traffickers and guerrillas simply coexist in these areas, or do they actually collaborate?

There are in fact points of contact between the cocaine industry and guerrilla organizations (see Chapter 4 for a detailed discussion). However, the evidence does not suggest the existence of a narco-guerrilla alliance—indeed, it points to a different conclusion. Drug dealers, especially the larger operators, hold some anti-establishment views; they are strongly anti-U.S., and they favor a more egalitarian social structure. However, as landowners, ranchers, and owners of industrial property (including cocaine laboratories), dealers are far more closely aligned with the traditional power structure than with the revolutionary left—indeed, they tend to perceive the latter as a mortal threat.

The narco-guerrilla relationship is complex and sometimes mysterious; little factual evidence is available on which to base an interpretation. The evidence that can be compiled, however, suggests the following conclusions.

First, most narcotics traffickers are not revolutionaries. They seek to buy into and to manipulate the political system, but not to change the system in any fundamental way. A 1984 manifesto of 100 top Colombian mafia leaders declared, "We have no connection with, nor do we accept any such connection with armed guerrillas. Our activities have never been designed to replace the democratic and republican form of government."[31] To be sure, cocaine traffickers and guerrillas both rely on violence in pursuit of their objectives. However, the objectives of cocaine traffickers are limited to influencing aspects of their law enforcement environment—

for example, judges' decisions on drug trafficking cases, the conduct of criminal investigations, or the Colombian government's extradition policy.

Second, the relationship between traffickers and the revolutionary left is probably more hostile than cooperative. The more mature and better funded the trafficking organization, the less likely it is to collaborate with guerrillas. Narco-guerrilla conflicts tend to revolve around issues such as territorial control, relations with the coca-growing peasantry, and the distribution of economic benefits from the drug trade. Guerrillas such as Colombia's FARC and Peru's Sendero Luminoso may sympathize with peasants, but they see cocaine dealers as part of the property-owning classes and hence as fair game for extortion. In Colombia, guerrillas have attacked traffickers' laboratories, ranches, and farms and have kidnapped members of their families. Traffickers have retaliated in a variety of ways: by organizing rural self-defense groups, by massacring peasant villagers who appear to support guerrillas, and by exterminating visible members of the extreme left in the cities.[32] In Peru's Upper Huallaga Valley, cocaine dealers and Sendero Luminoso guerrillas have clashed repeatedly; the issues focused on Sendero's attempts to gain control of coca-growing regions, raise the price of coca leaves, and regulate coca paste markets.[33]

Third, some insurgent organizations finance their activities in part by taxing the cocaine industry. However, they have been more successful in taxing the upstream phases of the industry (cultivation and low-level processing) than the more lucrative downstream phases (refining and exporting). Guerrilla organizations such as Colombia's FARC in effect control the dregs of the cocaine trade; the more profitable end is mostly in the hands of powerful trafficking syndicates. Such syndicates apparently have the resources and the weaponry to protect their refining and export operations against predatory guerrilla groups.

Fourth, the financial relationship between the cocaine industry and the insurgent groups has been characterized as an alliance, but that is an overstatement. Guerrilla groups attempt to exploit all production assets in territories under their control. They shake down ranchers, farmers, merchants, and even foreign multinationals whenever they see the opportunity. Furthermore, the cocaine industry supports entire regional economies in Colombia and Peru—guerrillas are just one of many groups that benefit from the industry.

Fifth, guerrilla organizations in Colombia and Peru built a base of political (as opposed to merely financial) support among the coca-growing peasantry. Guerrilla organizations such as Colombia's FARC and Peru's Sendero Luminoso play on growers' hostility toward U.S.-favored eradication campaigns, which directly threaten the livelihood of many campesinos. Guerrillas also exploit the peasantry's resentment against cocaine middlemen, who by many accounts bully farmers into accepting rock-bottom prices for their coca leaves and coca paste.

The cocaine industry on balance probably functions as a conservative political force. Cocaine traffickers, if not exactly pillars of society, share significant common interests with established groups. One interesting exception to this pattern is Carlos Lehder, who recently was convicted in a Jacksonville, Florida, court of 11 counts of drug smuggling and was sentenced to life in prison plus 135 years. Lehder espoused a radical fascist-populist ideology that called for sweeping changes in Colombia's political landscape. Lehder, never part of the inner circle of Colombia's cocaine elite, sought the overthrow of what he called the Colombian "monarchical oligarchy." He proposed replacing Colombia's two-party system with mass popular congresses. He also sought the expulsion of "North American imperialism" from South America. He viewed drug money as a "revolutionary weapon" for accomplishing his task.[34] Ideologically ambidextrous, Lehder was compatible with extremists of any political stripe: A DEA official in Bogotá called him the Colonel Muammar Qaddafy of the international drug trade. In fact, Lehder maintained ties with at least two Colombian revolutionary organizations: the M-19 and the Quintin Lamé Movement. Lehder may have helped to finance the M-19's raid on Colombia's Palace of Justice in November 1985—a raid culminating in a holocaust in which 11 Colombian Supreme Court justices and scores of other people were killed.

A significant accumulation of circumstantial evidence suggests that Lehder's radical politics made his colleagues in the Colombian mafia extremely uncomfortable. For most cocaine barons, the narcotics industry represents a way to acquire wealth and social status, not an instrument of revolutionary change. Conceivably, the mafia's inner circle thought that Lehder gave the cocaine industry a bad image. Some knowledgeable Colombian observers believe that leaders of the Medellín syndicates—eager to remove the narco-guerrilla stigma and to create a pro-establishment image—betrayed Lehder to the authorities.

Publics and Governments

The problems of narcotics control in the Andean countries stem largely from the power of entrenched narcotics interests. However, such problems also are attributable to other factors: weak central governments, the absence of strong public support, and tension between civilian and military authorities.

The governments of Colombia, Peru, and Bolivia have never exercised full control over their national territories. Vast sections of northern

Bolivia, eastern and southeastern Peru, and southern Colombia have always been a political no-man's-land. In these remote jungle regions, traffickers established coca plantations, laboratories, airstrips, and storage facilities. In some regions—for example, the Bolivian Beni and the Peruvian Upper Huallaga Valley—traffickers or alliances of traffickers and coca growers at times challenged the authority of the central government, behaving much as warlords. Yet, the lack of strategic reach is merely one aspect of the problem. Where governments do not exercise control, officials frequently fall prey to the blandishments of narcotics traffickers. For example, cocaine laboratories are located in the environs of Medellín, Cali, Cochabamba, and other major South American cities. Medellín's old Olaya Herrera International Airport in the center of the city for several months was the site of a major cocaine smuggling operation—police outposts at the airport were simply paid to look the other way.[35]

Public opinion imposes an additional constraint on drug control programs in Latin American countries. Top national leaders affirm their commitment to the war against drugs, but opinion polls taken in Colombia and Peru show that drug trafficking and drug abuse rank at the bottom of concerns of Latin American publics, well below problems such as inflation, unemployment, crime, and terrorism. (See discussion in Chapter 5.) Furthermore, there is a widespread belief in Latin America that the drug trade is good for the economy, even if it is harmful in other respects. Peru's Alan García, for example, once called the cocaine traffic the only successful multinational that has emerged in the Andean countries.[36] The crises of debt, economic stagnation, and rampant unemployment that haunt most countries in the region reinforce this perception. In addition, U.S. efforts to control drug cultivation and production in Latin America often impinge on nationalist sensitivities. The controversies over the extradition of Colombian drug traffickers to the United States and over the U.S. military intervention against cocaine laboratories in Bolivia ("Operation Blast Furnace") clearly demonstrate the political limits to U.S. antidrug policies in the region.

Finally, Latin American leaders question why the United States does not do more to control consumption of illicit drugs at home; they view demand, not supply, as the driving force behind the international narcotics traffic. The United States, they feel, is approaching the problem backwards. For example, Peru's Ambassador to the United States, Cesar Atala, says that the U.S. effort to eradicate the coca plant "reminds me of what happened to a fellow who one day went to his home and found his wife dillydallying with a stranger on his living room sofa. So, at the height of his outrage and humiliation, the fellow decided to solve the problem by selling the sofa."[37] Similarly, many North American politicians would like to see the war against drugs fought as far away from national borders as possible—hence, the continuing preoccupation in the United States with controlling cocaine at the source.

In the Andean countries, the attitude of military establishments constitutes an obstacle to narcotics control efforts. Corruption, strategic considerations, ideology, and institutional self-interest all affect the military's posture vis-à-vis the war against drugs. Military factions in Colombia, for example, have been linked to cocaine traffickers through common membership in right-wing vigilante organizations. In Peru, where the government faces a threat from Shining Path guerrillas, military commanders claim that drug eradication programs complicate counterinsurgency operations. As one Peruvian army commander put it, "We have to have popular support to fight terrorism—we have to be a friend to the population, and you can't do that by eradicating coca."[38] In Bolivia, the cocaine establishment and the military have been linked by an array of financial ties and by a common hostility toward democracy. Moreover, throughout the Andean countries, acute rivalry and tension aggravate relations between military establishments and national police forces, the recipients of most U.S. antidrug aid. The military, for its own institutional reasons, seeks to keep the police as ill-armed and as immobile as possible. In other words, military opposition has prevented the United States and civilian leaders in South America from building the police into an effective drug-fighting force.

In sum, many factors account for the Andean governments' difficulty in taking decisive action against the illicit drug trade. Crackdowns could cause serious repercussions in countries such as Peru and Bolivia, where prices for licit exports have collapsed, and more than one-half of the population is unemployed or underemployed. Antidrug policies can generate massive popular discontent and add to government political troubles. Imagine, for example, what would happen to democracy in Bolivia if 200,000 dispossessed coca farmers decided to march on La Paz! Some Colombian and Peruvian leaders think that eradication campaigns create new converts to revolutionary movements in their countries. Governments do not possess a popular mandate for carrying out a major antidrug initiative; furthermore, the drug issue clearly constitutes a source of conflict in civilian-military relations.

Scope and Organization

This book is about the South American cocaine industry—its socioeconomic dimensions, organization and logistics, survival strategies, and political setting. Chapter 1 describes the main features of the production-logistics chain for cocaine—from the cultivation of coca leaves to the export of the finished drug (cocaine hydrochloride) from South America. This chapter also discusses in some detail the impact of the cocaine trade on South American economies. Chapter 2 analyzes the evolution, the composition, and the strategies of pro-coca organizations—the coca lobby—in the Andean countries. Chapter 3 reviews the structure and operation of cocaine trafficking syndicates and discusses how these entities participate in the political systems of the Andean countries. Chapter 4 explores the complex relationship between the cocaine industry and guerrilla organizations in Colombia and Peru and briefly examines the participation of communist regimes (Cuba and Nicaragua) in international drug trafficking. Chapter 5 addresses the political and bureaucratic determinants of drug law enforcement in the cocaine-exporting countries; it also analyzes recent public debates and institutional alignments on drug policy in these countries. Finally, a concluding chapter considers the dilemmas that the United States confronts when trying to implement antidrug programs in South American source countries.

Notes

1. U.S. Department of State, *International Narcotics Control Strategy Report (INCSR)* (Washington, D.C., 1988). See appendices: "FY 1988 Estimate for U.S. Economic and Military Assistance" and "U.S. Economic and Military Assistance, FY 1984 Program."
2. Interview at U.S. embassy in La Paz, October 6, 1987.
   Joel Brinkley, "Bolivia Asks U.S. for Big Loan to Make Up Lost Cocaine Income," *The New York Times*, July 31, 1986.
3. National Narcotics Intelligence Consumer's Committee (NNICC), *The NNICC Report, 1985–1986*, pp. 15, 26, 35, 70.
4. F. Marian Chambers, Congressional Research Service, *Narcotics-Related Foreign Aid Sanctions: An Effective Foreign Policy?* (Washington, D.C., 1987), Report for the Caucus on International Narcotics Control, U.S. Senate, p. 20. *INCSR*, 1988, p. 8.
5. Author's estimate: reflects assumptions about export volume; direction of international sales (United States versus Europe); and percentage of cocaine sold at Latin American, U.S. wholesale, and U.S. distribution prices.
6. Interview with Jorge Alderete, Ministry of Interior, in La Paz, October 6, 1987. Interview with Alexander Watson, U.S. Ambassador to Peru, in Lima, October 15, 1987.
   Interviews with U.S. narcotics experts in Bogotá, October 21, 1987.
   Victor Masquera Chaux (Colombia's Ambassador to the United States), "The Drug Economy: An Introduction," speech delivered at the Woodrow Wilson Center in Washington, D.C., December 14, 1988, p. 2.
7. "Governments' Sweetheart Deals and Subsidies Attempt to Stop Widening the

Gaps in the Financial Circuit," *The Andean Report*, October 1986, pp. 141–142.

8. Hernando José Gómez, "La economía ilegal en Colombia: tamaño, evolución, características e impacto económico," *Coyuntura Económica*, September 1988, pp. 101–108.
9. See the discussion of Pablo Escobar's life style in "Quién fue," *Semana*, January 25, 1988, p. 24.
10. Fabio Castillo, *Los Jinetes de la Cocaína (Los Jinetes)* (Bogotá: Documentos Periodisticos, 1987), pp. 124–148.
11. Field trip to the Barrio Pablo Escobar, March 2, 1988.
 Field trip to Pacho, March 5, 1988.
 Hernán Gaviria Berrio, letter to Fabio Castillo, Medellín Cívico, April 1987, p. 13.
 "Civismo En Marcha," *Medellín Cívico*, March 1984, p. 2.
 "A Self-Styled Robin Hood," *Time*, February 25, 1985, p. 33.
 Warren Hoge, "Bolivians Find a Patron in Reputed Drug Chief," *The New York Times*, August 15, 1982.
 Jorge Eliecer Orozco, *Lehder . . . El Hombre* (Bogotá: Plaza y Janes, 1987), pp. 60, 120.
12. Kevin Healy, "Bolivia and Cocaine: A Developing Country's Dilemma," *British Journal of Addiction*, 1988, p. 20–21.
13. Government of Bolivia, "Triennial Program of the Battle Against Drug Trafficking" ("Triennial Program"), November 1986, pp. 5–6.
 Bradley Graham, "Bolivia Runs Risk in Drug Drive," *The Washington Post*, July 17, 1986.
14. "Bolivia," *Latin American Regional Reports*, March 3, 1988, p. 8.
 Inter–American Development Bank. *Economic and Social Progress in Latin America: 1988 Report* (Washington, D.C.: Inter-American Development Bank, 1988), pp. 352, 480.
15. R. W. Lee, "Drugs," in Richard Feinberg and Gregg Goldstein (eds), *The U.S. Economy and Developing Countries: Campaign 88 Briefing Papers for Candidates* (Washington, D.C.: Overseas Development Council, 1988), p. 2.
 Congressional Research Service, *Combatting International Drug Cartels: Issues for U.S. Policy*, Report for the Caucus on International Narcotics Control of the U.S. Senate (Washington, D.C.: U.S. Government Printing Office, 1987), p. 32.
16. Raul Gonzalez, "Coca and Subversion in the Huallaga" ("Coca and Subversion"), *Quehacer*, Lima, September–October 1987, pp. 55–72.
17. *INCSR*, 1988, p. 109.
18. R. W. Lee, "The Drug Trade and Developing Countries," *Policy Focus*, Overseas Development Council, Washington, D.C., No. 4 (June 1987), p. 7.
 "Triennial Program," pp. 5–6.
19. *INCSR*, 1988, p. 73.
20. Interviews with U.S. narcotics experts in Bogotá, October 19, 1987.
 Los Jinetes, pp. 41–110, 118.
 David Henry, "How to Make $7 Million in 7 Years" ("$7 Million in 7 Years"), *Forbes*, October 5, 1987, p. 154.
21. Interviews with U.S. and Bolivian narcotics experts in La Paz and Cochabamba, October 1–5, 1987.
22. *Los Jinetes*, pp. 37–38.

Small independent operators rely mainly on mules to smuggle cocaine. Major trafficking organizations ship cocaine in large loads, relying primarily on general aviation aircraft.

23. *Los Jinetes*, pp. 41–110.
24. Harold Seneker, "The World's Billionaires," *Forbes*, July 25, 1988, p. 90. "$7 Million in 7 Years," pp. 153–155.
25. "The Drug Flames Rise Higher," *The New York Times*, March 3, 1988. Bradley Graham, "Impact of Colombian Drug Traffickers Spreads," *The Washington Post*, February 24, 1988.
26. "El dossier de Medellín," *Semana*, January 27, 1987, p. 25.
27. "Estupor por sobornos de la mafia," *El Tiempo*, January 10, 1988, p. 9A.
28. "Libre capo de la mafia porque ningún juez quiso procesarlo," *El Tiempo*, February 9, 1988, p. 24.
29. See, e.g., "La patria acorralada," *Quindío Libre*, October 1, 1983, p. 2A. "No a la Extradición," *Medellín Cívico*, March 1984, p. 7. Gilberto Zapata, "El Triunfo Es de Colombia," *Medellín Cívico*, July 1987, p. 3.
30. Hernán Gaviria Berrio, "Letter to Fabio Castillo," *Medellín Cívico*, April 1987, p. 13.
31. "Text of Drug Traffickers' Terms for Ending Activities," *El Tiempo*, Bogotá, July 7, 1984.
32. For a good discussion of the mafia's links to the right, see Merrill Collett, "Colombia's Drug Lords Waging War on Leftists," *The Washington Post*, November 14, 1987, pp. 14A, 22A.
33. "Coca and Subversion," pp. 55–72.
34. Mario Arango Jaramillo and Jorge Child Velez, *Los Condenados de la Coca* (Medellín: Editorial J. M. Arango, 1985), pp. 141–142.
35. "El dossier de Medellín," p. 25.
36. Alan García, "Debt or Democracy: Latin America's Alternative," in Alan García, *Three Speeches for History* (Lima, 1988), pp. 68–69.
37. Cesar Atala, "The Latin American Drug Trade: A Peruvian View," paper presented at a conference on "The Latin American Narcotics Trade and U.S. National Security," Mississippi State University, Biloxi, Mississippi, June 17, 1988, p. 4.
38. Jackson Diehl, "Model Anti-Drug Drive Fails in Peru," *The Washington Post*, December 29, 1984.

1

Coca and Cocaine

Making money in a capitalist society is not a
crime but rather a virtue.
—Pablo Escobar, 1982

Characteristics of the Coca Trade

Geography of Cultivation

Cocaine is one of 13 alkaloids produced from the coca leaf, which has
been cultivated in South America for at least 2,000 years. Coca grows in
at least six South American countries: Argentina, Bolivia, Brazil, Colombia, Ecuador, and Peru. Small coca plantations also have been found in
the Darien region of Panama. Bolivia, Colombia, and Peru now account
for 99 percent or more of the world's coca production. Cultivation of the
plant is legal in Peru and Bolivia, although formally subject to controls,
but is outlawed everywhere else.

There are four major varieties of coca: *Erythroxylum (E.) coca,* which
grows on the eastern slopes of the Andes in Peru and Bolivia; *E. coca
ipadu,* which grows in the lowland rain forest of southeastern Colombia
and Amazonian Brazil; *E. novogranatense,* which is cultivated in highland
regions of western Colombia; and *E. novogranatense truxillense,* which is
found on the desert coast of northern Peru and in the dry Upper Marañon
Valley, which parallels the Peruvian coast. Coca grows in a wide range of
ecological conditions: in poor soils and fertile soils, in wet tropical climates
and in seasonally dry climates, on flat land and on steep slopes, and at
altitudes ranging from 200 meters to 2,000 meters above sea level. Outside
of high mountain ranges and the Andean altiplano, most of the tropical
land areas of Central and South America are probably suitable for coca
cultivation. The coca species characteristically grown in Colombia today
has been found in tropical parts of the Old World: India, Ceylon, Africa,

21

and what is now Indonesia. Indeed, around the turn of the century, a coca and cocaine industry thrived on the island of Java.[1] From a law enforcement perspective, the coca plant constitutes a moving target: Even if political conditions permit eradication in one or two traditional zones (for example, the Chapare or the Upper Huallaga Valley), containing the spread of cultivation may prove impossible.

Probably four-fifths or more of all South American coca originates in Peru and Bolivia. Colombia is generally ranked as the world's third largest producer, with an estimated 25,000 hectares under cultivation in 1987. Coca is grown in 14 of Peru's 24 departments, but 5 departments—Cuzco, Ayacucho, San Martín, Huanuco, and La Libertad—are responsible for substantially more than 90 percent of both cultivation and production. The two most important growing areas are the Upper Urubamba Valley in the La Convención province in Cuzco department and the Upper Huallaga Valley, a region of roughly 10,000 square kilometers bounded approximately by the towns of Panao in Huanuco department (at the southern end) and Campanilla in San Martín department (at the northern end). U.S. narcotics experts believe that the Upper Huallaga Valley now accounts for most of Peru's coca output. Within the Valley, coca represents 90 percent or more of total farm income.

In Bolivia, most coca production occurs in the Chapare and Yungas regions, located, respectively, in the departments of Cochabamba and La Paz. The Chapare, a vast subtropical rain forest, has no clearly defined geographical boundaries—but the region that contains coca cultivation is estimated at roughly 25,000 square kilometers, an area about as large as Vermont. The region produces an estimated 75–80 percent of Bolivia's coca output; moreover, in the Chapare, as in the Upper Huallaga Valley, coca is by far the most important cash crop. A new and increasingly important coca-growing area—there are eyewitness accounts of several thousand hectares under cultivation—lies in the Yapacani region of Santa Cruz department, immediately to the east of Cochabamba.

In Colombia, the coca plant is cultivated mainly in the remote llanos (plains) and jungle regions of southeastern and southern Colombia. Several departments and commissariats are responsible for most of Colombia's production: Meta, Guaviare, and Vaupes in the eastern Llanos, Caqueta in the south, and Putumayo along the Ecuadorian border. Yet, coca can also be found in the Sierra Nevada de Santa Marta, near the Colombian coast, in Boyaca department northeast of Bogotá, in the hilly regions of Cauca department in the southwest, and in the swamps of the Amazon basin.

The quality of Colombian coca is generally poor; its cocaine content is one-half or one-third that of leaves grown in Bolivia or Peru (0.25–0.30 percent compared to 0.50–0.75 percent).[2] Also, Colombia is not a major traditional producer. The vast majority of cultivation originated in the mid-1970s or later, possibly because of a strategic decision by Colombian trafficking syndicates to "integrate backward" by developing domestic alternatives to Peruvian and Bolivian leaf.

The quantity of coca that actually grows in Bolivia, Peru, and Colombia is largely a mystery. In general, U.S. government estimates are lower than those of producer-country governments. For example, the U.S. State Department's 1986 estimate for coca cultivation in Peru was 107,500 hectares,[3] but the figures used by Peru's Multisectoral Committee for Control of Drugs (COMUCOD) ranged from 135,000 hectares to 180,000 hectares. Peru's Minister of Interior, Abel Salinas, claimed in 1987 that 380,000 hectares of coca grew in Peru.[4] (The United States and Peru do agree on an average yield of 1 ton per hectare in that country.) By 1988, the U.S. estimates for Peru seemed to be in disarray—on a visit to the U.S. embassy in Lima in October 1988, available figures ranged from 110,000 hectares to 200,000 hectares. In Bolivia, the picture is similarly confusing. For 1988, the Ministry of Agriculture's Sub-Secretariat for Alternative Development and Substitution of Coca estimated that 155,452 tons of coca were produced on 60,011 hectares. (The estimate excluded a few thousand hectares grown outside of La Paz and Cochabamba departments.) However, the State Department's estimate is 56,400 tons on 40,300 hectares. The disparity obviously is enormous, especially on the subject of yields.[5]

Evidently, different estimates employ different data sources, methods of collection, and statistical assumptions. The United States, for example, relies heavily on aerial photography, but the frequently cloudy Andean weather and the cultivation of some coca under the tree-cover affect the reliability of this technique. Political factors also play a role. Producer countries may exaggerate the dimensions of the problem to improve their negotiating position when it comes time to bargain for more U.S. foreign aid. In the view of Andean leaders, coca farmers need generous compensation (cash payments, credits, technical assistance, and development works) for not growing coca, and the United States should foot most of the bill. Conceivably, the State Department might be inclined to understate production and thus minimize compensatory payments, prevent the cocaine issue from dominating diplomatic relations, and avoid alarming Congress. Given the uncertainties and the political pressures inherent in estimating coca cultivation and yields, no single set of figures should be considered truly reliable.

Coca Leaf Markets

What happens to all the coca that grows in South American countries? Coca leaves flow into three principal markets: a traditional market, a legal industrial market, and an illicit cocaine market. For all practical purposes, the traditional market and the legal industrial market are confined to Peru and Bolivia. Over the past 2 decades, the illicit cocaine market has become the dominant consumer of leaves in Peru and Bolivia, and virtually all leaf production in Colombia is destined for this market.

Use of the coca plant is deeply woven into the ways of life of highland Peruvians and Bolivians. The Inca kings and nobility chewed coca leaves, and the practice became widespread among the people of the high Andes after the Spanish conquest. Today, an estimated three to four million peasants and miners in the Andean altiplano chew coca, a mild narcotic, to suppress the effects of hunger, fatigue, and cold. In addition, coca is widely used as a medicine, and not just in the altiplano. In Bolivia, some 70 different folk remedies include coca, sometimes in combination with other plants. An estimated 87 percent of the inhabitants of small towns and rural communities use the coca leaf for health-care purposes.[6]

The amount of leaf consumed in Andean societies is hard to determine. The State Department estimates three million coca users in Peru and 300,000 in Bolivia, but consumption in both countries is put at 10,000 metric tons[7]—which would mean that the average Peruvian chewer makes do with one-tenth as much leaf as his Bolivian counterpart, a rather unlikely contention.

Parallel licit and gray markets for coca leaves seem to operate in Peru and Bolivia. Most leaves, in fact, apparently flow outside of official channels to reach consumers. Wages, for example, are often paid in coca, and coca is bartered to highland farmers for potatoes, maize, and other altiplano crops.[8] Peru's national wholesale agency for coca, ENACO, which buys leaves from coca farmers and sells them to registered retailers, only purchased 4,300 metric tons of coca in 1986—less than half of the 10,000-ton reference figure for traditional consumption. Similarly, the Bolivian government's marketing and distribution agencies, which until recently were run by the National Directorate for the Control of Dangerous Substances (DNCSP), only captured 3,800 tons of leaves in 1985.[9]

In Peru, a small percentage of leaf production, 2,000 tons according to an AID estimate, is used for commercial purposes. Between 1980 and 1985, Peru exported 1,434 metric tons of coca leaves to the United States for use in manufacturing Coca Cola extract. (The leaves are shipped to the Stepan Chemical Company in New Jersey; Stepan removes the cocaine from the leaves and sells de-cocainized residue to Coca Cola.)[10] Bolivia also exports an indeterminate quantity of coca leaves to the United States for making Coca Cola. Moreover, Peru converts leaves into licit cocaine for export. From 1980 to 1985, according to ENACO statistics, Peru exported about 2.25 metric tons of cocaine base (92 percent pure) to pharmaceutical companies in industrialized countries—mainly in Germany, Belgium, and the United Kingdom.[11]

ENACO, incidentally, has ambitions to build a much larger commercial industry that would take advantage of the supposed medicinal and nutritional properties of the coca leaf. Commercialization (or "industrialization") also has strong support in Bolivia. There is a widespread belief in Andean countries—one not based on much empirical evidence—that coca chewing regulates blood pressure and blood sugar levels, prevents tooth decay, and cures many stomach ailments. In addition, coca reputedly is an excellent source of nutrients such as protein, calcium, phosphorus, and B-vitamins. The commercial strategy would be to convert these benign essences of the coca leaf into products—medicine, tonics, elixirs, and so on—and to sell them in world markets for hard currency. The United States has strongly discouraged the commercialization movement and would basically prefer to see all coca production in Peru and Bolivia declared illegal. The commercialization movement probably will go nowhere in these countries without some outside financial support for research and development. U.S. government support is virtually out of the question, although funding by private U.S. pharmaceutical and food processing companies remains a possibility.

Finally, the bulk of South American coca leaves is used in manufacturing illicit cocaine. The illicit cocaine market and the traditional markets are to some extent competitors, and the competition favors the traffickers. Traffickers typically, although not always, pay a premium over the price paid by government wholesalers. The ratio of the illicit to the licit price in Peru has ranged from a low of 3:1 to a high of 15:1. Moreover, drug dealers pick up the leaves at the farm gate, saving the peasants the trouble of transporting their crops to government collection centers. The traffickers' demand almost certainly raises prices in the parallel gray market for leaves, although precise information on this point is unavailable. Hence, a fair amount of pressure is exerted on traditional markets in Peru and Bolivia; highland peasants and miners sometimes face a shortage of leaves at affordable prices, which in turn pressures wages to rise and produces social discontent.

There are certainly some countervailing factors. According to many estimates, to meet the new international demand, coca production has expanded, especially in traditional areas of cocaine manufacture such as the Upper Huallaga Valley and the Bolivian Chapare. In addition, law enforcement can disrupt coca markets; crackdowns in the cocaine industry can force buyers temporarily out of the market. When this happens, the price of leaves drops, sometimes to a level below the cost of production, and more than enough coca is available through licit wholesale and distribution channels. Moreover, Andean tradition may work against the development of a completely free market in coca. The age-old Andean custom of chewing coca leaves affords a convenient cover for the illicit coca trade. Politically, it makes good sense for coca farmers and middle-men to keep highland dwellers supplied with coca, even if the leaves change hands at prices lower than those that the traffickers would pay. Yet, the balance between traditional coca and illicit cocaine markets is clearly a delicate one. A radical reduction of coca cultivation in Peru and Bolivia—that is, the U.S. objective—would upset this balance. Traffickers would simply bid away dwindling supplies of leaf from licit consumers. Work and cultural patterns centered around chewing coca would begin to disappear, and Andean civilization as it exists today probably would collapse.

Why Coca?

For many farmers in Peru, Bolivia, and Colombia, coca is the sole cash crop, and for some—especially the newer migrants to the Chapare and the Upper Huallaga Valley—coca constitutes the only crop, because it offers what is in many respects the complete package for farmers. The coca plant produces three to six harvests each year for up to 40 years. Although market conditions vary, coca is typically much more profitable than licit cash crops in Peru, Bolivia, and Colombia. The high profits associated with cultivating the plant mean that a farmer who wants to start a coca farm can obtain financing, fertilizer, seed, and even technical assistance from drug traffickers or their intermediaries. The plant is easily cultivated and seems to flourish in agronomic, climatic, and topographical conditions that are unsuitable for most other crops. Another important consideration: Coca tends to grow in remote regions where the costs incurred to move traditional crops (in raw and unprocessed form) to market frequently approach prohibitive levels. For all these reasons, coca growers are cool to the idea of cultivating anything else. As one Chapare farmer put it, "We produce only coca, because it is the only profitable crop."[12]

The statistics on relative returns from coca all point in the same direction. According to Peru's *Andean Report*, a coca farmer in the Upper Huallaga Valley could earn a maximum gross income of $12,350 per hectare per year at leaf prices prevailing in October 1985; of this sum, 60 percent was profit. A coca farmer's net per-hectare earnings were 10 times those of a cacao farmer and 91 times those of a rice farmer.[13] By late 1984 in the Bolivian Chapare, a farmer cultivating coca could net $9,000 per hectare per year, 19 times as much as a farmer cultivating citrus, the next most profitable crop in the region.[14] Prices of South American coca leaf have dropped significantly from their peak levels, primarily because of the overproduction of leaf and the intensified enforcement pressure against cocaine laboratories. However, the general pattern still holds. According to a December 1986 AID report, a coca farmer in the Bolivian Chapare could net about $2,600 a year from a single hectare of coca—more than four times the return from a hectare of oranges or avocadoes (the most competitive traditional crops) and more than four times Bolivia's 1986 per capita income.[15] In addition, coca yields relatively quick returns. Coca can be harvested 18 months after planting. Many alternative cash crops—for example, oranges, rubber, tea, and coffee—require 4 years or more from planting to the first harvest. In sum, coca cultivation presents a very superior cash-flow option for the Bolivian, Peruvian, or Colombian farmer.[16]

The agronomics of coca, like its economics, do not favor substitution. Throughout South America, coca apparently thrives in conditions that other crops find inhospitable: heavy rainfall, rugged terrain, and soils high in acid and low in nutrients. In Peru, coca is grown mostly on steep slopes—as of 1986, such cultivation accounted for about 60–70 percent of total coca production in the Upper Huallaga Valley—and there is no suitable agricultural alternative for hillside coca land. Said a rural development official talking about the ecology of coca cultivation in the Valley, "That land should be allowed to grow back into the forest."[17] Similar conditions prevail in the Yungas region of Bolivia. In the Chapare, the terrain is flatter, but—as in most coca-growing areas—soils are generally poor, and the extremely heavy rainfall makes for a short growing season. Some U.S. experts believe that if coca were not cultivated in the Chapare, the fragile ecology of the region could only support about one-third of the families now residing in the region. Similarly, much of the land now devoted to coca growing in the Amazon and Llanos regions of Colombia probably would not be suitable for purposes other than pasture or forestry.

Within areas of coca cultivation, of course, some lands are more marginal than others. The flat, alluvial lands along river beds, which are suited to growing traditional crops, contrast with the humid jungle hillsides, which are not. Farmers in some cases may have shifted land out of food production (rice, bananas, yucca, and the like) and into coca cultivation. Resubstitution, however, is not easy. The coca plant robs the soil of essential vitamins and nutrients. Even when the soil might be salvageable (and this constraint probably rules out hillside coca land, according to

most experts), extensive reconstitution of the land would be required. AID
now has a special project underway for reclaiming eradicated land in the
Upper Huallaga Valley. The idea, according to AID's project director in
Lima, is to "change the prejudice of local farmers that former coca-
producing land cannot be replanted in legitimate crops."[18] AID might be
able to prove a point in a few demonstration plots, but, one wonders, at
what cost in fertilizer and other inputs.

A third constraint on developing profitable alternatives to coca arises
from the relative remoteness of the regions that produce the plant. In
Colombia, such regions are hundreds of miles from urban centers and are
not connected to them by roads or commercial air transport. Peru's Upper
Huallaga Valley lies 400 to 750 miles from the capital—a 10-hour drive
from Lima to the closest point (the town of Tingo María) at the southern
end of the Valley. Bolivia's Yungas begins roughly 75 miles from La Paz,
but is linked to the capital by a miserably maintained road that is frequently
blocked for days by mudslides and repair work; the average driving time
is about 6 hours. Possibly the most accessible region is the Chapare, whose
largest town, Villa Tunari, is located about 100 miles northeast of Cochabamba, 3 to 4 hours by road on a good day. Extremely heavy rainfall,
however, can render the road impassable for days on end.

Distance can best be conceptualized as the cost required to ship commodities to market, and in the coca-growing areas of Bolivia, Peru, and
especially Colombia—where the southeastern third of the country has
almost no roads to speak of—these costs are likely to be very high.
Consequently, peasants find themselves at a competitive disadvantage. In
the Medio Caguan, a coca-growing region in Caqueta department, peasants
pay more just to transport typical crops—rice, maize, yucca, and bananas—to market than they can receive from selling these crops. Hence,
virtually all agriculture other than coca cultivation focuses on subsistence—that is, farmers consume what they grow.[19] Similarly, transportation costs to Lima—650 km to 1,200 km distant—impose a major constraint
on the commercial development of the Upper Huallaga Valley. In Bolivia,
according to various rural development experts, even imported coffee,
oranges, and pineapples sell more cheaply in Bolivia's major cities than
the same cash crops grown in the Yungas or the Chapare.[20] Furthermore,
even where a theoretical market exists, the peasant is likely to lose much
of his crop before he can consummate a sale. As a commentator in the
magazine *Perú Económico* remarked in 1984:

> Coffee, tea, citrus, soybeans, pineapples, and tobacco have been acclaimed
> successively as the magic harvests that would make jungle agriculture profitable.
> But farmers later saw how their harvests were rotting in the fields, waiting to be
> loaded for shipment to markets.

The bottlenecks created by the absence of infrastructure for sale and transport led many campesinos to think that coca constituted a solution to their problems.[21]

In sum, the economic advantages of growing coca appear compelling when compared to alternatives. Coca yields relatively high returns, agricultural conditions do not favor substitution of other crops, and coca-growing regions are distant from and poorly linked to the outside world. Cultivation of alternative crops on any commercial scale would doubtless require massive government subsidies—hardly an appealing prospect for poverty-stricken Andean nations.

This scenario poses some dilemmas for U.S. policy. The United States supports multimillion-dollar development programs in both the Upper Huallaga Valley and in the Chapare. These programs originally were designed to shift farmers from coca cultivation into other lines of agricultural work. But the constraints on crop substitution in coca-growing regions have proven too formidable—the proverbial silk purse cannot be made out of a sow's ear. As a result, the programs are being redefined. U.S. AID officials interviewed in Lima and La Paz clearly see little future in crop substitution; they want to concentrate resources on high-visibility public works projects, such as building schools and roads and digging water wells.[22] Such projects, however, obviously benefit coca farmers along with everybody else—indeed, they may facilitate cocaine traffic. Roads, for example, make it easier for farmers to transport coca leaves to traffickers' laboratories. Consequently, developing coca-growing regions probably will be a waste of money. These regions are probably best suited to their current task—producing coca.

There may be better solutions. U.S. and Bolivian development experts claim that it would make more economic sense to put the $40 million or so now earmarked for Chapare development into areas with established agricultural potential, for example, the Upper Cochabamba Valley and the fertile plains around Santa Cruz. The argument is that successful agricultural and agribusiness development in these areas would lure at least some of the migrant farmers out of the Chapare. The idea has some theoretical merit. For example, a U.S. agricultural expert interviewed in La Paz in May 1986 reported that a tomato cooperative in Santa Cruz grossed between $7,000 per hectare and $10,000 per hectare in 1985, which compared not unfavorably to the $10,000 to $13,000 in gross income earned by a coca farmer that year. This suggests that if substitution is to work at all, it must be conducted on a broad geographical scale and involve a significant relocation of coca farmers (and others dependent on the coca trade) to better land and better working conditions.[23]

Cocaine Trafficking

From Coca to Cocaine

Coca becomes cocaine via a three-step process. In the first step, coca leaves are mashed, then soaked in a solution of kerosene and sodium carbonate to precipitate out the alkaloid. The product, a compound called coca paste (in South America, *sulfato* or *pasta básica cocaína*), is about 40-percent pure cocaine. In the second step, the paste is treated with sulfuric acid and potassium permanganate to form a cocaine base or "washed paste" (*pasta lavada*), which is 90- to 92-percent pure cocaine. In the final refining stage, ether and acetone are used to convert the base into cocaine hydrochloride (CHCL), the purest form of the drug. The cocaine is then usually diluted or "cut" with some inert ingredient, for example, sugar or lactose, before being snorted or otherwise ingested. Street cocaine, the final retail product, has a purity ranging from 10–20 percent in 1980 to 55–65 percent in 1986—the more saturated the market, the higher the purity.[24]

Cocaine is not hard to make. The relatively straightforward refining process does not require elaborate equipment or exotic chemicals. Moreover, a range of possible substitutes exist for most of the materials used in manufacturing (gasoline can replace kerosene, for example). There are some dangers: Two of the essential chemicals—acetone and especially ether—are extremely combustible and must be handled and stored very carefully. Ether emits vapors at room temperature and boils at 95 degrees Fahrenheit. If enough vapor mixes with the air, any spark—striking a match, dropping a tool on a concrete floor, or even turning on a light switch—can ignite an explosion. Yet, by and large, cocaine processing technology is simple, costs are low, and entry barriers are minimal compared to those in traditional manufacturing sectors. In all, the industry's characteristics fit well with the general conditions of peasant life in the Andean countries.

The conversion of coca leaves to cocaine is characterized by a tremendous reduction in the volume of the product and by an even more spectacular increase in its price. In Peru and Bolivia, 300 kilos to 500 kilos of leaves typically make 1 kilo of cocaine. (The ratio is probably higher in Colombia, because the cocaine content of Colombian leaves generally measures one-half or less than that of Peruvian or Bolivian leaves.) A hectare of coca in the Bolivian Chapare can produce 2,400 kilograms of leaves, worth roughly $5,000 to $6,000 at 1987 prices.[25] At a 500:1 ratio, this hectare's production would be worth $600,000 to $800,000 at prevailing U.S. street prices. The farmer, in other words, receives only a minuscule fraction of the total value of his product; however, he is doubtless not too concerned, because he earns much more by cultivating coca than he could by raising almost any other crop.

The Trafficking Chain

The story of cocaine begins at or near the farm site. Middlemen acting for traffickers pick up coca leaves from the farmer and transport them to nearby laboratories. Sometimes leaves are conveyed on the backs of hired laborers (known in Bolivia as *zepes*), who travel down hidden jungle trails to avoid detection by the authorities. A few of the larger coca growers have developed forward linkages into the production of paste and maintain clandestine laboratories on their farms. Paste laboratories are numerous; in 1985, an estimated 5,000 such laboratories operated in the Chapare region—about one for every eight coca-farming families.[26] Similar to the transport of leaves, paste production is labor intensive. Laboratory owners hire so-called *pisadores*, literally "tramplers," to stomp on the leaves before they are immersed in the kerosene solution, because crushing expedites the process of leaching out the cocaine. Stomping usually occurs at night, and the process, according to the American sociologist Kevin Healy, sometimes possesses an almost ritual quality.

> Over the course of their 12 hours of nighttime work, the pisadores become animated as they "dance" on the leaves to the accompaniment of piped-in regional music. . . . To further arouse positive work spirits for their tedious routine, pisadores are encouraged to consume large quantities of chicha [corn beer] and coca paste, which are often mixed together in an unusual and potent concoction.[27]

An obviously high level of integration exists between paste manufacture and coca cultivation. Coca growers, laborers hired to pick leaves at harvest time, illicit wholesalers, leaf carriers, laboratory owners, and *pisadores* all constitute more or less a single socioeconomic unit. Differentiation does occur, however, at the more advanced stages of cocaine manufacture. Converting base to hydrochloride tends to occur far from the farm site. Peru's advanced processing capability, such as it is, concentrates largely around Lima; Bolivia's capability centers in the Beni and Santa Cruz regions, respectively in the northern and eastern parts of the country, hundreds of miles from the centers of coca cultivation. Most Colombian CHCL laboratories, at least in recent years, have been located outside of coca-growing areas; for example, in ranches in the departments of Antioquia and Cordoba or deep in jungles along the Colombia-Brazil-Peru border. (One reason for such laboratory siting is that the traffickers do not

like dealing with the FARC, which controls many zones of coca cultivation.)

Moreover, cocaine production is "spread out" by country. Following
the general pattern, Peru and Bolivia supply semiprocessed cocaine to the
Colombians for refining and subsequent export to the United States. For
example, most of Peru's cocaine exports take the form of cocaine base
(produced in the Upper Huallaga Valley or in the Peruvian Amazon),
which is sold to Colombian buyers. Bolivia's cocaine industry is somewhat
more developed than Peru's. The "King of the Beni," Roberto Suarez,
pioneered the development of cocaine hydrochloride production in Bolivia, and his organization was able to market some CHCL in the United
States. Still, Bolivia's cocaine industry functions mainly as a supplier of
cocaine base to Colombian refiners. Colombians also purchase much of
Bolivia's CHCL production, which they then smuggle to Colombian
wholesalers in the United States.

Colombian trafficking organizations dominate the higher value-added
stages of the production-logistics chain: refining, smuggling, and wholesaling. This chain is described in Table 1.1. The National Narcotics Intelligence Consumers' Committee (NNICC), the federal coordinating committee for drug matters, estimates that 75 percent of the cocaine entering the
United States in 1985 and 1986 was refined in Colombia, 15 percent in
Bolivia, and 5 percent in Peru.[28] Moreover, according to the NNICC,
Colombian syndicates dominate both cocaine smuggling to the United
States and the wholesaling of cocaine in the United States. (In the 1970s,
the Colombians grabbed control of the wholesale traffic from Cuban-
Americans and from the traditional U.S. mafia.)[29] The Colombians' role
diminishes as the drug moves through the wholesale and retail distribution
network. Yet, their dominance at the upper levels of this network enables
Colombian dealers to capture some of the huge profits to be made by
selling to the U.S. market.

Peruvian and Bolivian dealers would like to "integrate forward" into the
more profitable ends of the business, but the Peruvians and Bolivians do
not pose a serious challenge to Colombian dominance of the U.S. market.
Although Peruvian and Bolivian dealers might be able to improve their
position in refining (and, in fact, have been doing so over time), making
inroads into operations further downstream will be difficult. Colombia's
formidable position reflects some natural advantages, such as geographic
proximity to the United States and the presence of a large Colombian
immigrant population in the United States. (Many more Colombians reside
in the United States than do South Americans of any other nationality.)
The resulting dense flow patterns of travel and commercial traffic between
Colombia and the United States create what U.S. economist Peter Reuter

TABLE 1.1
Cocaine in the 1980s:
The Structure, the Channels, the Profits

LOCATION	DISTRIBUTION	ACCOUNTING	GROSS PROFIT ON TRANSACTION
Colombia	Colombian **refiner** produces a load of 300 kg at an average cost of $3,000/kg.	Cost to refiner: $900,000	
	Refiner agrees to pay a **pilot**, who doesn't take possession, $3,000/kg to transport the load to the Bahamas by air and from there to Miami by yacht and car.	Cost to refiner: $900,000	
Miami	Pilot delivers shipment to the Colombian's Miami-based **wholesaler**, who divides the 300-kg load into packages of 5-10 kg. He sells one 5-kg package to a buyer from Atlanta for $23,500/kg, receiving a commission of $2,000/kg, which may be split with the person who arranged the transaction.	300 kg at $23,500= $7,050,000 for refiner, less costs of $2,400,000	**Refiner:** $4,650,000 **Pilot:** $900,000 **Wholesaler:** $600,000
Atlanta	The Atlanta **distributor** dilutes each kg to 42 oz from 35 and sells it in multi-ounce packages for an average of $1,500/oz.	210 oz at $1,500/oz= $315,000, less $117,500 for purchase	**Distributor:** $197,500
	A **dealer** in an office building buys 4 oz from the distributor. He dilutes each ounce to 36 grams from 28 and sells each gram for $60.	144 grams x $60= $8,640, less $6,000 for purchase	**Dealer:** $2,640
	A **consumer/dealer** buys 5 grams from the dealer, sells 4 grams to co-workers for $75 per gram, and consumes 1 gram.	4 grams at $75 each= $300, less $300 for purchase	**Consumer/dealer:** $0

Source: "The Cocaine Business: Big Risks and Profits, High Labor Turnover." *The Wall Street Journal.* June 30, 1986. Source cited as interviews with DEA officials, pilots, distributors, and lawyers.

calls a broad "pipeline" within which to "hide the movement of drugs."[30] Moreover, the large number of Colombian immigrants increases the probability that cocaine trafficking organizations can find Colombian distributors for their product.

Colombia's cocaine syndicates also draw on that country's long tradition of smuggling—in fact, the so-called Medellín syndicates evolved largely from families of *contrabandistas* that used to ply their trade in and out of the Gulf of Uraba, on Colombia's Caribbean coast. Colombia's criminal syndicates are noted for their business acumen and also for their ruthlessness. Colombians are unlikely to welcome the presence of Bolivian and Peruvian wholesalers in, say, Miami, Jackson Heights, and Los Angeles; they will no doubt resort to violence to eliminate the competition.

For all these reasons, Colombians have a stranglehold on the U.S. cocaine market. The best opportunity for the other Andean countries (especially Bolivia, because of geography) is to market refined cocaine in the West European market, where the Colombians are not so well established. By all indications, however, the Medellín and Cali organizations are moving quickly to establish wholesaling networks in Spain, England, West Germany, and other countries. The Colombians therefore apparently will call the shots on international cocaine traffic for some time to come.

A Note on Narco-Economics

In the mid-1980s, South American cocaine traffickers probably earned a minimum of $5 billion to $6 billion yearly from sales in international markets. For 1987, this figure can be calculated at about $5.1 billion, assuming that 250 tons of cocaine were exported (net of seizures) from South America. Of this total, an estimated 25 tons were sold at a South American export price of $5,000 per kilo; 25 tons were sold in Europe at $40,000 per kilo; and 200 tons changed hands in the United States at an average price of $20,000 per kilo. These assumptions are arbitrary, but they represent a composite of the best guesses of many U.S. and South American narcotics experts.

For example, the 250-ton figure is derived from the upper-bound U.S. estimate of potential cocaine production in South America—422.8 metric tons, processed from 211,400 metric tons of coca leaves. (The upper-bound figure is used to compensate for the difference between U.S. and South American estimates of coca cultivation.) From the maximum figure, 100 tons can be subtracted for worldwide seizures in 1987 and for domestic consumption in South America (mainly in leaf equivalent). The residual is accounted for by coca leaf that is not converted to cocaine because of losses, spoilage, or labor shortages. Such calculations, however, may still underestimate the level of South American cocaine exports. For example, there is some uncertainty about the quantity of coca leaves necessary to produce a given amount of cocaine. The United States applies an average conversion factor of 500:1 for all of South America. Yet, government sources in Peru and Bolivia, where most of the world's coca is produced, use ratios ranging between 350:1 and 300:1. Similar ratios were applied by the Earth Satellite Corporation in a 1981 report prepared for INM.[31] One key variable in such conversions is the cocaine content of the leaf. For some limited leaf samples obtained by DEA, the average cocaine content of the leaf is 0.72 percent in Bolivia, 0.53 percent in Peru, and 0.28 percent in Colombia. The efficiency of the manufacturing process represents another key variable in conversion ratios and depends on the skill of the processor and the quality of the chemicals and equipment used.

Colombia, of course, is the most important national actor in the cocaine trade. By their own estimates, the larger Colombian organizations account for 70–80 percent of the cocaine exported from Colombia.[32] Because they handle some Peruvian and Bolivian exports, these organizations probably control 60–70 percent of the world trade in cocaine. The profits of these organizations cannot be estimated with any certainty, in part because the prices of key inputs—chemicals and raw materials—fluctuate considerably. However, narcotics experts in Colombia and the United States believe that the rate of profit ranges from 50 percent to 80 percent. Few if any products are as profitable as cocaine.

The Cocaine Trade and South American Economies

Colombia, Bolivia, and Peru are all, to a greater or lesser extent, economically dependent on the cocaine industry. The industry is not by any means the most effective source of revenue for the economies of these nations; in fact, the wealth that it generates is not converted very efficiently into economic growth and may even retard growth in certain areas. The majority of narco-dollars are probably banked or invested abroad, and traffickers' domestic spending priorities certainly do not coincide with those of national economic planners (core economic activities seem to be shortchanged). A recent article in *The Economist* reported, "The economic impact of $1 billion spent bribing politicians and buying status symbols will usually be less than that of $1 billion spent building roads and electricity generators."[33]

Yet, cocaine earnings clearly add to a country's foreign exchange reserves, and cocaine production obviously constitutes a significant source of employment. The industry apparently has transformed the economic life of specific localities and communities that either are centers of illicit drug cultivation or are near such centers. Perhaps most important, the cocaine traffic may serve as a safety valve of sorts for countries or regions experiencing economic decline or stagnation. For example, according to a Bolivian government document, "Triennial Program for the Battle Against Drug Trafficking," Bolivia's gross national product declined by 2.3 percent per year from 1980 to 1986, but coca production annually grew an estimated 35 percent during those years. The official unemployment rate more than tripled from 1980 to 1986 (from 5.7 percent to 20 percent), but so did the number of families reportedly growing coca.[34] During 1986, more than 20,000 Bolivian miners lost their jobs, and as many as 5,000 may have sought work in the coca fields.[35] Cocaine exports can compensate for the loss of foreign exchange from traditional sources, a phenomenon illustrated from 1983 to 1987, when Bolivia's exports shrank by 38 percent and Peru's by 15 percent, primarily because world prices for traditional Andean commodities—oil, natural gas, and tin—declined precipitously during the same period. As the head of Peru's Investigative Commission on Narcotics remarked in a 1986 interview, "The price of copper goes down, the price of oil goes down, the price of oil products for export goes down, and the only price that increases is that of cocaine."[36]

In Colombia, the rise of the cocaine industry paralleled and partly compensated for the decline of Medellín in the 1970s as a major industrial center. Medellín's leading industrial sector, textiles, nearly collapsed because of Asian competition and punitive import tariffs. The depression lingered into the 1980s: From 1980 to 1985, the unemployment rate in Medellín was consistently higher than that of the other three major cities (Cali, Bogotá, and Barranquilla). In 1986, only Barranquilla suffered from a higher unemployment rate. Consequently, many Medellín residents were drawn into the cocaine traffic: "owners of small or middle-sized companies that were bankrupt or on the verge of bankruptcy, unemployed professionals, housewives who had no income, and other unemployed persons, skilled and unskilled."[37] The Colombian economist Mario Arango estimates that approximately 60 billion pesos ($313 million) of proceeds from illegal exports—mostly cocaine exports—flowed into Medellín's economy in 1987, producing local inflationary effects, but also stimulating a miniboom in textiles, construction, and other industries. As a result, 28,000 new jobs were created in Medellín that year. From 1983 to 1987, Medellín's unemployment rate as a percent of the national rate dropped from 140 percent to 98 percent.[38]

If the cocaine industry does not operate as an efficient engine of economic progress, it still provides an escape from abject poverty and misery for many inhabitants of the Andean world. Moreover, for rural dwellers especially, the cocaine industry offers a kind of instant introduction to modern life styles—the chance to enjoy color television, videocassette recorders, high-tech sound systems, and the latest-model Toyota landcruiser or Datsun car. Consequently, coca cultivation and cocaine trafficking have created radically new expectations and aspirations within Andean societies. If revolutions truly are born of frustrated expectations, the prospect of the sudden destruction or collapse of the cocaine industry should give nightmares to South American leaders—and to leaders in Washington as well.

Financial Aspects

Most of the billions of dollars earned by cocaine traffickers stay abroad in offshore havens such as the Cayman Islands or Panama or in investments in foreign real estate, securities, and businesses. A former money launderer for the Medellín drug syndicates claimed that in 1983 he was handling $10 billion to $11 billion worth of assets in the United States for these organizations.[39] A DEA official interviewed in late 1987 estimated that the Medellín syndicates' real estate holdings in southern Florida were in the neighborhood of $400 million, and traffickers reportedly own half of the approximately 200 highrises along Panama City's oceanfront.[40] Whether traffickers invest their money at home or abroad depends on several conditions in the source country: investment opportunities, interest rates, political stability, and—perhaps most important—government policy toward the drug trade. (The collapse of Colombia's extradition treaty with the United States may have encouraged Colombian traffickers to repatriate more of their capital.) Profits that return or remain at home may add to a country's official reserves or may circulate in the underground dollar economy. Traffickers' funds also return home in the form of contraband, diamonds, gold, and other valuables, which are then sold or exchanged for local currency.

Whatever their prevailing policies toward the drug traffic, Latin American governments generally try to encourage the repatriation of narcodollars and the flow of this money into the legitimate banking system.

In Bolivia, under the Siles Zuazo regime, central banks and commercial banks could not buy dollars freely, but exchange controls were lifted when Paz took office in the summer of 1985. From the second quarter of 1985 to the third quarter of 1986, official reserves climbed from $144.4 million to $252.1 million, possibly because of an influx of drug money into the banking system.[41] Bolivian authorities believe that most drug dollars are still exchanged on the black market. In Peru, the Belaunde government in 1983 enacted a law (which the García administration let stand) that allowed Peruvians to repatriate foreign exchange from any source, no questions asked, without assuming liability for back taxes or criminal penalties.[42] Except for very large transactions, Peruvian banks do not usually ask even for proof of identity when exchanging dollars for soles, the local currency.

The Colombian government periodically cracks down on the nation's drug traffickers, but generally has maintained at least an unofficial policy of welcoming their money. In the 1970s, lax drug enforcement and liberal banking rules helped propel a rise in the nation's net international reserves from about $150 million in 1970 to nearly $5 billion in 1980. (Other factors, such as high coffee prices for much of the period, also contributed to the increase.)[43] Every new Colombian president taking office since Alfredo Lopez Michelsen has decreed some kind of tax amnesty. For example, Belisario Bentancur's administration declared an "immediate, wide, and generous amnesty" on illegal income, including that from the lucrative drug trade. The amnesty was designed, in Betancur's words, to "attract hidden capital, from wherever it comes, without looking back at its origins, without the application of any kind of sanctions."[44] Some of the nation's top drug traffickers apparently responded to the call. Carlos Lehder, for instance, said he took advantage of Betancur's offer to repatriate $170 million of illegal income earned in his Bahamas smuggling operations.[45] (See Chapter 3, "The Cocaine Mafia.")

In mid-1984, the Colombian government's general posture toward the illicit drug industry hardened considerably. After the assassination of Justice Minister Rodrigo Lara Bonilla in April 1984, Betancur declared drugs "the most serious problem that Colombia has had in its history" and called for a "great national mobilization" against traffickers.[46] A plausible argument can be made that the increasingly unfavorable political climate prompted drug dealers to withdraw some of their money from the country and to repatriate a smaller proportion of their earnings. From the second quarter of 1983 to the third quarter of 1984, international reserves dropped by more than 70 percent, from $2.8 billion to about $800 million. (They subsequently recovered nicely, reaching $2.7 billion at the end of 1986 and $3.5 billion by mid-1988.)[47] The government's financial policies, however, seem to remain relatively constant. By mid-1986, any amount of dollars, at least theoretically, could be exchanged at the Banco de la República under the categories of "tourism," "personal services," and "transfers and donations"—and not even the name of the transactor was required. (Another common technique for laundering the proceeds of drug sales relies on overinvoicing exports: The trafficker inflates the value of export earnings from a legitimate business to account for narco-dollar earnings.) Moreover, the Barco administration announced its own tax amnesty shortly after Barco took office. As one Colombian observer remarked, "All elected presidents allege that this is the only way that they can finance their new four-year term."[48]

The cocaine dollars that return to the exporting country may represent only a small fraction of traffickers' total earnings, but their impact is significant in financial markets, especially in Peru and Bolivia. (Colombia enjoys a much larger and more diversified economy than Peru and Bolivia, as well as a flourishing export sector that earned $5.3 billion in 1987— twice the value of Peru's exports and more than 10 times the value of Bolivia's.) Any successful crackdown on the cocaine industry would put noticeable pressure on these countries' finances, seriously devaluing the currency and possibly triggering an uncontrollable wage-price spiral. A massive expansion in international loans could compensate in part for these effects; however, because the countries are not particularly credit-worthy—Peru's recent nationalistic stance on debt repayment has aggravated its already poor relations with the international financial community—such loans may be difficult to arrange.

What Happens to Cocaine Money

Large infusions of dollars from any source are of great potential value to a developing nation, and narco-dollars are no exception. Drug earnings stabilize a country's currency, help finance needed imports, and may even enhance a country's creditworthiness. Yet, establishing a link between drug money and economic growth, at least in the conventional sense of the term, is difficult. During the cocaine boom of the 1980s, Bolivia's formal economy actually shrank. The gross domestic product declined by an estimated 14 percent from 1980 to 1986.[49] A good argument can be made that the cocaine economy has functioned as a hedge of sorts against economic disaster, absorbing labor from moribund economic sectors (the Bolivian tin industry, for example) and becoming a vital source of hard currency when world prices for traditional exports—oil, gas, copper, and tin—collapse. But that argument is not the same as saying that the cocaine industry constitutes a positive factor in a country's development. Such a conclusion might be warranted, but much depends on whether coca growers and cocaine traffickers spend their money locally in economically productive ways.

Evidence on this point is vague—people in the drug trade do not publish balance sheets or release annual reports. Yet, accounts from a variety of sources—journalists, U.S. DEA and State Department officials, and government authorities in producer countries—suggest that cocaine money (earned at all stages of production and distribution) flows into the following activities.

- **Direct Capital and Operating Expenses:** seeds and fertilizer, farm tools, laboratory equipment, chemicals, raw materials, means of transport (aircraft, boats, and trucks), and labor (*pisadores,* chemists, pilots, couriers, and the like)
- **Security:** private armies, "enforcers," and contract assassins; automatic and semiautomatic weapons (for example, Uzis, AR-15s); state-of-the-art radio equipment; scramblers and coding devices; and computerized navigation systems
- **Critical Services:** lawyers, accountants, bank employees, investment counselors, and the like
- **Protection and Intelligence:** payoffs to politicians in office, law enforcement officials, judges, and the military; and maintenance of an informant network in government agencies and in U.S. embassies overseas
- **Political Participation:** contributions to political campaigns, public relations and image-building (for example, promotion of prodrug positions in the media), sponsorship of candidate slates and political movements, and running for political office
- **Private Welfare Activities:** housing projects, sewer repair, medical services, roads, schools, and charitable donations
- **Legitimate Capital Investment:** typically ranches (cattle breeding and horse farming); commercial agriculture; banks; hotels; restaurants and discothèques; real estate and construction companies; apartment complexes; sports clubs; radio stations and publishing ventures; and various retail outlets, such as gas stations, car dealerships, and drug stores
- **Luxury Consumption:** for example, yachts, Mercedes-Benzes, beach-front condos, color televisions, videocassette recorders, gold chains, and antiques.

Cocaine earnings are largely recycled in the cocaine industry itself, expended on capital and operating costs—plant labor, equipment, and raw materials—and on the creation of a secure environment for the industry. Some of the money spent on inputs for the industry may not enter the local economy at all—for example, when Colombian traffickers buy ether and acetone (precursor chemicals) from Brazil or coca paste or cocaine base from Peru or Bolivia. Protection expenses provide employment and salary supplements, but little else. Private armies guard cocaine shipments, laboratories, and key industry executives. (In Colombia, traffickers' security companies are more or less legal and are licensed by the Ministry of Defense.) Traffickers also make huge outlays to buy off local police or military commanders, cultivate friends in high places, and express their points of view to the general public.

Mafia money does flow into legitimate businesses, although it does so selectively. The Colombian mafia as a whole invested an estimated $5.5 billion in urban and rural real estate between 1979 and 1988; real estate has probably absorbed most of the mafia's repatriated funds.[50] In Bolivia, the well-known cocaine "king" Roberto Suarez reportedly owns 22,000 head of cattle.[51] In fact, many Bolivian traffickers also are large landholders who engage in ranching and commercial farming. They plow some of their drug proceeds into developing those businesses, for example, into cross-breeding cattle or improving cotton or sugarcane yields.

Service industries such as hotels, travel agencies, real estate firms, transport companies, and banks also absorb trafficking funds. In Cali, the Orejuela family at one time controlled a financial empire that comprised a Chrysler dealership; a construction firm; a number of drug stores; a toy company, Mundo de los Niños; an automobile race track; various real estate companies; 28 radio stations in Colombian cities; and one of Colombia's largest banks, the Banco de los Trabajadores. (The Orejuelas recently divested themselves of the radio stations and their shares in the troubled bank.)[52] In Peru, Reynaldo Rodríguez Lopez, a trafficker who was a trusted adviser to Peru's top police officials, owned a travel agency (International Tourist Services) that served as a cover for his cocaine smuggling operations. Similarly, the suspicion is that aerial-spraying companies belonging to Gonzalo Rodríguez Gacha and an executive airline service (Pilotos Executivos) controlled through intermediaries by the Ochoa family are being used to transport cocaine.

Mario Arango, the aforementioned Colombian economist, offers some empirical evidence of these financial flows. In late 1987 and early 1988, he interviewed 20 medium- and high-level cocaine capos in Medellín about their legal investment preferences. Although the sample is small, successfully conducting the interviews was an impressive feat in itself. The number-one investment preferences of the capos are detailed below.[53]

Preference	Number	Percent
Real estate (rural and urban)	9	45
Cattle ranching	4	20
Commerce (wholesale, retail)	3	15
Construction of high-rise office buildings, luxury condominiums	2	10
Services and recreation (sports, gymnasiums, hotels, restaurants, discothèques, clinics)	2	10

All this does not add up to a very balanced investment picture. Traffickers are not captains of industry like the Rockefellers, Harrimans, and

Carnegies of yore. Relatively little narcotics money flows directly into core industries such as mining, oil, power generation, and manufacturing. Such enterprises are either government-owned or dominated by established economic elites who make it a point to exclude drug dealers and other parvenus. Moreover, the economics of some drug trafficking investments are suspect. For example, the enormous Posada Alemana hotel complex built by Carlos Lehder in Armenia—at a cost of roughly $5 million—was touted as a future "tourist epicenter" in Colombia's coffee-growing zone, but lost more than $1 million in its 3-year existence.[54] Moreover, traffickers' businesses are sometimes just fronts for money laundering: They operate consistently at a loss, but they may thereby force legitimate ventures out of business. For all these reasons, the mafia's legitimate investments are unlikely to catalyze the economic take-off of drug-producing countries in Latin America.

Cocaine trafficking, however, clearly has transformed the social fabric of many South American communities. The creation of a new subculture devoted to personal consumption and entertainment certainly represents one of the major effects. As a 1981 *Wall Street Journal* article on the city of Santa Cruz in Bolivia—a center of both commercial agriculture and cocaine trafficking—noted:

> Today, Santa Cruz has become Bolivia's largest city, with thriving shopping centers, expensive restaurants, luxury hotels, and enough discothèques and bawdy houses to entertain revelers until dawn. But an up-and-down business such as agriculture could hardly have supported such a meteoric rise. The real reason behind Santa Cruz' sudden prosperity is that it has become the cocaine capital of the world.[55]

At the same time, conspicuous consumption constitutes a virtual hallmark of the illicit narcotics trade in both its rural and urban phases. In South American cities such as Medellín, Colombia, and Santa Cruz, Bolivia, cocaine capos flaunt ostentatious life styles, buying luxury high-rise apartment buildings, Mercedes-Benzes and BMWs, helicopters, and antiques. After an enormous bomb exploded in January 1988 in front of one of Pablo Escobar's Medellín buildings ("Monaco"), police discovered in the wreckage a veritable treasure trove of paintings, including works by Botero, Obregon, and (according to one informed U.S. source) Van Gogh. Also found were Ming dynasty vases, Greek sculptures, and a collection of 30 antique cars in the basement.[56]

In the remote jungle regions where coca is cultivated, the new-found wealth of coca farmers has produced an almost schizophrenic development pattern. Governments do not possess the power to tax the very considerable inflow of narco-dollars or to direct these dollars toward general social needs such as health, education, and transport. Hence, private wealth tends to coexist with public squalor. The town of Tocache in the Upper Huallaga Valley typifies this pattern. A coca boom town, Tocache has no paved streets and no drinking water or sewage system, but it boasts six banks, six Telex machines, several stereo dealerships, and one of the largest Nissan outlets in Peru.[57]

The residents of areas such as the Upper Huallaga and the Chapare desperately want the social services that the coca trade apparently cannot provide. Indeed, some coca growers' organizations in these regions have offered to reduce coca cultivation voluntarily if the government proposes a comprehensive program of rural development: roads, schools, clinics, agricultural processing plants, and the like. So far, however, there has not been a meeting of the minds. Coca farmers have made excessive demands, and South American governments have not been able to commit extensive resources to rural modernization projects.

To be sure, countervailing influences exist: Major cocaine chieftains have themselves assumed the responsibility for delivering social services to the population, usually in their home towns or provinces. These activities are a key part of the mafia's overall political strategy, which involves building a basis of mass support "below" as well as corrupting those in authority "above." The importance of these activities should not be underestimated; however, the mafia's largesse does not usually extend to coca-growing regions. Here, greedy and untutored peasants pursue their squalid visions of the good life with virtually no concern for the public good.

Working for the Industry

The cocaine industry is an important employer, directly hiring peasant growers, seasonal part-time laborers who plant and harvest, and various cogs in the production-logistics machine: leaf merchants, truck drivers, *pisadores*, chemists, couriers, small aircraft owners and pilots, laborers who build clandestine airstrips, armed guards for airstrips and laboratories, and the heads of trafficking organizations. The bulk of these people probably are engaged in the agricultural end of the business. Bolivian government sources estimate that approximately 70,000 to 80,000 coca growers farm in that country. Peru's COMUCOD gave a figure in 1986 of "slightly over 100,000 families involved in coca production" in all of Peru.[58] Less coca is cultivated in Colombia than in Peru and Bolivia, so there are fewer growers—a very rough estimate might be 25,000 farmers, or one family per hectare. Coca farming does not necessarily constitute a full-time occupation. In Bolivia, for example, many peasants float back and forth between the Chapare and the Upper Cochabamba Valley; from May to September, they work in the coca fields, and from October to January, they plant and harvest corn, wheat, and other traditional crops in the Valley.

Most Peruvian and Bolivian sources assume a family size of five to six persons per producer. The Peruvian coca expert Edgardo Machado estimates that, on average, there are three working members per family. Using this assumption, the estimate is that some 210,000 to 240,000 people are employed in cultivating coca in Bolivia, more than 300,000 in Peru, and 75,000 in Colombia—a total of 585,000 and 615,000 workers. Another scholar, Ethan Nadelmann of Princeton University, estimates that 2.2 farmers are required to cultivate each ton of coca leaves, which would translate into about 465,000 farmers by using the upper-bound U.S. estimates of South American production in 1987.[59] There is a legal market for coca leaves in Peru and Bolivia, but a relatively small percentage of farmers—perhaps 10 percent—produces solely for that market.

Estimates vary widely on the number of people engaged in downstream functions—transporting leaves, converting leaves to cocaine, smuggling cocaine products, guarding laboratories, and so on. A 1986 study by the Bolivian Senate's Special Committee on Drug Trafficking and Drug Addiction projected 80,000 coca proprietors—this would mean 240,000 people who cultivate coca—and an additional 45,000 workers involved in the illicit cocaine market (see Figure 1.1). This calculation yields a 5.3:1 ratio of coca producers to traffickers. Nadelmann's work suggests a 2.7:1 ratio, and a 1987 State Department report on Bolivia estimates that there are 200,000 coca producers and another 100,000 "involved in precursor smuggling, coca maceration, the construction and guarding of maceration pits, and the buying and selling of coca leaves, paste, and CHCL."[60] (Some narcotics experts put the total number of coca producers and cocaine traffickers in Bolivia at 350,000.) In Colombia, which has a large cocaine refining industry, the ratio is probably higher—1:1 might be a reasonable estimate.

Using these admittedly tenuous assumptions, the total employment in the South American cocaine trade can be calculated at between 500,000 and 1 million workers. But this figure only represents direct employment; the dimensions of the problem are really much larger, because the industry generates substantial indirect employment by increasing the demand for goods and services. Sectors such as real estate construction, banking, and entertainment—as well as sales of cars, consumer electronics, antiques, and other luxury goods—apparently have thrived on the influx of narco-dollars. Lawyers, investment counselors, and others who provide consulting services to traffickers have seen their businesses boom in recent years.

FIGURE 1.1
Structure of the Bolivian Cocaine Industry

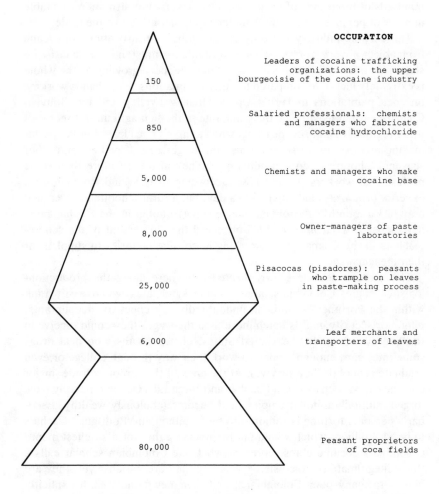

OCCUPATION

150 — Leaders of cocaine trafficking organizations: the upper bourgeoisie of the cocaine industry

850 — Salaried professionals: chemists and managers who fabricate cocaine hydrochloride

5,000 — Chemists and managers who make cocaine base

8,000 — Owner-managers of paste laboratories

25,000 — Pisacocas (pisadores): peasants who trample on leaves in paste-making process

6,000 — Leaf merchants and transporters of leaves

80,000 — Peasant proprietors of coca fields

Source: Bolivian National Senate. ''Informe Preliminar Sobre Narcotrafico.'' La Paz: 1986 pp. 23–24.

And companies that supply the drug trade, such as manufacturers of farm equipment or precursor chemicals, have undoubtedly benefited as well. In other words, an immense and pervasive cocaine constituency thrives in South American countries, a constituency that encompasses not just hundreds of thousands of farmers and traffickers, but also an incalculable number of persons who profit from the multiplier effects of the trade.

The cocaine industry not only creates jobs, but also offers an escape from abject poverty for many and a veritable fortune (and even quasi-elite status) for a few. Although leaf prices fluctuate, coca growing on the whole is extremely lucrative compared to other occupations. Field hands working on coca plantations in Peru's Upper Huallaga Valley and the Bolivian Chapare earn at least twice the going rate in the licit agricultural sector of these regions. *Pisadores*, peasants who stamp on coca leaves in the paste-making process, make several times the wages of leaf pickers and other seasonal laborers in coca production.[61] They also earn more than some professional workers: In mid-1986, according to U.S. and Bolivian coca experts, *pisadores* made up to $40 a day, but a rural schoolteacher earned only $23 a month![62] A Bolivian police report quoted in the Cochabamba newspaper *Los Tiempos* in 1985 observed that 70 percent of the school-teachers in the Chapare were working in cocaine factories to supplement their meager wages.[63]

This pattern doubtless is replicated elsewhere along the production-logistics chain. Colombia's large cocaine syndicates would easily rank within the Fortune 500 and can undoubtedly pay chemists, accountants, pilots, or security guards much more than the wages they could receive in the licit economy. In the United States, ghetto youths who deal drugs sometimes earn enough money to work their way through college or even graduate school (if they survive). At the apex of the narcotics trade, major cocaine capos such as Pablo Escobar and Jorge Luis Ochoa reputedly have forged multibillion-dollar empires and become fabulously wealthy. Escobar's personal fortune is rumored to be $3 billion and Rodríguez Gacha's to be $1.3 billion, which would put them among the world's richest men.[64] Colombia's cocaine elites represent what one Colombian scholar calls a "new illegitimate bourgeoisie."[65] Socially they are pariahs; yet, they are heroes to many poor Colombians, and their newfound wealth explicitly challenges traditional class structures and social mobility patterns.

The Cocaine Economy: A Mixed Blessing

Like any boom crop or product, cocaine creates undesirable economic side effects. The drug bonanza—similar to the California gold rush of the last century or the Nigerian oil boom of the early 1980s—generated inflationary pressures in some economic sectors. Housing markets have been especially affected. For example, inflows of narco-dollars into Colombia in the late 1970s and early 1980s reportedly drove prices of luxury housing up by more than 500 percent. (In 1984, prices slumped—a sign that narco-dollars were leaving the country—but they rose again between 1985 and 1988.)[66] The result is a distorted pattern of growth. Cities that are epicenters of the cocaine trade, Medellín and Cali, for example, exhibit exceptionally high rates of construction, as measured by new housing permits during the 1980s.[67] Moreover, traffickers in effect have bid away resources from government programs to provide housing for lower- and middle-income citizens. As former Colombian President Belisario Bentancur explained in a 1986 speech, such plans "have virtually failed because the existence of buyers with money from drug trafficking has led to the construction almost exclusively of luxury homes, causing shortages where the greatest need exists [and] greatly increasing the price of real estate."[68]

Furthermore, the drug trade affects price structures in the countryside. As a United Nations Fund for Drug Abuse and Control (UNFDAC) memorandum stated about Bolivia, "Coca and cocaine cause inflation, because they introduce a huge monetary mass into the system and, besides, raise the price of goods in coca growing areas, especially the Chapare."[69] A few examples follow. According to American sociologist Kevin Healy, prices of kerosene and toilet paper in 1985 were, respectively, two to three times and nine times the prices in Bolivia's major cities. (These articles are used for making cocaine as well as for household purposes.) Healy reports that the daily cost of living in the Chapare town of Sinahota was as high as $100 in the mid-1980s; the average wage in Bolivia, however, is approximately $40 a month. The inflationary pattern in the Chapare is reflected in the neighboring urban center of Cochabamba. In 1984, Cochabamba ranked as one of the least expensive Bolivian cities in which to live; by 1986, it had become the most expensive.[70]

Traditional agriculture, however, is the biggest loser from the cocaine industry, especially subsistence agriculture in the zones where coca is grown. Peasants substitute coca for less profitable food crops. The Cochabamba newspaper *Los Tiempos*, for example, refers to the "systematic suppression" of subsistence crops such as rice and yucca in the Chapare region. Shortages are so acute, said the newspaper, that hungry peasants are systematically stealing yucca from the few remaining fields. According to Kevin Healy, the Chapare now imports food, although this dependency may just be regional; that is, production elsewhere in Bolivia may have increased.[71] A representative of Peru's National Coca Enterprise (ENACO) interviewed in Tingo María said that food production in the Upper Huallaga Valley decreased during the coca boom of the 1980s; peasants, he said, shifted land or other inputs (labor, tools, and fertilizer) into cultivating coca. Shortages of labor—at least at affordable prices—during planting or harvesting season contributed to the decay of traditional agriculture. For example, rice farmers in the department of San Martín (in the Upper Huallaga region) almost lost their harvest in 1985, because coca farmers had bid away nearly all available supplies of labor. These coca jobs paid daily wages of 50,000 soles to 100,000 soles, compared to the 15,000 soles to 20,000 soles paid by the rice industry. Such unfair competition has almost put licit farmers in the Valley out of business.[72]

Coca-growing regions exert a pull on other parts of the country, causing population shifts. In Bolivia's Upper Cochabamba Valley and in parts of the Peruvian and Bolivian altiplano, farmers have simply abandoned their plots and moved to the coca fields. Moreover, workers, miners, and even professionals such as engineers and schoolteachers have gravitated to coca-growing areas in search of a better life. Because of the explosive growth in the coca economy, the Chapare's population swelled from 80,000 to 120,000 between 1981 and 1985; the province of Tocache in the Upper Huallaga Valley grew more than 600 percent from 1977 to 1987, from 7,000 to 50,000.[73] These migration patterns are to some extent a response to hard times and unemployment; however, they arguably drain the licit economy of labor, talent, and services. As a lawyer in Cochabamba declared, "Now there aren't any carpenters or bricklayers, because they've all gone off to stamp on coca. They're leaving us without craftsmen and workers."[74]

Such patterns are not immutable. Aggressive antidrug campaigns can temporarily alter the economics of farming illicit crops. Unfortunately, in Bolivia, Peru, and Colombia, the governments exercise little real authority in coca-growing zones, and eradication programs have suffered as a result. Bolivia and Peru are now trying a new enforcement approach: depriving peasants of buyers for their leaves by concentrating attacks on the next links in the production chain, the laboratories that convert the leaves into cocaine. Results so far are mixed. In mid-1986, Operation Blast Furnace, a combined U.S.-Bolivian campaign against cocaine laboratories in the Beni and Santa Cruz regions, drove the price of leaves from $125 per 100-pound bale to under $20—less than the cost of production. Cocaine farmers no longer made profits growing coca. Yet, after the U.S. forces left Bolivia in October-November 1986, prices rose again, exceeding $100 per hundredweight in mid-1987; they dropped to between $20 per hundred-weight and $30 per hundredweight in January 1988, but rose to more than $100 per hundredweight in the summer of 1988.[75]

Lasting changes occur only when peasants can find alternative ways of making a living. As argued above, the prospects for large-scale crop substitution in coca-growing areas are very dim. The solution, if there is one, seems to lie in stimulating reverse migration. The Bolivian government's new "Triennial Program for the Struggle Against Drug Trafficking," for example, says, "We plan to carry out programs of integral development in those regions where the expulsion of the population originated. The object of this is to attract those farmers who emigrated to the Chapare so that they will return to their lands."[76] This is probably a reasonable strategy for both Bolivia and Peru. Yet, integral development—the creation of economic alternatives to the cocaine industry—will require the extensive overhaul of Andean economies and (very probably) billions of dollars in foreign aid and private investment from the United States and other industrialized countries.

Net Assessment

Conspicuous waste, uneven development, and schizophrenic life styles are the hallmarks of the cocaine economy. As a renegade industry, the cocaine sector contributes nothing (at least directly) to the public treasury and to government development programs. Obviously, the sector's spending priorities are inferior to those of national planners—key economic sectors are shortchanged, and substantial money is frittered away on nonproductive private consumption. From a purely economic (as opposed to political or moral) standpoint, it is unfortunate that governments do not control the cocaine trade; if they did, narco-dollars might be a real boost for development.

Still, the cocaine trade produces benefits: Cocaine is a vital source of hard currency, especially in Peru and Bolivia. Some cocaine profits are invested in the legal economy, albeit primarily in agriculture, ranching, and services. Even apparently unproductive expenditures create myriad economic linkages—in economic parlance, multiplier effects—that affect the economy in several ways. For example, the traffickers' demand for luxury housing has been a boon for building contractors and, indirectly, for domestic producers of construction materials such as cement, bricks, and glass. (This pattern has been especially pronounced in Colombia.) Local industrialists may have created new manufacturing capacity to meet the cocaine industry's requirements for farm equipment, chemicals, generators, filters, centrifuges, and other tools of the trade. In other words, the cocaine trade creates reciprocal patterns of activity in the economy, and these interactions can work over time to facilitate economic growth in Colombia, Bolivia, and Peru.

Whether or not the cocaine industry generates advantages or disadvantages for Andean economies—and the case can be made both ways—it indisputably has gained a powerful economic foothold, especially in Peru and Bolivia. The industry attracts labor from economic sectors that have fallen on hard times. For example, the collapse of world tin prices forced many Bolivian tin mines to shut down, and many unemployed miners went to the coca fields looking for work. In the Andean highlands, farm incomes have been damaged by low prices for traditional crops, by heavily eroded soils, and by the increasing fragmentation of land ownership. Consequently, many Andean peasants, too, are migrating to coca-growing areas. "Probably before they cultivated coca leaves, they were starving," remarked Bolivia's Ambassador to the United States, Fernando Illanes, in a July 1986 interview.[77] So, in a sense, the cocaine trade acts as an important safety valve for the troubled economies of these Andean nations, even if such economic dependence is not healthy in the long term. Political leaders in these nations fear, with some justification, that economic and political chaos would result if the industry shut down tomorrow.

The greatest obstacles to a successful crackdown on drugs, however, stem from political rather than economic concerns. Powerful constituencies have developed around the various phases of the cocaine traffic, and these constituencies have amassed enough money and power to effect major changes in the Andean political landscape. The following chapter will discuss one aspect of this phenomenon: the political organizations of coca farmers that have emerged in the Andean countries in recent years.

Notes

1. Timothy Plowman, "Botanical Perspectives on Coca," in F. R. Jeri (ed), *Cocaine 1980: Proceedings of the Interamerican Seminar on Coca and Cocaine* (Lima: Pacific Press, 1980), pp. 90–91, 97, 99.
   Peter White, "Coca—An Ancient Herb Turns Deadly," *The National Geographic*, January 1989, p. 24.
2. Drug Enforcement Administration, *Special Report: Worldwide Cocaine Trafficking Trends* (Washington, D.C., 1985), p. 5.
3. Department of State, *International Narcotics Control Strategy Report (INCSR)* (Washington, D.C., 1988), pp. 78, 92, 109.
4. Comité Multisectoral de Control de Drogas (COMUCOD), *Plan Nacional de Prevención y Control de Drogas: Mediano Plazo 1986-1990 (Plan Nacional)* Lima, 1986, pp. 38, 64.
   "Coca, ese becerro de oro," *Actualidad Económica*, No. 88 (March 1987), p. 3.
5. Telephone conversations with the U.S. embassy in La Paz and with the Sub-Secretariat of Alternative Development in La Paz, January 1989.
6. Kevin Healy, "The Cocaine Industry in Bolivia—Its Impact on the Peasantry," *CS Quarterly*, Vol. 9, No. 4 (1985), p. 28.
7. *INCSR*, 1988, p. 70.
   INCSR, 1987, p. 125.

8. Edmundo Morales, "New Trends in Coca and Cocaine Economy in the Andes of Peru" (Narcotics and Drug Research, Inc., 1985), pp. 7–14.

9. Empresa Nacional de la Coca (ENACO), "Compras Mensuales," February 1987.
   Interviews with U.S. narcotics experts in La Paz, May 20–22, 1986.

10. ENACO, "Verificación de ventas por exportación de hoja de coca y cancelaciones abonadas periodo 1980–1985," Lima, December 1985.

11. ENACO, "Exportación de cocaína rendimiento de transferencias pasta básica cocaína y utilización periodos 1978–1985," Lima, December 1985.

12. "Narcotráfico supone movimiento de dos mil millones de dólares," *Presencia*, August 5, 1984.

13. "U.S. AID Project Wins Few Friends and Fails to Match the Drug Industry's Complete Package," *The Andean Report*, Lima, December 1985, p. 244.

14. Organization of American States, "Socio-Economic Studies for the Inter-American Specialized Conference on Drug Traffic," Washington, D.C., February 12, 1986, p. 14.

15. Gerald Owens, "Costs of Production: Coca," unsolicited report to AID, December 31, 1986, pp. 5–6.

16. Coca farming, incidentally, seems to be more profitable than farming opium, the raw material for heroin. In Thailand, according to State Department sources, an opium grower can actually earn greater returns by cultivating some traditional crops and consequently may be more receptive to crop substitution schemes.

17. See note 13.

18. Agency for International Development, "Project Field Operations" (part of a 1987 project status report), 1987, p. 128.

19. Jaime Jaramillo et al., *Coca, Colonización y Guerrilla* (Bogotá: Universidad Nacional de Colombia, 1986), p. 107.

20. IRI Research Institute, "Huallaga Valley Agribusiness and Military Study," May 1985, p. 375.
    Interviews with U.S. and Bolivian agricultural officials, May 1986 and October 1987.

21. "Coca en Perú," *Perú Económico*, January 1984, p. 50.

22. Interviews with U.S. AID officials in Lima and La Paz, March 1986 and May 1986.
    See also note 13.

23. Interviews with U.S. AID officials and officials of the Secretariat for the Development of the Bolivian Tropics, May 12–21, 1986.
    "Triennial Program," p. 15.

24. National Narcotics Intelligence Consumers' Committee (NNICC), *The Supply of Drugs to the U.S. Illicit Market from Foreign and Domestic Sources in 1980* (*Supply of Drugs in 1980*) (Washington, D.C., 1980), p. 49.
    NNICC, *The NNICC Report 1985-1986* (*NNICC Report*) (Washington, D.C., June 1987), p. 28.

25. Secretaría de Desarollo del Trópico Boliviano, "Intento de approximación al flujo de ingresos en el comercio de la coca," Cochabamba, May 1980.

26. "La lumpen burguesia de la coca," *Meridiano*, La Paz, November 13, 1985.

27. Kevin Healy, "The Boom Within the Crisis: Some Recent Effects of Foreign Cocaine Markets on Bolivian Rural Society and Economy" ("The Boom Within the Crisis"), in Deborah Pacini and Christine Franquemont (eds), *Coca*

and Cocaine (Peterborough, New Hampshire: Transcript Printing Company, 1986), p. 123.

28. *NNICC Report*, p. 36.
29. *Supply of Drugs in 1980*, p. 48.
30. Peter Reuter, "Eternal Hope: America's Quest for Narcotics Control," *The Public Interest*, No. 79 (Spring 1985), p. 91.
31. *Plan Nacional*, p. 18.
    Bolivian National Senate, "Preliminary Report," p. 8.
    Unidad de Análisis de Políticas Económicas (UDAPE), "La económica informal en una visión macroeconómica," La Paz, September 1985, p. 93.
32. "Text of Drug Traffickers' Terms for Ending Activities," *El Tiempo*, July 7, 1984, pp. 1A, 1C.
33. "Colombia: The Drug Economy," *The Economist*, April 2, 1988, p. 63.
34. "Triennial Program," pp. 5–6.
35. "Bolivia," *Latin American Regional Reports*, March 3, 1988, p. 8.
36. "Casi todo está corrompido por narcotraficantes," *El Nacional*, Lima, February 1, 1986, p. 12.
37. Mario Arango Jaramillo, *Impacto del Narcotráfico en Antioquia* (*Impacto del narcotráfico*) (Medellín: J. M. Arango, 1988), p. 96.
38. *Impacto del Narcotráfico*, pp. 137–141.
    Hernando Gomez, "La Economía ilegal en Colombia: tamaño, evolución características e impacto económico," *Coyuntura Económica*, September 1988, p. 109.
39. Committee on Foreign Relations, U.S. Senate, *Drugs, Law Enforcement and Foreign Policy: Panama* (Washington, D.C.: U.S. Government Printing Office, 1988), Hearings, February 8–11, 1988, p. 245.
40. "Fighting the Cocaine Wars," *Time*, February 25, 1985, p. 29.
    "De 100 mil milliones calculan bienes de la mafia en Florida," *El Tiempo*, December 2, 1987, p. 3A.
41. International Monetary Fund (IMF), *International Financial Statistics* (Washington, D.C.: IMF, November 1987), pp. 122–123.
42. "Sí tienen que investigar los coca dólares," *El Nacional*, February 2, 1986.
43. Mario Arango Jaramillo and Jorge Child, *Narcotráfico Imperio de la Cocaína* (Medellín: Editorial Percepción, 1984), p. 9.
    International Financial Statistics, November 1987, p. 162.
44. Javier Brena, "President Will Allow Drug Dealers to Declare Income," The Associated Press, International News, December 24, 1982.
45. "Lehder cuenta como se hizo millionario con bonanza de la droga," *El Espectador*, June 29, 1983.
46. "Betancur Addresses Nation," Bogotá, Radio Cadena Super, May 1, 1984.
47. *International Financial Statistics*, August 1988, p. 173.
    International Financial Statistics, December 1986, pp. 162–163.
48. Fabio Castillo, *Los Jinetes de la Cocaína* (*Los Jinetes*) (Bogotá: Editorial Documentos Periodisticos, 1987), p. 175.
49. UDAPE, "Información económica," 1986, p. 1.
50. "El Narco Agro," *Semana*, November 29–December 5, 1988, p. 34.
51. "El rey de la coca," *Hoy*, Santiago, July 13, 1983.
52. *Los Jinetes*, pp. 124–131.
53. *Impacto del Narcotráfico*, p. 126.
54. Jorge Eliecer Orozco, *Lehder . . . El Hombre* (Bogotá: Plaza y Janes, 1987), p. 101.

55. "Cocaine Wealth Comes to Bolivian City, Creating Wealth, Eroding Agriculture," *Wall Street Journal*, March 25, 1981.
56. "Quién fué," *Semana*, January 25, 1988, p. 4.
    Interviews with Medellín businessmen, March 5–10, 1988.
57. Scott L. Malcolmson, "Cocaine Republic," *Village Voice*, August 26, 1986, p. 18.
    "Tocache: Some Things Go Better With. . . ," *The Andean Report*, December 1985, pp. 242–243.
58. "Triennial Program," p. 5.
    Bolivian National Senate, "Preliminary Report," p. 26.
    Plan Nacional, p. 260.
59. "Coca Growing, Cocaine Consumption Seen as National Problems," interview with Edgardo Machado, *El Comercio*, June 16, 1985.
    "La economía de la cocaína en America Latina" (chart by Nadelmann), *Los Jinetes*, p. 174.
60. Bolivian National Senate, "Preliminary Report," p. 26.
    INCSR, pp. 122–123.
61. "The Boom Within the Crisis," p. 122.
62. Interviews with U.S. and Bolivian agricultural experts in La Paz and Cochabamba, May 13–20, 1986.
63. "The Boom Within the Crisis," p. 124.
64. "The Americas," *Forbes*, October 5, 1987, p. 155.
    "The Americas," *Forbes*, July 25, 1988, p. 121.
65. Alvaro Camacho Guizado, *Droga Corrupción y Poder* (Cali, Colombia: Universidad de Valle, 1981), p. 98.
66. R. W. Lee, "The Latin American Drug Connection," *Foreign Policy*, No. 61 (Winter 1985–1986), p. 148.
    William R. Long, "Billionaire Drug Traffickers Rules: Powerful Medellín Cartel Safe in its Colombian Base," *Los Angeles Times*, February 21, 1988.
67. The measure used in yearly housing permits as a percentage of population. The ratio is about three times that of Bogotá and twice that of Barranquilla. Statistics provided by Departmento Administrativo Nacional de Estadística (DANE).
68. "President on Drug Trafficking as a Destabilizing Factor," *Cámbio*, Madrid, February 10, 1986, pp. 72–75.
69. United Nations Fund for Drug Abuse and Control (UNFDAC), "Bolivia," unpublished memorandum, 1986, p. 3.
70. "Boom Within the Crisis," pp. 117–118, 127.
71. Ibid., p. 128.
    "La yuca en vez de coca?" *Los Tiempos*, Cochabamba, August 24, 1984.
72. "Rice Pickers Prefer to Harvest Coca for High Wages," *El Comercio*, May 19, 1985, p. A–12.
73. "Boom Within the Crisis," p. 102.
    Interviews with U.S. narcotics experts in Lima, October 15, 1987.
74. "In a Land of the Poor, Coca Producers Drive BMWs," *Miami Herald*, December 1, 1985.
75. Bureau of International Narcotics Matters, Department of State, *Mid-Year Update, INCSR* (Washington, D.C., September 1987), p. 10.

Interviews with U.S. narcotics experts in La Paz, October 11, 1988.

76. "Triennial Program," p. 15.

77. Henry Gottlieb, "Bolivian Peasants Are Cocaine's Victims," The Associated Press, Washington Dateline, July 26, 1986.

2

The Coca Lobby

Coca is responsible for the sad history of our people.
— Bolivian historian H. Fajardo, 1981

We will gladly lay down our lives to protect our coca fields.
— Chapare peasant leader, April 1987

Basic Characteristics

Structure and Origins

In Peru and Bolivia, where coca has been cultivated for centuries, coca farmers (*cocaleros*) have organized to protect their interests. What may be called the "coca lobby" in these countries comprises, first, federations or committees that represent growers; for example, regional organizations in Peru's Upper Huallaga Valley and in the Yungas and Chapare regions of Bolivia. Second, Bolivia also has two nationwide coca producers' associations, which include national campesino and labor unions as well. The leaders of these mass membership organizations consistently support the goals of Bolivian coca farmers in their confrontations with the government. Third, the lobby can be considered to comprise elected representatives of coca-growing areas, from mayors and assemblymen to deputies or senators in national law-making bodies. (Deputies and senators from Bolivia's Cochabamba department, for example, act as a kind of coca caucus within the Bolivian Congress.) However, the boundaries of the coca lobby are fluid: People from all sections of society—intellectuals, military officers, government bureaucrats, jurists, and political leaders—at different times have taken up the cause of coca farmers.

The coca lobby is unique to Peru and Bolivia; there is nothing comparable in other South American countries, because coca growing is

55

entrenched in the history, culture, and economy of these two Andean countries. The coca leaf played a central role in the commercial and religious life of South American Indians for thousands of years.[1] Moreover, several million people in the Andean altiplano and in parts of the Amazon basin still consume coca leaves—mainly through the practice of chewing or *acullico*—to combat hunger, fatigue, and assorted circulatory and intestinal ailments. The cultivation of coca is legal, although formally subject to government controls, in Peru and Bolivia. Bolivia's new coca law (enacted in July 1988) established 12,000 hectares of licit cultivation to meet licit demand; the rest is targeted for eventual eradication. In Peru in 1985, there reportedly were about 25,000 officially registered producers cultivating nearly 18,000 hectares of legal coca.[2] The traditional market provides a justification and cover for the illegal market; it is hard to say where one market leaves off and the other begins. For example, many of Peru's registered producers sell part or all of their coca leaves to traffickers, who typically pay a much higher price than the government marketing agency, Empresa Nacional de Coca (ENACO).

Finally, because cultivation has expanded greatly to meet illicit demand, coca growing is important to the rural economies of Peru and Bolivia. The Bolivian government estimated the aggregate value of coca production at $230 million in 1986; coca thus accounted for more than 20 percent of total national farm income in that year.[3] In areas such as the Chapare and the Upper Huallaga Valley, that proportion runs well over 90 percent. Including farmers and their families (and calculating five persons per family), the coca trade supports 2–3 percent of Peru's total population and 5–6 percent of Bolivia's.

This combination of factors exists nowhere else in South America. Colombia, the third largest producer (generating an estimated 20,000 metric tons), might serve as a point of comparison. Coca growing in Colombia carries little social legitimacy. Only a few scattered Indian tribes chew coca, and—with the exception of some small plantations in Cauca, Huila, and Magdalena departments—nearly all production dates from the mid-1970s or later and is completely illegal under Colombian law. Finally, coca cultivation does not represent an important economic activity by national standards, probably sustaining well under one percent of Colombia's population. For these reasons, Colombia's growers exert very little political clout; when they do articulate interests, they tend to do so through Fuerzas Armadas Revolucionarias de Colombia (FARC) revolutionaries, who exercise political and military control in some coca-growing areas.

Agenda

Core Objectives.   The coca lobby is not, formally speaking, a cocaine lobby. As a slogan of the Bolivian Labor Congress (COB), one of the umbrella organizations for coca growers in Bolivia, puts it, "Liberty in the production of coca, radical struggle against narcotics trafficking."[4] Regional growers' federations in Bolivia have promised to cooperate with the government in "a frontal and decisive struggle" against the cocaine trade and the "mafias" responsible for it.[5] Reality, however, never works quite so simply. Coca farmers profit by selling to drug dealers, so attacks on the cocaine processing infrastructure damage farmers by disrupting the market for their leaves. Furthermore, thousands of farmers have integrated forward into the production of coca paste, and drug trafficking syndicates reportedly stand behind a number of pro-coca federations and fronts. Yet, the coca lobby's formal agenda largely (although not exclusively) addresses the needs of the farmer—most fundamentally by trying to protect the farmers' coca crops against eradication and destruction by governments.

The coca lobby has been a determined foe of coca reduction programs worked out by national governments and the United States. The coca lobby attacked these agreements on nationalist and populist grounds. For example, a leader of a pro-coca splinter party in Bolivia says, "It is criminal and unacceptable to obligate campesinos to eradicate their coca plants in order to comply with the dictates of the North American government."[6] The Congress of Bolivian Workers accuses the United States of pressuring Bolivia to meet eradication targets and thus trying to convert Bolivia into a "Yankee colony."[7] Coca nationalism is rhetorically combined with an incessant stress on the socioeconomic importance of the coca trade. Coca is the "sustenance of thousands of our peasant comrades," reports a leader of Bolivia's National Campesino Federation.[8] The former mayor of Tingo María, Peru, says about coca growing, "Perhaps it is wrong, perhaps they are guilty, but the peasants must live, mustn't they?"[9] A pro-coca journalist in Bolivia notes that coca "is perhaps the only wealth in all our history that benefits an important sector of the Bolivian population."[10]

The coca lobby campaigns against eradication less because it sees coca growing as good per se than because it views Latin American governments and the U.S. government as offering no satisfactory alternatives to growers. However, the coca lobby's conceptions of reasonable alternatives tend to be extreme and unworkable. First, spokesmen for cocaleros want substitute crops that can yield comparable returns—an impossible demand. Because of their poor soil, rugged terrain, and distance from major markets, coca-growing regions are poorly suited to commercial agriculture. No single crop or combination of crops in those regions is ever likely to match the return from coca.

The coca lobby also presses for an increase in direct compensation for the destruction of coca fields. Farmers in Peru and Bolivia now are promised, respectively, $300 and $2,000 for each hectare eradicated. (Why Peruvian farmers are offered such a lower payment remains a mystery.) Peasant spokesmen contend that these figures are far too low, and with good reason. If leaf prices are $100 per carga (hundredweight), a Bolivian peasant can net about $2,600 in a single year; at a rock-bottom price of $50 per carga, the farmer can still earn twice as much income per hectare as he could from growing any traditional crop. Bolivian peasant leaders in 1987 demanded compensation of $6,000 per hectare, which agricultural experts believe is approximately the start-up cost for converting to another marketable crop such as tea or oranges. In 1988, a "cultural adviser" for the COB, Filemon Escobar, claimed that to persuade Bolivian peasants to abandon the cultivation of coca bushes, "We will need $1 billion a year." The money would be used for "investments such as the construction of roads and health care posts, rural electrification, and production diversification."[11]

Third, the coca lobby calls for massive agro-industrial development, supported by new infrastructures such as electrification, sanitation, educational facilities, and roads. Moreover, the lobby insists that the transformation and modernization of their communities precede the eradication of coca. Such projects would cost hundreds of millions if not billions of dollars, and some of them actually would promote the illicit narcotics trade. New agricultural institutes would unintentionally teach peasants how to grow better strains of coca. Electrification, as former Ambassador to Bolivia Edwin Corr once remarked, "will allow narco-traffickers to work also at night."[12] A new $90-million highway that the Inter-American Development Bank is building through the Chapare rain forest was correctly criticized by a U.S. official in the following terms: "If coca leaf production is not controlled in the lands being opened up by the highway, this is going to be the golden turnpike of cocaine."[13]

The coca lobby also vigorously promotes the commercialization or industrialization of coca leaves (now diverted to illicit markets) as a partial alternative to eradication. The idea of creating legitimate industrial uses for coca attracts broad support in Peru and Bolivia—even at the government level. Proponents of industrialization argue that coca leaves possess special nutritional and medicinal properties and can be converted to entirely new products, especially food and pharmaceuticals, that will sell in international markets. "The coca leaf is wonderful," says the research director of Peru's State Marketing Agency for Coca, ENACO. ENACO manages an active research and marketing program for coca-based products, including tea, soft drinks, mouthwash, toothpaste, diet pills, and medicine to regulate blood sugar.[14] Bolivian organizations such as the Medical-Pharmaceutical Research Society (SMIMFA) talk about building a new cocaine-based pharmaceutical industry that would "produce medicines of high quality for combatting a range of illnesses."[15] Even the Bolivian Vice President under Siles Zuazo, Jaime Paz Zamora, advocated industrialization, calling on the United States to create a fund for investigating the medicinal properties of coca and for marketing products extracted from the plant.[16] The Coca Industrialization Council (COINCOCA), which is subordinate to the Yungas and Chapare peasants' federation, has trial-manufactured several coca products with the authorization of the Ministry of Social Security and Public Health. Such products include a coca syrup that "is good for physical and sexual fatigue," a compound called "cocabetes" that supposedly lowers blood sugar, a weight-reducing drug, and a wine made from coca that "does not create the headaches typical of other kinds of wines."[17]

Not everyone is enthusiastic about the idea of industrialization. A Bolivian writer argues that a cocaine-based pharmaceutical industry would not survive competition from synthetic drugs. Anaesthetics such as novocaine and xylocaine, he says, are one-fourth as expensive to produce as cocaine. A U.S. embassy official in La Paz scornfully remarked in a 1984 interview, "The idea that coca could become a legal competitive product is almost impossible. They say it has nutrition, but dirt has nutrition, too. Just pick some other weed and decide you are going to compete with barley and oats and corn, the foods God gave us. It's absurd."[18] In general, U.S. officials are suspicious of industrialization, seeing it as a convenient smokescreen for cocaine trafficking. Also, U.S. drug laws prohibit the sale of most coca-based products in the United States. Yet, given the longstanding importance of the coca leaf in Andean cultures—and the widespread popular aversion to destroying the coca plant—the idea of industrialization is unlikely to disappear any time soon.

Aside from opposing eradication—or demanding massive rural change as the price for eliminating coca—the coca lobby defends farmers' interests in other ways. In Peru's Upper Huallaga Valley, local defense fronts in the provinces of Tocache and Leoncio Prado sought legalization of thousands of hectares of coca planted in the early and mid-1980s. Such cultivation violates Peruvian law, which defines legal cultivation as only that cultivation registered by the 1978 deadline. In Bolivia and Peru, growers opposed government attempts to regulate the sale of coca leaves.

Free sale of coca is equivalent to legalizing the production of cocaine, because farmers, if left to their own devices, are more likely to sell to traffickers than to the government wholesalers who buy for the traditional market. Free sale, however, is the reality in Bolivia and Peru. In Bolivia, almost 100 percent of the leaves in the Chapare, the main growing area, ends up in the hands of traffickers. In Peru, ENACO's purchases of coca leaf in 1986 were only 4,400 tons out of the 100,000 tons that the United States estimated were produced in Peru in that year.[19]

Peasant organizations in coca-growing zones such as Peru's Upper Huallaga Valley and the Bolivian Chapare have campaigned hard against the presence of antidrug police in their zones. Police are accused of violating personal and property rights of coca farmers—for example, stealing or killing livestock, raping peasant women, stealing money from peasants' homes, and confiscating coca leaves and reselling them to traffickers. In Bolivia, DEA advisers accompanying UMOPAR (rural mobile police detachments) have also come under fire. For example, peasant spokesmen have attempted to link DEA agents to "a series of outrages" in different parts of the Chapare, including two thefts (of $6,800 and $5,900) from Chapare peasants that allegedly occurred in May 1988.[20] The coca lobby's antipathy toward police, however, reflects more than a simple concern with the rights of farmers. Coca farmers, as noted above, have integrated forward into the production of coca paste, and paste laboratories are a primary target of law enforcement officials operating in coca-producing zones in Bolivia and Peru.

A Consumers Lobby?   The coca lobby basically constitutes a producers lobby and as such is concerned mainly about the impact of eradication and of other coca-control programs on the livelihood of farmers. Growers' organizations sometimes make the case for coca in terms of the ancestral tradition of chewing leaves. Yet, the grower and chewer are basically concerned about different matters: The grower wants to sell his leaves to the highest bidder, and the chewer wants to buy leaves at an affordable price. The rare advocates for coca consumers in Bolivia and Peru tend for the most part to be pro-Indian intellectuals—people concerned with preserving the coca-centered culture and tradition of the altiplano.

For example, the Peruvian writer Fernando Cabieses argues that eradication of coca would trigger the "apocolypse" of Andean culture; it would "drive the point of a lance through the heart of the Andean way of life." He notes, "The profound mystical, religious, mythological, and cultural significance of coca is not replaceable by any other element in the Andean world." Cabieses rhetorically asks whether the "utopian and uncertain goal of eliminating U.S. drug addiction justifies a cultural aggression against an oppressed people."[21]

Likewise, the Bolivian writer Amado Canelas strongly criticizes the coca "abolitionism" that prevails both in Western culture and within the dominant white and mestizo strata of his own society. The epitome of abolitionism, in Canelas' view, is the so-called Single Convention on Narcotics Drugs. This multinational agreement, signed by Peru and Bolivia in 1961, obligated the two countries to phase out coca chewing over 25 years. Canelas points to a "paradox": Although "coca production is perhaps ten times greater than the requirements of legal demand," a "notorious shortage" of leaves plagues the mines and other consuming centers. Government wholesale agencies that purchase leaves for resale to chewers, Canelas explains, cannot obtain leaves at the official price, which falls far below the price that traffickers pay. When the government sets a higher "extra-official" price to compete with traffickers, the chewing population is, in effect, forced out of the market. In Canelas' view, both the eradication of coca and the "pull" of the cocaine industry represent serious threats to coca chewing, "one of the most precious and important legacies of the ancestral Andean culture."[22]

Canelas' main points seem particularly valid. The U.S. government is basically hostile to traditional coca markets, seeing them as camouflage for illicit cocaine production. Strong abolitionist sentiment exists in Bolivia and Peru, as the signing of the Single Convention suggests. (The Single Convention is a major target of the coca lobby; recently, the Bolivian government nearly repudiated the agreement. See the section later in this chapter on "Milestones.") Finally, the demands of the drug traffickers are taking their toll on traditional chewing markets—farmers would rather sell their leaves to traffickers. In sum, the Andean way of life is under considerable attack in one guise or another from Western civilization.

Successes

The coca lobby tries to influence public opinion through the media. In general, its demands received more attention in the media in Bolivia than in Peru, because Bolivian coca growers exercise more political clout nationally than their Peruvian counterparts. Yet, in both countries, newspapers, magazines, and radio stations serve as important outlets for pro-coca propaganda.

In addition, and with much greater effect, the coca lobby has demonstrated its political muscle by organizing a variety of mass actions such as the following illustrative roadblocks, strikes, and attacks on police:

- In April 1983, Bolivia's Confederation of Peasant Workers called a national strike in reaction to a U.S.-Bolivian communique announcing a coca-reduction plan. The strike blocked highways and stopped the supply of food and other necessities to major cities.[23]
- In 1984, Bolivian coca growers sealed off the city of Cochabamba on two occasions: once to protest a planned military-police invasion of the Chapare and once to demand the lifting of a government ban on marketing coca leaves.[24]
- In January 1986, 17,000 growers surrounded 245 "Leopards"—members of a Bolivian antidrug strike force—near the Chapare town of Ivirgarzama, isolating the detachment for 5 days.[25]
- In April–May 1986, militant pro-coca groups in Peru's Upper Huallaga Valley, demanding a halt to eradication programs, staged a general strike that cut roads and paralyzed economic activity throughout the Valley. For good measure, the strikers also laid siege for several days to a U.S.-supported aid mission in the town of Aucayacu, about 60 miles north of Tingo María.[26]
- In May 1987, some 10,000 peasants mobilized by the COB and the regional coca growers' federations blockaded Cochabamba and cut the road leading from La Paz to the Yungas. The action targeted a U.S.-Bolivia plan to eliminate 90 percent of coca cultivation in the Chapare by the end of the 1980s.[27]
- In August 1987, coca farmers (possibly spurred on by Sendero Luminoso guerrillas) virtually shut down the jungle highway between Tingo María and Tocache. They destroyed bridges, dug trenches, and erected barricades made of rocks and logs. The peasants apparently were protesting an invasion of Tocache the month before by the Peruvian government (in an attempt to reassert police control in the region).[28]
- In June 1988, 4,000 to 5,000 coca farmers occupied the offices of the Coca Reduction Agency (DIRECO) in Villa Tunari, the administrative center of U.S. antidrug programs in the Chapare. The action responded in part to rumors that DIRECO, which is responsible for eradication, was testing herbicides against coca in the Chapare region. UMOPAR units stationed in Villa Tunari mounted a counterattack, and 10 to 15 peasants and 1 policeman were killed in the ensuing battle.[29]
- In August 1988, coca farmers and Sendero Luminoso guerrillas collaborated in a general strike that shut down businesses and paralyzed traffic throughout the valley for 5 days. The strike reflected both the goals of Sendero's Popular War strategy and the concerns of coca growers. As a Sendero leaflet picked up at the site of one of the roadblocks stated, "Down with the Fascist, Corporatist APRISTA government. Down with the Genocidal Armed Forces. Down with the eradication of coca plantations."[30]

The mass mobilization tactics of the coca lobby have kept governments on the defensive. In Bolivia, the eradication that does occur is the product of a complex process of bargaining with regional growers' federations and their component *centrales* and *sindicatos*. Involuntary eradication is probably impossible, at least in the immediate future. In Peru, the CORAH eradication program financed by the United States continues, but its effectiveness declined precipitously in recent years, from eradicating 4,830 hectares in 1985 to 2,575 in 1986 and finally to 355 in 1987.[31]

The demise of eradication as a drug control strategy may be imminent. Governments simply cannot wield the clout necessary to stop farmers from cultivating coca—the farmers are too numerous and too well organized. Governments in Peru and Bolivia now hope to sever links between the grower and the processor by attacking traffickers' laboratories and lines of communication to drive leaf prices down to the point where farmers will find it unprofitable to grow coca. In Peru, the new approach was signalled by a series of anti-cocaine operations called "Condor" that the García government initiated in August 1985. Peru's top narcotics policeman, Colonel (now General) Juan Zarate said of Condor, "We're planning to limit the traffic by making life difficult for smugglers so there are no buyers for coca."[32] In Bolivia, the 1986 Operation Blast Furnace (which employed U.S. troops) and simultaneous operations against coca paste laboratories in the Chapare temporarily disrupted the market for coca leaves. Since Blast Furnace, aggressive enforcement by Bolivian police (with substantial help from the DEA) has kept the price of leaves below pre-Blast Furnace levels. However, although the new strategy makes the economics of coca farming less attractive, the United States did not anticipate one by-product: Peasant farmers have been driven to integrate forward into the production of coca paste, until recently the preserve of major cocaine traffickers. The resulting rise in growers' profits and in their economic stake in drugs intensified rural opposition to the Bolivian government's eradication programs.

Specific Cases

Differences Between Peru and Bolivia

The coca lobby in Bolivia maintains a higher political profile than does its counterpart in Peru and, overall, has enjoyed more success. Peruvian organizations, however, seem to be growing in strength. Several key comparisons should be made. First, coca growing represents a more important economic activity in Bolivia than in Peru and employs a higher proportion of the economically active population. Estimates point to 100,000 coca growers out of Peru's population of 20 million and 70,000 to 80,000 growers out of Bolivia's population of 6.4 million.

Second, coca growers in Bolivia and Peru work through regional organizations, but the Bolivians are also well organized nationally. Bolivia has both a National Coca Producers Association (ANAPCOCA) and a National Coordinating Committee of Coca Producers (CONCOCA). Bolivian growers held three National Congresses, one in 1983 and two in 1988. The 10 grower federations in the Yungas and the Chapare sponsor a Coca Industrialization Council (COINCOCA). Moreover—and critically important—Bolivian coca growers command the support of key umbrella organizations: the 1.3-million-member Congress of Bolivian Workers (COB) and the Confederation of Bolivian Peasant Workers (CSUTCB), which has between 900,000 and 1,000,000 members and is the main component of the COB. In other words, the Bolivian coca lobby theoretically includes about 20 percent of the country's population of 6.4 million.[33] Furthermore, growers can count on the backing (primarily for ideological reasons) of several far-left political parties in the Bolivian Chamber of Deputies. These parties together constitute a bloc of roughly 35 to 40 deputies out of a total of 120 deputies in the Chamber.

Third, eradication program results differ. Peru has an eradication program in place, the so-called Coca Reduction Agency in the Upper Huallaga (CORAH) project. Recently, strong resistance by growers and extremely difficult security conditions in the Valley forced CORAH activities to a standstill. Yet, between 1983 and 1987, CORAH teams eradicated nearly 12,000 hectares of coca in the Valley. Moreover, the Peruvian government remains officially dedicated to a policy of eliminating illicit coca fields, by force if necessary. In contrast, the Bolivian government has yet to mount a successful eradication program. From 1983 to 1987, roughly 1,700 acres of coca were destroyed in Bolivia, nearly all during 1987.[34] Bolivian officials say privately that forcible eradication would precipitate a civil war between coca farmers and the government and possibly would lead to the demise of Bolivia's fledgling democratic system.

Finally, since early 1987, the organizations representing coca farmers in the Upper Huallaga Valley have been infiltrated and in some cases even supplanted (at least temporarily) by guerrilla organizations, the Tupac Amaru Revolutionary Movement (MRTA) and the Sendero Luminoso. Sendero, which perceives coca cultivation as a social problem and as an economic necessity for the time being, has been especially successful in cultivating ties with coca farmers. During 1988, Sendero propagandists had a field day denouncing U.S.-Peruvian plans to spray herbicides on coca plants. The guerrillas mobilize peasants to defend themselves against CORAH and also to resist exploitation by narcotics dealers. (The price of leaves stands as a major issue in relations between traffickers and the coca-growing peasantry.) As peasant communities have fallen under the spell of Sendero's Marxist-Leninist-Maoist line, the coca lobby in the Upper Huallaga has acquired a distinctly revolutionary tinge.

The following sections explore in detail the political activities of coca farmers and their allies in Bolivia and Peru. The record is sobering. U.S. policymakers have long been enamored with the idea of eliminating the U.S. cocaine problem by exterminating the coca plant, but they may not have adequately factored peasant resistance into their calculations. (A former U.S. Assistant Secretary of State for Narcotics Matters once confidently asserted that $1 spent overseas on crop reduction is worth $10 spent domestically on drug enforcement.[35]) However, the power of the coca lobby and the economic realities discussed in the previous chapter suggest that crop reduction will not be a cheap solution and, indeed, may be prohibitively expensive for the United States and its Latin American allies.

The Politics of Coca Control in Bolivia

Pro-Coca Organizations.   The coca lobby in Bolivia incorporates an extensive organizational structure. First, as of mid-1988, six regional federations were operating in different parts of the Chapare region: the Special Federation of Campesinos of the Tropical Region of Cochabamba (referred to in later discussions as FEAT), the Single Federation of United Centrales, the Federation of Colonizers of Chimore, the Federation of Colonizers of Tropical Carrasco, the Independent Federation of Tiraque, and the Federation of the Traditional Yungas of the Chapare. The Chapare organizations encompass, in a line of hierarchical subordination, 54 *centrales,* over 600 *sindicatos,* and at least 36,000 affiliated peasant families. In addition, several thousand peasant families are not affiliated with any of the federations. There are also four growers' organizations in the Yungas: the Single Federation of Peasant Workers of the North Yungas, the Single Federation of Peasant Workers of the South Yungas, the Federation of Colonizers of Caranavi, and the Special Federation of Choquechaca-La Asunta.[36] However, the Chapare federations have been most active politically, because that region produces most of Bolivia's illegal coca, and the coca there has been targeted for eradication in accords between Bolivia and the United States.

In addition, several national organizations actively support the interests of coca growers, who can join their own national organizations, CON-COCA and ANAPCOCA (mentioned above). Growers also count on the direct support of the mass-membership worker and peasant unions, the COB and the CSUTCB. The National Colonizers Confederation, comprising 600,000 members, occasionally takes stands favoring coca growers.

Other groups deserve brief mention, such as SMIMFA, which strongly supports the industrialization of coca and also favors legalization. SMIMFA asserted in a television program in 1982, "Coca dollars, good or bad, are Bolivian. The nationalization and the legalization of coca will allow money to be moved from secret bank accounts into our national banks . . ."[37] The Assembly of Human Rights rejects eradication of "rational cultivation" and requests the removal of antidrug police from growing zones, because "they commit abuses against campesinos and their human rights."[38] Furthermore, various splinter parties of the Revolutionary Leftist Movement (MIR) at various times take strongly pro-coca positions.

The Bolivian coca lobby is not monolithic. For example, some groups take a stronger hard-line stand on eradication than other groups—that is, disagreement over the terms under which eradication should take place do occur. By and large, however, the lobby opposes crop-control policies promoted by the Bolivian government and its U.S. backers. The following sections describe the politics of coca control in Bolivia, specifically analyzing instances of confrontation between the coca lobby and the Bolivian government.

Milestones.   In May 1982, the military government of Celso Torrelio, seeking a resumption of the U.S. economic and military aid cut off under the García Meza administration, decided to demonstrate Bolivia's good faith in the war against drugs by using herbicide on coca. The spraying focused on a nontraditional and apparently illegal growing area in the Yapacani region of Santa Cruz department. Approximately 100 hectares of coca were sprayed manually with the herbicide 2-4-D, a component (although by no means the most toxic component) of the notorious defoliant Agent Orange, which was used in Vietnam. By almost every standard, "Operation Yapacani" was a disaster. First, it did not work. The peasants simply cut the leaves and the tops off their coca bushes before the spray could kill the entire plant, so little coca was actually destroyed.[39] Second, the operation precipitated a major political outcry. Predictably, the coca lobby—the COB, the CSUTCB, and the regional growers' federations—condemned the action. The well-known Bolivian drug trafficker Roberto Suarez wrote an open letter to the media, accusing the United States of forcing the Bolivian government to "use the horrendous herbicide 'Agent Orange' to destroy fields and to assassinate indiscriminately hundreds of peasants in the Chapare."[40] Most important, key Bolivian institutions such as the armed forces, the scientific establishment, the church, and the news media objected strongly to the spraying. Facing such opposition, the Bolivian government issued a communiqué declaring that chemicals would not be used in future actions against illegal or excess coca plantations. Later, under the Siles administration, a prohibition against the use of chemicals or fire to kill coca plants was written into Bolivia's antidrug law. The coca lobby clearly won the first round.[41]

Under the Siles Zuazo government, which came to power in October 1982, Bolivia and the United States sought a mutually agreeable formula for reducing excess coca crops and for controlling the drug traffic. A visit to Bolivia by U.S. Attorney General William French Smith in mid-April 1983 culminated several months of U.S.-Bolivia discussions on the coca problem and produced a joint communiqué in which the Bolivian government promised, among other things, to reduce coca production to the level of legitimate demand. Several days after the Attorney General's visit, Bolivia's national peasant union, the CSUTCB, called a nationwide strike that blocked roads and shut off food supplies to major cities. The CSUTCB halted the strike after exacting a promise from the Siles government to reconsider its agreement with the United States. Throughout the spring and summer of 1983, peasant federations in the Chapare placed full-page advertisements in the national press to defend the production of coca. All to little avail: In August 1983, the Bolivian government signed a formal accord with the United States that called for some tough new drug enforcement initiatives in Bolivia.[42]

This agreement included the reduction of coca cultivation in the Chapare by 4,000 hectares by the end of 1985; a program for permanent control of the legitimate transport, purchase, and sale of coca leaf; and the establishment of a "substantial police presence" in the Chapare to eliminate trafficking in coca paste. To minimize the adverse impact of these controls on farmers, the United States agreed to help fund an agricultural and socioeconomic development program for the Chapare.[43] In addition, rumors of secret accord provisions surfaced: One provision reportedly pared down coca plantations to a maximum of one-half hectare per farmer. A second provision created a new system of criminal investigations and "a judicial system under which judges will accept proofs and sentence lawbreakers in such a way that they will not dare to break the law again." A third provision sought the development of a network of agents and informants—"one paid member in each sindicato"—in the various peasant organizations in the Chapare.[44]

The formal terms of the accord were not announced until January 1984, 5 months after the signing—no doubt because the United States and Bolivian governments feared an adverse public reaction. When the response came, it was, indeed, negative. In February, a group of parliamentarians from Cochabamba department (which includes the Chapare region) called the accord unconstitutional, harmful to the Bolivian economy, and a violation of national sovereignty and demanded that the agreement be reviewed by the Bolivian Congress.[45] In March, 2,000 Chapare farmers arrived in Cochabamba in 50 trucks to protest the signing of the agreement and paraded around the city, chanting, "down with Edwin Corr [the U.S. Ambassador]," "down with democracy," and other anti-U.S. and anti-Bolivian slogans. Farmers also tried to take over the local offices of the National Directorate for the Control of Dangerous Substances (DNCSP), the superordinate agency for the antidrug police. In May 1984, a congress of coca growers in the Chapare threatened to appeal to Bolivia's Supreme Court for an annulment of the agreements.[46]

At the end of July 1984, the Siles government took action to implement one of the major points in the accords: the establishment of a political presence in the Chapare. The Chapare had fallen outside government control for some time: Government police were expelled from the region years before and replaced by the self-appointed police of drug traffickers. In parts of the area, a free market thrived, not just in coca leaves but in cocaine. The town of Sinahota—dubbed by some Bolivian commentators the "Chicago of Cocaine"—organized Sunday fairs at which coca paste was sold (usually for dollars) or bartered for electrical appliances and household necessities. Between 4,000 and 5,000 people "of every class and color" attended these weekly events.[47]

On July 31, the government issued a decree establishing a military zone in the Chapare and announcing a joint army, navy, air force, and police invasion of the area "to combat drug trafficking" and "to establish the rule of law." The decree was somewhat unclear on the status of coca plantations in the Chapare, not specifically ruling out the possibility of eradication, but stating that the government would not use herbicide against plants.[48] The government's plan was attacked by all national and regional campesino organizations. The Confederation of Settlers declared a national "state of emergency" in view of the government's decision to "militarize the Chapare region." One Chapare peasant leader, Eudoro Barrientos, voiced the concerns of many growers: "We will not permit the entrance of the police units into the zone, because the abuses committed by police against innocent people and the protection that they offer drug traffickers are still fresh in people's minds."[49]

The immediate reaction to the decree was another demonstration of peasant power. Peasants from the Chapare and the Cochabamba Valley blockaded the city of Cochabamba and cut the main highway with the Chapare. In the first week of August, the government and campesino leaders conducted some hard bargaining. A complex deal finally was struck: The government promised not to destroy Chapare farmers' coca crops and not to interfere in the commercialization of coca. In addition, the government may have agreed to exclude the antidrug police

(UMOPAR) in the Chapare from the occupation force. In any event, the "Leopards," as the police units were popularly called, accompanied the invasion, but were withdrawn from the Chapare about 3 weeks later. The deal also included benefits for the Cochabamba farmers who had joined the coca growers in the blockades. The government promised to raise the purchase price of wheat and to provide the farmers with 50 new tractors.[50]

The peasants agreed to disband, and government forces entered the Chapare on August 10, 1984, beginning a military occupation that would last for 6 months but would not achieve its real aims. The announcement of the invasion precipitated a mass exodus of drug operators and other fortune-seekers from the Chapare, so no major traffickers were arrested. Many paste-producing sites were abandoned, and the more notorious cocaine markets, such as Sinahota, ceased to function (between August and September 1984, the population of that town reportedly dropped from 10,000 to 400). However, the military occupation did not eliminate the cocaine trade, it just displaced it. New paste laboratories soon appeared outside the Chapare, especially in the Upper Cochabamba Valley. Peasants began shipping their leaves to "New Sinahotas" in the Valley, such as Toco, Punata, and Chiza.[51]

In October 1984, the government banned shipments of coca leaves from the Chapare and stepped up efforts to control the circulation of leaves within the region. The stage was set for a new confrontation with the Bolivian government. In early November, campesinos again sealed off Cochabamba and blocked the Chapare highway, demanding the "free sale of coca" and an end to the military occupation. The coca growers won a partial victory: The government lifted controls on transporting coca leaves, and the military left the Chapare later that month.[52]

In February 1985, however, the government began redeploying UMOPAR and other police units into the Chapare, and UMOPAR's active strength by the end of 1986 totaled 300 personnel in the zone. By the end of 1987, the outpost had increased to 313, and an estimated 25 DEA agents and 14 U.S. military advisers were stationed in the zone.[53] These forces encountered stiff peasant resistance—one dramatic example was the 5-day siege of the Leopards' camp at Ivirgarzama in January 1986. The ostensible reason for the peasants' actions was an incident in which two members of the UMOPAR detachment allegedly raped a local woman. Many observers felt, however, that the siege represented a generalized protest against attempts by UMOPAR to suppress the manufacture of coca paste or to shake down paste producers. In late June and early July 1987, a similar incident occurred. Hundreds of peasants surrounded an encampment of DEA agents in Chimore province and demanded that the agents leave the area. According to a leader of the Chimore growers' federation, the peasants "fear that U.S. officials will destroy their coca plantations and are fed up with the outrages that they are enduring."[54] The incident prompted a formal Bolivian government request that all U.S. DEA and military personnel withdraw from the Chapare temporarily "for security reasons." The Americans left on July 3, but apparently returned to the region 3 weeks later.

In late June 1988, in another more serious confrontation, some 4,000 to 5,000 coca growers occupied UMOPAR barracks in Villa Tunari, more or less taking control of the town, the administrative center of U.S. antinarcotics programs in the Chapare. Police reinforcements, backed by three U.S.-made assault helicopters on loan to Bolivia, regained control of Villa Tunari, but 10–15 peasants and 1 policeman were killed in the incident. The attack on Villa Tunari apparently was precipitated by two factors: the imminent passage of the antinarcotics law (referenced later in this section) that would outlaw most coca production in the Chapare, and a rumor—apparently false—that the Bolivian government planned to use herbicides against coca plantations in the zone. Following the incident, the COB demanded that all U.S. narcotics officials be expelled from Bolivia and called a 48-hour strike that reportedly shut down many factories, mines, trains, and domestic airline flights.[55] The Bolivian government's hold on the Chapare region in July 1988—even with U.S. help—appears tenuous, so the outlook for a successful drive against cocaine trafficking there remains highly uncertain.

Furthermore, the Bolivian government and the Chapare federations are at an impasse over eradicating coca. In November 1985, the Ministry of Interior signed a coca production agreement with the two peasant federations in the Chapare region that represent Chapare and Chimore provinces. The agreement stipulated that peasants represented by the federations would eradicate voluntarily any coca in excess of 2 hectares that they owned, and the agreement also called for eliminating at least 1,000 hectares by December 15, 1985. In return, the Bolivian government (with U.S. funds) would pay peasants $350 for each hectare of coca destroyed. In addition, the Bolivian government promised to provide new social services to Chapare farmers—especially roads, schools, electrification, and credits to grow alternative crops—once eradication targets were met.[56]

The Bolivian government hoped that the agreement somehow would forestall the partial cutoff of U.S. economic and military aid to Bolivia that was threatened by the U.S. Foreign Assistance Act of 1986. (The hope was unrealistic: The act required that Bolivia eliminate 4,000 hectares of coca, not just 1,000, by the end of 1985 to receive its full appropriation for FY 1986.) President Paz Estenssoro proclaimed that the reduction was "indispensable for the international relations of our country, especially our relations with the United States." He also noted that "U.S. aid is vital to Bolivia," because "our economy has deteriorated sharply," and that the peasant leaders who signed the agreement were "putting national interest above personal interests and making it possible for us to receive the aid."[57] Peasant leaders such as FEAT's Eudoro Barrientos argued a different case—that the agreement would reduce excess production and prop up the price of coca leaves, which in late 1985 was at $200–$400 per carga, well below the peak levels of $800–$850 per carga prevailing in the spring and summer of that year.[58]

The agreement, however, turned into a fiasco. Key national organizations such as the COB, the CSUTCB, and ANAPCOCA rejected it. An important Chapare growers' organization, the Federation of Colonizers of Carrasco, would have nothing to do with the arrangement, denouncing in a communiqué the "pseudo-leaders" who signed the pact with the government "behind the backs of the genuine producers and contrary to the true aspirations" of the colonizers.[59] The pact did not garner much rank-and-file support within FEAT. According to an informal poll by *Opinión* (a Cochabamba newspaper), 80 percent of the membership of the Federation opposed the reduction plan. There was open talk of a sellout by the Federation's leaders, and some campesinos even put a price on Barrientos' head.[60]

Opponents phrased their objections in familiar terms: that the plan violated national sovereignty, that the $350 per hectare offered to farmers was too low (the CSUTCB demanded $3,000 in compensation), that "integrated development" of the Chapare would have to precede eradication, and (perhaps most important) that destruction of coca fields was impossible unless substitute crops were available that would yield returns equivalent to those of coca. Other arguments also were launched: For example, ANAPCOCA declared that eradication should be tied to the cancellation of Bolivia's foreign debt, and the Carrasco Federation suggested that the United States should simply buy up the Bolivian excess crop instead of pressuring Bolivia's coca farmers.[61]

Under the circumstances, nothing much could happen. By the end of April 1986, fewer than 100 hectares of coca bushes had been eradicated—mainly, according to Bolivian officials, old and diseased plants that the peasants wanted to uproot anyway. Only 200 hectares were eradicated in all of 1988. Again, the coca lobby won a victory of sorts against the government.

The Bolivian government had to find new ways of pressuring coca farmers. The introduction of 170 U.S. Army personnel and six Blackhawk helicopters into Bolivia in July 1986 finally signalled the beginning of a new phase in Bolivia's narcotics control strategy. The U.S. forces were dispatched to help the Bolivian police raid laboratories and clandestine airstrips in the Beni and Santa Cruz regions—major trafficking strongholds. The operation, dubbed Blast Furnace, was accompanied by a stepped-up Bolivian effort to destroy coca paste laboratories in the Chapare. The strategy was to wipe out the market for coca leaves, and the market was, in fact, in turmoil for a period of time. The price of leaves in some parts of the Chapare reportedly plummeted from $125–$150 per carga to between $10 and $20 per carga—well below the cost of production (thought to be around $30–$40 per carga).[62] This experience drained off some of the Chapare's floating population, as farmers started returning to their home areas. A rash of telephone calls to AID offices in Cochabamba asked for help in planting new cash crops: Never before had farmers shown any interest in crop substitution. Yet, immediately following the departure of U.S. troops in November, the average price rebounded to $40–$50 per carga and by mid-1987 had climbed to more than $100 per carga. Business, in other words, was returning to normal.[63]

Blast Furnace could be considered a technical success, because it not only disrupted the market for coca leaves, but also significantly reduced Bolivia's cocaine exports. However, the presence of U.S. forces dropped the Paz government in a pot of political hot water, provoking bitter opposition in Bolivia, not just from the coca lobby, but also from academics, journalists, and key congressmen. The COB organized a demonstration of 20,000 workers, peasants, students, teachers, and housewives in La Paz to demand the expulsion of U.S. troops from Bolivian territory. In the far-off Beni town of Santa Ana de Yacuma (the home of Bolivia's "King of Cocaine," Roberto Suarez), a mob of angry villagers forced U.S. and Bolivian forces to cancel an operation to arrest drug traffickers. According to one account, "The police and the Blackhawks left the town after being surrounded by hostile crowds of up to 3,000 people shouting, 'Yankee go home.' "[64] The president of the Bolivian Chamber of Deputies, Gaston Encinas, condemned the U.S. intervention as illegal and as a violation of "national security." The former president of the Bolivian Senate and current Senator Oscar Zamora charged the government with "high treason" for allowing the entry of U.S. troops. The head of Paz's own National Revolutionary Movement (MNR) in the city of Santa Cruz resigned to form a new party and called for the president's impeachment, saying that Paz had "betrayed all the MNR principles, programs, and guidelines."[65] The Bolivian government also had to endure intense criticism from other South American countries for allowing a highly visible U.S. military presence. This storm of political protest almost certainly hastened the departure of U.S. Army units, which left between late October and mid-November 1986.

A new round in the ongoing political warfare over coca began in early 1987 with the government's start-up of a so-called "Three Year Plan for the Struggle Against Narcotics Trafficking." The plan—an unrealistic document that reflected intensive behind-the-scenes pressure by the United States—called for eliminating 50,000 hectares of illicit coca in Bolivia by 1990, specifically including 35,000 hectares of the estimated 40,000 hectares of coca cultivation in the Chapare and 15,000 hectares of the estimated 30,000 hectares in the Yungas. The plan was backed by a draft law that declared all coca cultivation outside of the provinces of the north and south Yungas to be nontraditional and subject to eradication. The plan envisioned a 12-month period of voluntary eradication; after that, the government would "proceed to eliminate through force the coca fields which still exist."[66]

Also included in the package was a $300-million fund for "agricultural conversion, economic reactivation, and regional development." This, said the government, would allow the elimination of coca fields "without destroying the social equilibrium in the producing zones"—that is, without destabilizing the countryside. Bolivia would provide 20 percent of the $300 million; the other $240 million would have to come from outside donors (that is, the industrialized countries). Of this fund, $100 million—$2,000 per hectare for 50,000 hectares—would be used to compensate farm families for the destruction of their fields. This sum was designed to help the farmer "change his way of life and become a part of society."[67]

At the end of February 1987, Bolivia and the United States signed a bilateral agreement to implement the plan (although the United States did not commit itself to funding the economic part of the package). Bolivia promised to eradicate a total of 1,800 hectares of coca by August 1988 and somehow to wipe out the other 48,200 in the subsequent 2 years. Given the alignment of political forces in the country, this objective was unrealistic if not laughable, and the reaction of the coca lobby was not slow in coming. In March, the COB declared a national "state of emergency" to oppose the plan. In April, the Chapare growers' federations formed a so-called Regional Committee for the Reform of Coca Plantations; the federations' leaders promised a fight to the death against eradication. At the end of May, the COB, the CSUTCB, and the regional federations mobilized an estimated 10,000 peasants to block roads in La Paz and Cochabamba departments, paralyzing the nation's highway system for several days.[68]

The Bolivian government thus confronted yet another demonstration of the coca lobby's power to disrupt national life. The government did not abandon its "Three Year Plan," but did make important concessions to growers. On June 6, 1987, several government ministries signed an agreement with the main organizations composing the lobby: the COB, the CSUTCB, and eight of the regional federations encompassing the Yungas and the Chapare. The agreement in effect committed the government not to use force in eradicating "excess" coca; the term voluntary substitution was used throughout the document, and the term eradication did not appear. Furthermore, the process of voluntary substitution would exclude the use of herbicides, chemicals, and biological agents (the most promising methods for eliminating large expanses of coca). According to another provision, substitution would proceed "simultaneously" with socioeconomic development in the countryside, and campesinos would receive "just compensation" for their crops. (In the eyes of most peasant leaders, the $2,000 per hectare offered by the government did not begin to cover the cost of switching to another crop.)[69]

Finally, under the agreement, cultivation of coca for traditional purposes—chewing, medicinal uses, religious rituals, and the like—would acquire a permanent juridical status. Coca grown for the traditional market would no longer be a "controlled substance." By signing the agreement, the Bolivian government turned its back on the Single Convention that had obligated signatories to phase out coca chewing over a period of 25 years (see above section, "A Consumers' Lobby?"). As already noted, the continued existence of the so-called legal market, whose exact dimensions never were clear, serves to perpetuate the illicit market. Peasants can always say that they are cultivating coca to meet traditional demand.

The agreement defused tensions between the government and the campesinos and ushered in a period of cooperation, although, as it turned out, this proved to be a short-lived cooperative phase. Negotiations over voluntary substitution continued during the summer months, and, beginning in late September, Chapare peasants began eradicating coca in what their leaders described as a good-will gesture to the government. Between September and mid-December, about 1,000 hectares were destroyed—a minor miracle for Bolivia, but still a minuscule percentage of that country's total cultivation. (Most of the eradication occurred in Corresco province, which has a number of relatively large—5 hectares to 10 hectares—plots of coca; for large farmers, the burden of reduction would have been relatively lower.) Campesinos received compensatory payments of $2,000 per hectare, but not much else. By November, peasant leaders were complaining that the government had reneged on the June 6 agreement. The agreement, said FEAT leader Alberto Vargas in a November 8 interview, "not only includes compensation," but also comprises other socioeconomic benefits such as electrification, roads, potable water, and agricultural credits of as much as $4,000 per farmer.[70] Quite obviously the honeymoon, such as it was, was coming to an end.

A "National Forum of Coca Producers," which represented the full force of the coca lobby (all the major organizations were in attendance), was held in Cochabamba from December 13 to 15, 1987. The Forum accused the government of bad faith and resolved to suspend immediately "the work of voluntary reduction of hectares of coca." The Forum also issued a resolution demanding the removal from coca-producing zones of topographers, measurers, and other workers associated with eradication. The reason (or pretext) for the coca lobby's harder line was the government's failure to keep its promise to improve living conditions in coca-growing zones and to help peasants convert to other crops.[71]

After complex negotiations with the government in early 1988, the Chapare farmers agreed to resume eradication. Between January and June, peasants destroyed about 990 hectares of coca. However, in mid-1988, relations deteriorated again. The occasion was the draft coca law that the government was pushing through the congress to implement the Three Year Plan. The peasants objected to the bill's definition of coca as a narcotic and a controlled substance. At the end of May, thousands of peasants from the Yungas and Chapare marched on La Paz and Cochabamba to demonstrate their opposition to the bill. On June 7, some 25,000 coca farmers set up roadblocks on the three main highways linking Cochabamba with the rest of the country, effectively sealing off the city for the fourth time since 1983. Police and military units cleared the roads the following day, but on June 9, a mob of several thousand peasants occupied the Cochabamba offices of the Subsecretary of Rural Alternative Development and of the Coca Reduction Agency (DIRECO), Bolivian government agencies charged with managing coca eradication and substitution programs. The peasants held 10 Bolivians and 2 North Americans—the latter apparently U.S. AID employees—for 7 hours. The peasants evacuated the offices and released the hostages after an "intense telephone conversation" with the Minister of Agriculture and Campesino Affairs and the Ministry of Interior. The government apparently promised to meet with the coca growers to hear their complaint.[72]

At the end of June, there was a very serious incident at Villa Tunari in the Chapare. A mob of several thousand peasants broke into the offices of DIRECO. The action was in part a protest against the new coca bill (which at that point had almost completed its passage through congress). However, there was a more specific objective. Narco-traffickers apparently had circulated reports that DIRECO and DEA were testing several herbicides against coca plantations in the Chapare. The peasants said that they were looking for evidence—documents, equipment, chemicals, and so on—that would support the rumors. The UMOPAR contingent at Villa Tunari called for reinforcements that arrived by helicopter. (It was widely reported in the media that the reinforcements included DEA agents.) The police counterattacked, and in the ensuing battle, as many as 16 people may have lost their lives. Three peasants were shot to death, and more than 10 others were pushed over steep embankments into the Chapare River, which runs alongside the DIRECO and UMOPAR compounds, where they drowned. One policeman reportedly was killed. The Villa Tunari incident became a cause célèbre for the coca lobby, precipitating a wave of protests and sympathy strikes throughout the country. Moreover, the incident apparently cast a pall over the voluntary eradication program. Farmers had eradicated almost 1,000 hectares between January and June 1988, but from July through September, eradication totaled only 120 hectares.[73]

In mid-July, congress passed the new coca law. The final version was, in fact, relatively favorable to the coca farmers. The law established 12,000 hectares as the maximum extension required to satisfy legal demand. The other 50,000 hectares to 60,000 hectares in the country, including almost all of that growing in the Chapare, was defined as excess production and hence was subject to eradication. The law also referred to "annual plans"—that is, targets—for reduction of 5,000 hectares to 8,000 hectares. Yet, eradication in most coca-growing zones was to occur voluntarily, and peasants would be compensated as envisioned in the Three Year Plan. Peasants would receive $2,000 per hectare in direct compensation plus several thousand dollars more in credits, technical assistance, and other benefits. There was no time limit for eliminating excess production—that is, all production above 12,000 hectares. The law also included a prohibition against the use of chemical herbicides against coca.[74]

Despite these very favorable provisions for the coca farmers, the coca lobby objected to the new law on various grounds: that the 12,000-hectare limit was too low, that the yearly reduction targets of 5,000–6,000 hectares were too high, and that the government did not have the money on hand to compensate farmers adequately for eradication. In August, the Coca Federation, the COB, and the CSUTCB held a "National Congress of Coca Farmers" in Cochabamba. The participants pledged noncompliance with the new law and called on farmers not to eradicate "a single coca plant" until the law was modified. A resolution was also passed to hold an "International Andean Conference" of coca producers from all South American countries, either in La Paz or Cochabamba at the end of 1988. The political ambitions of the coca lobby were clearly acquiring a new dimension.[75]

Voluntary substitution may well constitute a lost cause; the economics of the process are mindboggling. Bolivian government officials now say that the per-hectare cost of substitution—what it will take to induce farmers to abandon coca cultivation—is $7,000 to $8,000.[76] Eradicating

50,000 hectares would thus cost $350 million to $400 million (the Three Year Plan initially envisioned a price tag of $300 million, or $6,000 per hectare). There is virtually no chance that the U.S. Congress, in the era of Gramm-Rudman and $200-billion budget deficits, will fund such a program. Congress only authorized $7.3 million in economic support funds (ESF) for Bolivia in FY 1988, 70 percent less than the State Department's request ($25 million).[77] ESF are ultimately the main source of the $2,000 per hectare-eradicated paid to Chapare farmers. The $7.3 million could theoretically pay for the eradication of 3,650 hectares. At a rate of 3,650 hectares per year, Bolivia would need 14 years to reach its target of eliminating 50,000 hectares of coca.

On the other hand, even the most generous agricultural reconversion program will not work as long as coca provides farmers with a better cash-flow opportunity than any other crop. Farmers will not abandon their own fields just because the government provides water wells, roads, generators, and clinics. As U.S. administrators in South America, Southeast Asia, and elsewhere have confirmed time and time again, development aid can help to perpetuate the drug traffic, encouraging farmers to stay in regions such as the Chapare and the Upper Huallaga Valley or stimulating more migration to these zones, which are not well suited agronomically, climatically, and geographically for cultivating most traditional crops. Moreover, compensating farmers to destroy crops seems to be a risky strategy. Persistent rumors claim that some Bolivian farmers have invested their $2,000 per hectare in planting new coca fields, either in more remote parts of the Chapare or in other regions of the country.[78]

The prospects for indirect eradication are not very good either. In early 1988, the government—in an extension and modification of the Blast Furnace concept—stepped up attacks on paste laboratories, trying to make it harder for farmers to sell their leaves. Combined Bolivian police-DEA raids reportedly destroyed 1,470 paste laboratories, mostly in the Chapare, from October 1987 to April 1988. The exercises drove down leaf prices in a few areas. For example, some coca fields in Chimore province were not harvested in the spring of 1988, and their owners reportedly left the area to look for other work—or perhaps to grow coca elsewhere.[79]

Yet, leaf prices rose dramatically in the summer of 1988. In January, prices ranged from $25–$40 per carga—a range that reflects average prices at three different locations in the Chapare—that is, they were near or less than the imputed cost of production. In June, prices were $50–$65 per carga. By August, per-carga prices had jumped to $120–$130, and in September they were only slightly lower, $95–$110. U.S. officials in La Paz are at a loss to explain these trends. One official theorized that traffickers may be artificially raising the price of leaves to keep farmers interested in growing coca.[80] Another possible explanation lies in the Bolivian authorities' inability to maintain sufficient enforcement pressure on coca paste laboratories to force leaf buyers out of the market.

The strategy of indirect eradication is probably the best that can be employed, all things considered, but the chances of success seem remote. There is no question that knocking out coca paste laboratories can temporarily deprive farmers of markets for their leaves. Yet, such a policy is likely to be self-defeating. In the face of uncertain leaf prices, every coca-farming family will have an incentive to become a paste producer or at least to develop such a capability. And paste laboratories—which require only a maceration pit, plastic sheeting, and some common chemicals—are simple to build and operate. Furthermore, as suggested above, the Bolivian police lack the means and probably the motivation to sustain an effective campaign against Bolivia's cocaine processing infrastructure.

Such, then, are the politics of coca control in Bolivia. The prognosis is for continuing U.S. pressure on Bolivia to make headway in eradication and for continuing confrontations between the Bolivian government and the coca lobby. With or without a coca law, the Bolivian government clearly does not possess the power to eradicate coca plantations. Furthermore, coca and cocaine are deeply ingrained in the economic, social, and political life of the country. Barring a U.S. military occupation of Bolivia and the sterilization of all plant life in the Yungas and the Chapare, Bolivia's status as a major coca producer is unlikely to change for many years to come.

The Peruvian Coca Lobby

The coca lobby in Peru represents a primarily regional phenomenon centered in the Upper Huallaga Valley, which is literally a sea of cocaine. The Upper Huallaga, one of Peru's two largest zones of coca cultivation (the other is in Cuzco department), has been the site of an active U.S.-financed eradication program, CORAH, which has been underway since mid-1983. Growers in the Upper Huallaga Valley can be divided roughly into two groups. One group is mainly centered in Leoncio Prado province in the department of Huanuco (the southernmost part of the Upper Huallaga zone). The second group is concentrated in Tocache province in the department of San Martín, directly north of Huanuco. Tocache now ranks as the largest and highest-density area of coca cultivation in the Valley and boasts the largest coca bushes, some between 12 feet and 15 feet tall. The Huallaga River runs through the capitals of Leoncio Prado and Tocache—respectively, Tingo María and Tocache (identified on maps of the region as Tocache Nuevo). Most coca cultivations in the immediate neighborhood of Tingo María have been destroyed by CORAH eradication teams. On the other hand, coca fields extend to the edge of the Tocache airstrip, which is within easy walking distance of the town.

Symbols of coca-induced affluence abound in the Valley: dish antennas (*parabólicos*) resting atop peasant huts; shiny Nissan trucks; discothèques; pornographic movie houses; houses of prostitution; and street markets crowded with VCRs, cameras, computers, and Seiko watches. In the Upper Huallaga, according to the Lima publication *Quehacer,* a maid earns more money than a schoolteacher, but in many schools, teachers are entitled to a special remuneration. The parents' association—more compassionate and understanding than such organizations in most parts of the world—provides teachers with at least a hectare for growing coca plants. Local peasants obligingly cultivate the plots and arrange for processing of the leaves into coca paste. Thus, says *Quehacer,* "Everyone has a place in the drug trafficking chain."[81]

In Leoncio Prado, there was at one time a coca growers' organization, the Regional Coca Producers Committee of Leoncio Prado Province (the full name was Comité Regional de Productores de Coca de La Provincia de Leoncio Prado y Anexos). The Comite was more or less defunct by 1987, but its interest-articulation function was assumed by the Front for the Defense of the Province of Leoncio Prado (FEDIP). The Leoncio Prado FEDIP, like other such "fronts" in Peru, is a loosely united coalition of local interest groups. Because cocaine is the mainstay of the economy, however, the FEDIP is especially sensitive to the demands of *cocaleros*— for example, it favors legalizing all coca cultivation in the Valley.[82]

As in Bolivia, Peru's coca lobby includes the elected officials from coca-growing regions. For example, the APRISTA (meaning affiliated with APRA, one of Peru's major political parties) mayor of Tingo María, Ciro Gallegos, was a staunch defender of the rights of coca growers and a vociferous opponent of both CORAH and the AID-financed Special Upper Huallaga Valley Project (PEAH). His predecessor, Tito Jaime Fernandez, for years fought various attempts by the Peruvian government to outlaw coca production in the Valley. (Gallegos retired in mid-1987; his successor, Carlos Rocas Chavez, although a less flamboyant personality, seems to share Gallegos' distaste for eradication.) In the Peruvian Congress, Huanaco Senator Andres Quintana Gurt has served as a leading critic of CORAH and of the antinarcotics program in the Valley in general. (Quintana Gurt is one of two APRISTA members of the Senate Investigation Commission on Narcotics, whose functions include reviewing antidrug legislation and investigating the atrocities of CORAH and PEAH.) A Huanaco Deputy, Huerto Milla, accuses CORAH of committing "acts of great injustice" against the peasantry, including embezzling funds earmarked to compensate peasants for eradicated plots.[83]

Moreover, by mid-1986, a Committee for the Defense of Human Rights based in Tingo María was offering partial and qualified support to coca growers, specifically on the issue of abuses by police. The Committee, headed until 1987 by a Catholic priest, Father Fortunato Lagarde, included most of the local power structure and was founded in 1982 by the then-mayor, Tito Jaime Fernandez. Fernandez was assassinated in April 1984 in what many Tingo María residents believe was a contract killing by Peru's most corrupt law enforcement agency, the Peruvian Investigative Police. During the Jaime and Gallegos administrations, a constant stream of letters flowed out of the mayor's office denouncing PIP and UMOPAR (the rural mobile police) for extortion, torture, robberies, assaults, rapes, and other outrages against the coca-producing peasantry. Typical of these was a letter from Jaime to the attorney general of Leoncio Prado attacking "outrages and violations of homes committed by the PIP (Peruvian Investigative Police) and UMOPAR in the course of the struggle against drug trafficking and illicit coca cultivation."[84] Finally, coca growers in Leoncio Prado received support from ENACO, the Peruvian government's wholesale agency for coca leaves. ENACO's purchase of leaves in the Upper Huallaga region dwindled over the past few years, and it blames CORAH's eradication policies in part for this situation. ENACO, as noted earlier, strongly supports the "industrialization of coca"—converting leaves into products with commercial value.[85]

The core constituency of the coca lobby in Leoncio Prado comprises so-called legal coca growers who hold plots registered as of 1978 (all other coca cultivated since 1978 is definitionally illegal under Peruvian laws). These growers are usually long-term residents of the Valley, and most cultivate several crops for food as well as growing small plots of coca, which provide the majority of the farmers' cash incomes. In addition, a number of recent immigrants to the Valley cultivate illegal coca—and usually little else—and may receive seeds and financing from drug traffickers. In fact, both groups sell coca to the illicit market and are considered fair game by CORAH. Political leaders who have represented the Valley (such as Mayor Gallegos and Senator Quintana Gurt) seem mainly concerned with protecting the interests of established growers rather than those of recent arrivals. The umbrella organization FEDIP, however, apparently speaks for all growers in the province by directly advocating legalization.

Leoncio Prado has borne the brunt of Peru's eradication effort: More than 8,000 hectares of the 8,700 hectares eradicated in the Valley between 1983 and 1985 were in that province. (The rest were in the Nuevo Progreso district of Tocache province.) Moreover, the CORAH eradication project has fallen hard on the established growers, eliminating about 60 percent of the registered hectarage in Leoncio Prado between 1983 and 1985. CORAH contends that, registered or not, virtually all *cocaleros* in the Valley sell leaves to traffickers, so there really is no such thing as legal cultivation. Yet, targeting registered owners created strong political pressures against eradication, in part because such owners tend to be long-term residents who, over time, have cultivated good connections with city hall. They can and have exerted substantial pressure on the mayor of Tingo María and on other elected officials of the region. Moreover, CORAH's policies have aroused ENACO's antagonism. ENACO buys virtually all of its leaves from "licit" growers, who, even if they sell much of their output to drug traffickers, continue to supply ENACO, if only for appearances' sake. The eradication of registered hectarage and the competition from drug traffickers have cut deeply into ENACO's operations. According to an ENACO spokesman interviewed in Tingo María in February 1986, its average monthly purchase of leaves in Leoncio Prado declined from 33 metric tons in 1983 to 11 metric tons in 1985.[86]

In the northern part of the Upper Huallaga region, growers were, until recently, represented by the Front for the Defense of the Interests of the People (FEDIP) of Tocache province. The "people" include tens of thousands of farmers who cultivate coca, in large part illegally, in that province. In other words, FEDIP's main constituents are not legal growers but rather outlaw migrant farmers. The agenda of the Tocache FEDIP and its subordinate organizations (such as the FEDIPs in the districts of Tocache, Uchize, and Nuevo Progreso) at various times has included legalizing coca cultivation, protecting coca growers' rights against abuses by UMOPAR, and promoting public works and agro-industrial development in the provinces. At the height of its power, in May 1986, FEDIP proposed carving out an entirely new Department of the Alto Huallaga that would encompass coca-growing areas in what are now the departments of Huanuco, San Martín, and Ucayali. The capital of the proposed new department—dubbed by some Peruvian reporters "The Independent Republic of Cocaine"—was to be Tocache City, the capital of the province of the same name. Such a scheme, needless to say, flouted the central government's authority and constituted a direct threat to Peru's territorial integrity.[87]

The Tocache FEDIP was, and perhaps still is, an amalgam of diverse forces. In early to mid-1986, it reportedly was heavily influenced by Peruvian and Colombian drug traffickers, who encouraged growers to arm themselves, patrol rivers, and in general discourage penetration of Tocache by law enforcement authorities. FEDIP also embraced a leftist element, which became increasingly important as time went on and included members of the Movement of the Revolutionary Left (MIR), a leftist splinter party that apparently has close ties with coca farmers. The Tupac Amaru Revolutionary Movement also was represented in the Front for a while; however, Tupac moved its base of operations north to the Central Huallaga Valley in March 1987, after losing a power struggle with its revolutionary rival, Sendero Luminoso.[88]

In late 1986 or early 1987, Sendero began infiltrating both the Leoncio Prado and Tocache FEDIPs, helping the movement to gain "a base of support among coca farmers in areas that were previously narco-controlled."[89] By mid-1987, FEDIP was clearly dominated by leftists of various stripes rather than by cocaine dealers. In July 1987, the Peruvian government invaded Tocache with a 1,800-man police force (which included squadrons of police paratroopers called *Sinchis*) to restore the government's authority in the province, which had teetered in a state of near-anarchy for more than a year. After the invasion, FEDIP temporarily faded into obscurity, but the Front (which was extensively restructured in late 1987) is still a voice for peasant interests. Its leaders belong to the MIR and other parties associated with the United Left (also true of the Leoncio Prado FEDIP leaders), but some of these leaders undoubtedly stand in for Sendero Luminoso.

Agenda. The coca lobby is too diffuse and too diverse politically to construct a unified agenda, but demands do overlap on certain issues. First, from Tingo María to Tocache, there is general agreement that eradication must stop. Mayor Gallegos wanted "the complete change or disappearance" of CORAH. The Tocache FEDIP sought the dissolution of the program and the transfer of its budget to "the sectors of education, health, agriculture, or urban affairs."[90] Sendero Luminoso—now a charter member of the coca lobby—exploits the eradication issue to gain converts among the coca-growing peasantry. By mid-1988, Sendero was also making political hay out of U.S.-Peruvian plans to use the herbicide "Spike" against coca plantations in the Valley. Sendero sees coca as a social problem. "For now," said a Senderista cadre interviewed in the Valley in August 1987, "peasants will continue to sow coca because coca is their livelihood." (He indicated that coca cultivation would no longer be permitted after the revolution, but added, "The date of our seizure of power is not fixed.")[91] Sendero also opposes crop substitution, which it views as akin to "dispossessing" the peasant. A party document captured in 1986 notes, "Through coca cultivation, the peasantry earns more because it is a product that has a ready market."[92]

Second, the coca lobby seeks the removal from the zone of UMOPAR, the Civil Guard's mobile detachment of antidrug police. UMOPAR's task is interdicting the drug traffic in rural areas: busting laboratories, confiscating cocaine, and arresting traffickers. UMOPAR also, however, provides protection for CORAH eradication workers, a function that creates more direct contact between antidrug police and coca-growing peasants in Peru than in Bolivia and that consequently entails greater potential for abuses. UMOPAR personnel reportedly maltreated peasants in a variety of ways: killing farm animals, breaking into homes, stealing cash and anything else of value—radios, watches, refrigerators, cameras, and so on—and even raping wives and daughters of coca growers. (The Catholic Church in Tingo María contains a file a foot thick of coca growers' complaints against UMOPAR and PIP personnel.) Police dismiss such allegations as disinformation, narco-propaganda, but some Ministry of Interior officials call them "partly self-interested and partly well-founded." The U.S. Ambassador to Peru, Alexander Watson, acknowledges that U.S. interests in protecting human rights and in prosecuting the war against drugs have sometimes been at odds in the Upper Huallaga Valley.[93]

Third, the coca lobby is, for the most part, aggressively prodevelopment. The exception is Sendero Luminoso, which adheres to "Marxist-Leninist-Maoist" doctrines of class warfare and peasant revolution and which—unlike rural-based guerrilla groups in Colombia—does not maintain a dialogue with the government. Sendero's peasant strategy is not development-oriented; rather, the movement seeks to polarize relations between coca farmers and the Peruvian government. (On the other hand, a more mature revolutionary movement, Colombia's FARC, lobbies for government assistance to support rural modernization in FARC-dominated areas.) Most pro-coca groups, however, are not at war with the system. They are calling on Peruvian authorities (and indirectly on the United States) to offer coca farmers new income opportunities and a better standard of living; they are interested in economic progress rather than revolution.

For example, the Tocache FEDIP in April 1986 presented a list of 54 demands to the Peruvian government, including a broad rural development agenda: for example, the establishment of four rice mills, six agricultural processing plants, seven agronomic institutes, colleges (including a National Coca Institute), a weather station, networks of roads and irrigation canals, a hospital and seven clinics, and a major hydroelectric power station. As a quid pro quo for these demands (which also included legalizing coca in the province and removing or dismantling CORAH, PEAH, and UMOPAR), FEDIP offered to ration coca plots to 2 hectares per family.[94] In Leoncio Prado, the local Defense Front, the mayor of Tingo María, and congressmen representing the region strongly condemned the effects of eradication campaigns on peasants' livelihoods. At least 9,000 hectares of coca have been eradicated in the province since 1983, and hundreds of angry farmers want to know what will replace what had been their most important (and in many cases their only) cash crop. The rhetoric of the coca lobby in Leoncio Prado thus focuses on the "profound poverty and misery" caused by eradication and on the need to find substitute crops for coca.[95]

The United States, specifically AID, supports the $41.8-million PEAH development project in the Upper Huallaga. In a sense, PEAH was envisioned as the carrot for coca farmers, while CORAH was the stick, but the project has not lived up to expectations—indeed, it generated tremendous resentment among Valley residents. Critics such as Ciro Gallegos complain that PEAH's approach was faulty; too much money was spent on showcase development projects and a bureaucracy and too little on assistance to farmers who had lost their coca fields to CORAH.[96] The accusations seemed in part justified. By the end of March 1986, PEAH had spent almost as much on project administration and development as on agricultural extension services: $1.3 million compared to $1.6 million. Another $3.4 million was expended on roads and potable water facilities, but the coca farmers wanted a quick-acting substitution package: When CORAH is pulling out coca plants, they reasoned, PEAH should be putting in new crops. However, PEAH has viewed its mission differently. Said one U.S. AID official interviewed in May 1986, "We are in the development business, not the crop substitution business."

PEAH still has a poor image in the Valley. "It is hard to see how the project has benefited farmers," said Carlos Rocas, Tingo María's current mayor, in an October 1987 interview.[97] To be fair, there is probably little that PEAH *can* do. As explained in Chapter 1, few agricultural crops can grow on the steep slopes and in the acid jungle soils that favor coca cultivation; fewer still can survive in the soils where coca has recently grown. However, the broader question is whether the United States should put development funds into regions that offer few advantages for commercial agriculture. The Peruvian government, echoing the demands of the coca lobby, wants the United States and other industrialized countries to bankroll a $750-million rural modernization program in the Upper Huallaga Valley. Such a scheme on the face of it seems impractical, that is, it is probably a waste of money to try to develop regions that produce coca.

Finally, although the coca farmers' interests are distinct from those of *narcotraficantes,* the farmers also dislike interdiction campaigns. From the farmer's perspective, attacks on paste laboratories and traffickers' lines of communication are bad for business; buyers of coca leaves become scarce, and the price of leaves falls. Peruvian farmers, unlike their Bolivian counterparts, have not seen prices fall below the cost of production; prices in 1987 ranged from $75 per carga to $230 per carga. However, the pre-1987 price was generally more than $300 per carga, so the economy in the Upper Huallaga Valley was, relatively speaking, depressed. Stepped-up attacks on paste laboratories, clandestine airstrips, and Colombian aircraft flying in and out of the Valley were responsible for some although not all of the decline.[98]

The resentment of farmers and others dependent on the coca economy focuses largely on the United States. The North Americans, of course, fund most of the interdiction, and, in certain respects, the drug war in the Upper Huallaga Valley has become increasingly Americanized. By late 1987, U.S. pilots who had flown for Air America in Laos and Vietnam were ferrying DEA agents and UMOPAR troops around the Valley on antidrug missions. (Both pilots and helicopters are leased to Peru by a company called Evergreen based in Portland, Oregon; the State Department pays for the contract.) A political cost is attached to the more visible U.S. presences—Peru's guerrilla movements find it that much easier to convey their anti-imperialist message to the coca-growing population. Sendero seems to be taking advantage of the opportunity; as one cadre said in an interview with Peru's communist daily, *El Diario*, "Here are the American advisers, their mercenary pilots, veterans of the counterrevolutionary Vietnam war, who were defeated by that small nation [pueblo]—here they will be defeated by the masses together with their Army of Popular Liberation."[99]

Impacts. The U.S.-backed anti-cocaine drive in the Upper Huallaga Valley proceeded in an atmosphere of continuing violence, terror, subversion, and peasant hostility. Between November 1984 and August 1987, the drug war cost the lives of 23 CORAH workers, 38 police officers (UMOPAR and PIP), and one Tingo María district attorney.[100] Coca-growing campesinos, cocaine traffickers, and unidentified "subversive delinquents" frequently block the main jungle highway, the *carretera marginal,* between Tingo María and Tocache. (Right now, the only reasonably safe way to travel through the Valley is by helicopter.) Finally, Sendero Luminoso has penetrated peasant communities in some parts of the Valley, in effect placing these zones off limits to CORAH eradicators. All these factors have taken their toll on eradication; only 355 hectares of coca were destroyed in 1987, compared to 2,575 the previous year and 4,830 in 1985.[101]

Some of the history of the drug war is worth recounting in detail. Violent opposition to the eradication program dates from November 1984, when 15 CORAH eradicators and four surveyors working for the organization were murdered while they slept in their camp at Corvinilla, a town on the west bank of the Huallaga River not far from Tingo María.[102] According to one version of the incident, CORAH was paid off by coca farmers or drug traffickers *not* to eradicate in the zone, but reneged; the killings were the retaliation.

In June 1985, the Tocache FEDIP organized a general strike, demanding the legalization of coca cultivation and the immediate suspension of antinarcotics activity. The strikers conducted mass demonstrations and marches and blocked road and river traffic throughout the province. During the strike, a crowd of 3,000 people surrounded and stoned an UMOPAR detachment, incinerating two CORAH trucks and damaging two police vehicles. An UMOPAR report—shedding some light on military-police relations in the Valley—stated that Peruvian marines stationed in Tocache under the state of emergency just stood by, showing themselves "complacent toward the aggressive and violent activities of the mob."[103] In November of that year, 200 armed coca growers captured a patrol of 10 UMOPAR members 15 km south of Tocache City, reportedly to prevent the confiscation of 15 tons of coca paste by the unit. The police were tied, beaten, and eventually turned over to the local military authorities. The growers simply moved their cache of paste to another location.[104]

In late April 1986, FEDIP orchestrated a massive general strike to press numerous demands on the Peruvian government, including legalization of coca; dissolution of CORAH, UMOPAR, and PEAH; massive new development projects in the Valley; and the creation of a new coca-growing Department of the Upper Huallaga. The strike spilled over into Leoncio Prado, and the entire jungle highway from Tingo María to Tocache was blocked in six places. For a time, the AID/PEAH encampment was under siege—the only way out was by foot or by river. FEDIP thus forced the government to negotiate. A government commission that included the Vice Minister of Interior, Augustín Mantilla, flew to Tocache to initiate a dialogue with the strikers. On his return to Lima, Mantilla denied making concessions to FEDIP. Yet, the strike (which began petering out in May) did result in the temporary withdrawal of UMOPAR and CORAH from the province.[105]

From May 1986 until July 1987, Tocache existed in a state of near-anarchy; the government exercised little political control in the province, the scene of a confused power struggle among cocaine dealers (both Peruvian and Colombian), the Tupac Amaru Movement (MRTA), and Sendero Luminoso. At stake in the struggle were at least 25,000 hectares of coca, a lucrative coca paste industry, and the allegiance of tens of thousands of peasants. MRTA, according to various accounts, moved into Tocache in the summer of 1986, and Sendero followed in December. (MRTA had long been active in Leoncio Prado, capitalizing on the

resentment of peasants against eradication.) Sendero proved more successful than its MRTA rival in organizing coca growers; Sendero's line was
that peasants were victimized not just by CORAH eradications but also by
narcotics traffickers, who, said Sendero, bullied peasants into accepting
low prices for their coca leaves.[106]

In March 1987, Sendero and MRTA fought a bloody battle outside of
Tocache City—between 40 and 60 people died, most of them Tupac—that
established Sendero as the predominant guerrilla force in the Upper
Huallaga Valley. Tupac retreated north, and its current stronghold lies
between the towns of Juanjui and Tarapoto in the Central Huallaga region.
In early April, Sendero briefly took over two radio stations in Tocache and
held antigovernment rallies in the town square, haranguing residents about
the virtues of "Comrade Guzman" (Ariel Guzman, the Movement's
leader). Sometime in mid-April, Senderistos torched the town hall of
Tocache, destroying municipal records and forcing the mayor and his
entourage to flee. (By late 1987, there was still no civilian authority in
Tocache.) Sendero never really occupied the town, however. By May and
June of 1987, according to various local accounts, the narcos dominated
Tocache and other larger towns in the province (such as Uchiza and Nuevo
Progreso), but much of the countryside was at least intermittently in the
hands of Sendero forces. For practical purposes, the province was divided
between "red" (revolutionary) and "white" (narco-controlled) zones—to
use the terminology of Sendero cadres.[107]

The Peruvian government—curiously passive in the face of these developments—finally decided to "re-establish the rule of law" in Tocache,
sending 1,800 police into the region on July 15. (See previous discussion
in this chapter.) In response, campesinos, probably with Sendero support,
established a major blockade of the carretera marginal in August. Peasants
blew up three bridges; erected barricades of bricks, rocks, and logs; and
dug trenches at 50-meter intervals along the 70-kilometer stretch of highway linking Tingo María and Tocache. By October, when the author flew
on a helicopter drug raid in the Valley, the highway was only partially
repaired. Moreover, traffic traveling along the road had to make its way
through numerous hostile checkpoints manned (according to different
versions) by coca farmers, drug traffickers, or Senderisto guerrillas.[108]

In August 1988, a repeat performance occurred. Coca farmers, in
obvious collaboration with Sendero, carried out a massive "72-hour"
general strike in the Upper Huallaga Valley that lasted 5 full days. Offices
and businesses shut down, and transportation throughout the region was
paralyzed. Thousands of peasants manned roadblocks of logs, boulders,
and burning rubber tires at several points along the jungle highway. The
stretch of highway between Tingo María and Bellavista (a town 25 km

north of Tocache) was completely impassable, and the road linking Tingo María and Huanaco (the department capital of the same name) was cut. The strike was a general demonstration against government authority, but one of the main aims was to protest U.S.-Peruvian plans to spray herbicide on coca. A Sendero leaflet found near one of the roadblocks read in part, "We repudiate and denounce the plan of CORAH, PEAH, UMOPAR, and DEA to eradicate plantations of coca; under the pretext of eliminating the drug traffic, these organizations are using insecticides (*sic*) of high destructive power—such as 'Spike'—which not only destroy coca, flora, and fauna, but also threaten the lives of people and animals throughout the entire Huallaga."[109]

The coca lobby's demonstrated ability to shut down the road system in the Upper Huallaga forced a change in eradication strategy. In September 1987, U.S. and Peruvian authorities set up a forward base for CORAH at Santa Lucia, 25 km north of Tingo María. From this encampment, teams of eradicators can be moved by U.S.-piloted helicopters into high-density coca zones in Tocache, Leoncio Prado, and other provinces. Yet, pervasive insecurity in these zones—most are patrolled by Sendero forces, guarded by well-armed cocaine traffickers, or protected by the coca farmers themselves—undermines both the morale and the effectiveness of CORAH teams. To add to the general insecurity, cocaine traffickers have offered a bounty of $500,000 for the destruction of each U.S. helicopter operating in the Valley. In other words, conditions could hardly be worse.

The Role of the Army. The Peruvian armed forces have played an important role in the Valley's cocaine wars. Under a state-of-emergency decree, the military exercised complete political, legal, and military control in the Upper Huallaga from August 1984 to December 1985. Political leaders in Huanuco (such as Ciro Gallegos and Andres Quintana Gurt) wanted the state of emergency to continue. In Tocache, some peasant leaders favored a joint exercise of power by the army and ordinary (that is, nondrug) units of Peru's Civil Guard.[110]

Why the army? Basically because the coca lobby (not counting Sendero Luminoso) saw the army as a friend to the coca growers and as a counterweight to the drug control establishment. Strong historical reasons account for this view. The military initially was called into the Valley to combat subversion. Sendero Luminoso guerrillas had opened up a second front in the Valley in the fall of 1983, possibly with the aim of exploiting popular resentment against CORAH and UMOPAR. There were reports that before the state of emergency, Sendero recruited between 1,000 and 1,500 disaffected Valley residents to its cause. Sendero's revolutionary message was especially well received in Leoncio Prado, where a once-thriving coca economy was depressed by extensive eradication. In any event, the political-military command (PMC) took the view that eradication and drug control generally were not particularly compatible with its counterinsurgency mission. As one army officer put it, "We have to have popular support to fight terrorism. We have to be a friend to the population. You can't do that by eradicating coca."[111] PMC did not halt the eradication program, but kept CORAH out of important zones of coca cultivation (for example, the Monzón district in Leoncio province and all of Tocache province were declared off limits). The military did nothing to combat drugs during this period (all of its missions were counterinsurgency-oriented). Moreover, the PMC virtually demobilized UMOPAR, confining the unit to barracks for the first several months of the emergency and severely restricting its operations thereafter. The state of emergency represented a kind of golden age for the cocaine industry, and individual military officers profited greatly. The commander of the zone, Brigadier General (now retired) Julio Carbajal and 31 other army officers are now under military investigation for taking bribes from cocaine dealers.[112]

The experience of military rule in the Upper Huallaga led the antidrug establishment (both Peruvian and North American) to downplay the Sendero threat in the Valley in 1986. A strong guerrilla presence, it was feared, would precipitate a "reimplantation" of the state of emergency and the concomitant suppression of antidrug activities. General Juan Zarate, the head of the Civil Guard's antidrug division (DIPOD) reported in February 1986 that there were almost no Sendero or other guerrilla units in the region. U.S. narcotics officials interviewed in Lima at about the same time thought that many supposed guerrilla activities—such as attacking police outposts, intimidating peasant villagers, and plastering revolutionary slogans on buildings in Tingo María and Tocache (and also on the marginal highway)—were really the work of cocaine traffickers. The idea, of course, was to draw the military into the region again. (Some U.S. officials contend that the Sendero "threat" before the 1984–1985 state of emergency was also a carefully orchestrated deception by cocaine dealers.) The Vice Minister of Interior, Augustín Mantilla, denounced what he saw as fake guerrillas operating in the Valley. In an April 1986 interview, he talked about "mafia" elements who "disguise themselves as subversives, possibly with the hidden aim of forcing the government to declare the zone under emergency and to put it back under the control of the army."[113]

The fake guerrilla theory undoubtedly had some basis in fact, but the theory caused both U.S. and Peruvian officials to overlook the political impact of the antinarcotics campaign and, by the same token, to underestimate the seriousness of the security situation. Sendero was dormant but not dead after the military operation of 1984–1985. After the military left, Sendero regrouped and resumed actively recruiting peasants in the Valley, extending its influence north from Tingo María to Tocache. Moreover, the Tupac Amaru established a foothold for a time in Tocache. (Some observers say that Tupac cultivated ties with narcos in the region, but others disagree strongly with this assessment.) By the early summer of 1987, the Peruvian government knew that it had to act to restore control in the Upper Huallaga. Before the invasion of Tocache on July 15, however, a fierce debate ensued about whether the armed forces or the native police should be in charge of the region. The government initially sought a compromise, giving the area east of the Huallaga to the military and the area to the west to the Civil Guard. The military, which despises the police (see the discussion in Chapter 5), wanted control of the entire region or nothing at all. The military took no part in the July operation beyond lending a couple of air force transport planes. The Upper Huallaga Valley was declared a police emergency zone, a decision that suggested the government was more interested in fighting drugs than in fighting guerrillas. The police are not well trained in counterinsurgency warfare—it is not their mission—and they generally fare badly in encounters with guerrillas.[114]

The uncertainty did not last very long, however. On November 10, the government again called in the armed forces, decreeing a broad military emergency zone that encompassed most of the Upper and Central Huallaga Valley. The government decree mentioned nine provinces in San Martín (including Tocache), Leoncio Prado province in Huanuco, and the Cholon district of Monzón province, also in Huanuco. Police were told to "place themselves at the disposal of the political-military command in these zones."[115] The government's decree apparently was prompted by a destructive attack in early November by heavily armed MRTA guerrillas on Junjui in the Central Huallaga—a fair-sized town of 50,000 people—and also by the continuing guerrilla violence in coca-growing areas to the south. The impact of the new regime remains to be seen. A State Department report in March 1988 observed that the military was neither interfering with nor assisting the antidrug effort.[116] The military has not confined UMOPAR to barracks or restricted the sphere of antidrug operations. On the other hand, army detachments in some areas (such as the Uchiza district) reportedly are sharing in the cocaine bonanza. According to one U.S. narcotics expert in Lima, they are collecting fees of $5,000 or more per airplane-load of cocaine base flown out of the Valley.

Prognosis

The coca lobby, backed at various times by guerrillas and *narcotraficantes*, has clearly frustrated U.S. eradication policies in South America.

In Bolivia and Peru, where the majority of the world's coca is produced, eradication may not be a viable policy. INM's former representative in Bolivia, Don Yellman, noted, "We have had to proceed with the eradication approach, because that's what Congress wanted. We tried it and it didn't work."[117] Compared to their Bolivian and Peruvian counterparts, Colombian coca farmers are fewer in number, less powerful, and not as well organized. However, the FARC gives some protection to growers (in return for payment of a tax), so little eradication can be expected in guerrilla-occupied areas. Indirect eradication—Blast Furnace and its various refinements—can create a temporary glut of coca leaves and depress farmers' profit margins. Yet, farmers in the Upper Huallaga Valley, the Chapare, and the Colombian Llanos continue to cultivate coca, because—despite fluctuating prices—it generates a better cash flow than any other crop.

Most coca eradication in South America to date has been by hand, but the process is labor-intensive, inefficient (20 workers require 1 day to clear 1 hectare of land), and hazardous. A faster and less dangerous (for the eradicators) method is killing the plant from the air with herbicides. The State Department supports spraying as the salvation of its failing narcotics assistance programs in South America: A recent strategy report claimed that aerial spraying in the Upper Huallaga Valley could destroy 10,000 hectares of coca a year.[118]

Spraying, however, is not a panacea, even where it does "work." The highly touted anti-marijuana program in Colombia, for example, reduced cultivation in traditional growing areas in the Sierra Nevada de Santa Marta and the Serrania de Perija, but cultivation simply moved elsewhere. Net cultivation of marijuana in Colombia actually doubled between 1985 and 1987. Furthermore, special problems are associated with coca: The coca bush, more like a small tree in parts of the Chapare and the Upper Huallaga Valley, is extremely difficult to kill. A herbicide sufficiently toxic to destroy coca from the air might also damage other crops, harm farm animals or wildlife, and pollute the waterways. No effective and environmentally safe herbicide for use against coca has yet been found. In addition, South American countries ultimately may refuse to take the spraying route—the issue is extremely sensitive politically (see the discussion in Chapter 5). Bolivia definitively rejected the use of "chemical means" of eradication. In Colombia, the National Council of Dangerous Drugs (NCDD) discontinued an experimental spraying program in 1986, and chances for resuming the tests seem only fair. As the 1988 State Department *International Narcotics Control Strategy Report* notes, "There is a great deal of reluctance to initiate a program that will leave the GOC [government of Colombia] open to criticism by environmentalists, the political opposition, and peasants involved in illicit drug cultivation."[119] Colombia's Minister of Justice and Chairman of the NCDD, Enrique Low Murtra, argued before the U.N. Commission on Narcotic Drugs in February 1988 that spraying has "destructive effects on the health of the population."[120] In Peru, a pilot program of spraying is underway, but there, too, concerns about ecological damage have surfaced. Environmentalists fear both the runoff of toxic chemicals onto crops cultivated downhill from coca fields and the eventual contamination of the Huallaga River. The State Department wants to use Eli Lilly's herbicide tebuthiuron (Spike) in Peru, but recent negative publicity—including the manufacturer's own refusal to sell the chemical to INM—has doubtless aggravated existing fears.[121]

South American concerns over the environmental consequences of spraying are real, but the central issue is not so much spraying as eradication itself. Even if a toxic but safe herbicide is developed, governments may prove reluctant to dispossess huge masses of peasants. Washington's 1-year eradication target in Peru, for example, could leave 50,000 peasants (assuming a family of five per hectare) without any means of livelihood. This development undoubtedly could wreak havoc on the economy of the Upper Huallaga and would increase the regional incidence of crime, subversion, and terrorism. For Peru and the other Andean countries, the main problem is not how best to destroy coca plants, but rather how to cope with the consequences of eradication.

Andean governments caught in a vise between the competing demands of the coca lobby (in its various guises) and the coca abolitionists in Washington are likely to adopt the form rather than the substance of a spraying policy. This development means a prolonged—perhaps an indefinite—period of tests and pilot projects and interminable official studies and reports that detail the conflicting opinions on the ecological effects of each promising new herbicide. Meanwhile, Andean countries will seek, as a condition for moving beyond the test phase, massive U.S. aid and unaffordable safety-net programs for coca farmers. The impasse probably will continue until the hundreds of thousands of peasants who now cultivate coca can be employed elsewhere in the economy. In turn, such employment will require very high rates of growth in Andean economies and intelligent government planning for industrial and agricultural development.

NOTES

1. Timothy Plowman, "Botanical Perspectives on Coca," in F. R. Jeri (ed), *Cocaine 1980: Proceedings of the Interamerican Seminar on Coca and Cocaine* (Lima: Pacific Press, 1980), p. 90.

2. Dirección de Policía de Drogas de La Guardia Civil de Perú, "Proyecto de Ayuda Específica del Gobierno de EE. UU. de NA. para La Guardia Civil de Perú," Lima, 1984, pp. 8-9.
Interviews with ENACO in Lima, May 1986.
"Ley De Sustancias controladas y otras disposiciones transitorias," *Presencia,* July 18, 1988.
3. Government of Bolivia, "Triennial Program of the Battle against Drug Trafficking" ("Triennial Program"), La Paz, November 1986, p. 6.
UDAPE, "Información económica," 1987, p. 1.
4. Walter Degadillo, "Pliego único," Radio Cristal, May 2, 1986.
5. "Acuerdo entre el gobierno constitucional, CSUTCB, y federaciones campesinos productores de coca sobre el plan integral de desarollo y sustitución de los cultivos de coca y la lucha contra el narcotráfico" ("Acuerdo entre el gobierno"), La Paz, June 6, 1987, p. 1.
6. "Decision de EE UU de suspender ayuda a Bolivia es prepotente," *Presencia,* March 4, 1986.
7. "No debe preocupar suspención de ayuda de Estados Unidos," *Presencia,* March 5, 1986.
8. "VIII ampliado campesino reafirma rechazo a eradicación de coca," *Presencia,* January 11, 1986.
9. William Montalbano, "Latins Push Belated War on Cocaine," *Los Angeles Times,* December 1, 1985.
10. "¿A quién beneficia la reducción de cocales?" *Meridiano,* December 2, 1985.
11. "Corruption Hampers Combat," *Polha de Sao Paolo,* Sao Paolo, June 11, 1987.
"COB's Escobar on coca substitution," *Presencia,* February 1, 1988.
12. Instituto de Estudios Políticos para América Latina, y Africa, *Narcotráfico y Política* (Madrid: Graficas Margaritas, 1982), p. 152.
13. Juan de Onis, "New Bolivian Road May Become Cocaine Turnpike," *Los Angeles Times,* December 2, 1985.
14. "Viva la coca," *Caretas,* January 13, 1986, pp. 38-39.
15. Anonymous, *Narcotráfico y Política II* (Cochabamba: No publisher identified, 1985), p. 81.
16. "Vice President on U.S. Role in Anti-Drug Campaign," *La Paz Cadena Panamericana,* June 27, 1984.
17. "Producers' Group Introduces New Coca Products," *Presencia,* October 8, 1988.
On industrialization see also "Club de la cocaína legal," *Presencia,* May 22, 1983.
18. Joel Brinkley, "Bolivia in Turmoil at Drug Crackdown," *The New York Times,* September 12, 1984.
19. See Chapter 1, note 9.
20. On these human rights issues, see "Colonos concedieron 48 horas para que agentes de la DEA abandonen el Chapare," *Presencia,* May 24, 1988.
"Productores de coca denuncian abusos," *Opinión,* May 23, 1988.
"Peasants Accuse UMOPAR of Selling Coca," *Presencia,* March 8, 1988.
Luis Morales Ortega, "Así se preparan los guerrilleros en la selva del Alto Huallaga," *El Diario,* Lima, September 18, 1987.
Interviews with Catholic Church officials in Lima, February 17–18, 1986.
21. Fernando Cabiesaes, *Etnología, Fisiología, y Farmacología de la Coca y la Cocaína* (Lima: El Museo Peruano de Ciencias de Salud, 1985), pp. 14–16.

22. Amado Canelas, *Bolivia: Coca, Cocaína; Subdesarollo y Poder Político (Coca, Cocaína)* (La Paz: Los Amigos del Libro, 1983), pp. 78–79, 83, 194, 197, 404.
23. "Bolivia: Riding High on Cocaine" ("Bolivia: Riding High"), *Latin American Regional Reports: Andean Group*, June 24, 1983, p. 7.
24. *Narcotráfico y Política II*, pp. 167–168.
    Alberto Zuazo, "Cocaine Producers Vow to Fight Back," United Press International, August 5, 1984.
    "Farmers Blockade Roads, Threaten Other Measures," *La Paz Cadena Panamericana*, August 2, 1984.
    "Peasants Isolate Cochabamba," Paris AFP, November 14, 1984.
25. "Leopardos enjaulados," *Opinión*, Cochabamba, January 19, 1986.
    "Coca Farmers Ending Siege of Bolivian Narcotics Officers," *The Washington Post*, January 12, 1986.
26. "Agricultores piden que una comisión especial vaya a Tocache y Uchiza," *El Comercio*, May 3, 1986.
    Interviews with U.S. and Peruvian agricultural officials, May 25–27, 1986.
27. Richard Craig, "Illicit Drug Traffic: Implications for South American Source Countries," *Journal of Interamerican Studies and World Affairs*, Summer 1987, p. 10.
28. "Marginal 70 km de destrucción" ("Marginal 70 km"), *Caretas*, September 7, 1987, pp. 31–35.
29. "Coca Violence," Latin American Newsletter Ltd., July 28, 1988, p. 8.
    "Workers Strike to Protest the Killing of Six Coca Leaf Farmers," Associated Press, International News, June 30, 1988.
30. Bases Huallaga, "Paro de 72 horas," August 1988.
31. *INCSR*, 1988, p. 109.
32. "Mixed Signals from the Cocaine Dollar Belt" ("Mixed Signals"), *The Andean Report*, December 1985, p. 241.
33. R. W. Lee, "The Drug Trade and Developing Countries," Overseas Development Council, *Policy Focus*, No. 4 (June 1987), p. 7.
34. *INCSR*, 1988, pp. 78, 109.
    INCSR, 1985, p. 117.
35. Peter Reuter, "Eternal Hope: America's Quest for Narcotics Control," *The Public Interest*, Spring 1985, p. 87.
36. *INCSR*, 1988, p. 70.
    "Acuerdo entre el gobierno," p. 5.
37. *Coca, Cocaína*, p. 392.
    "Club de la Cocaína Legal," see note 17.
    "Asociación Nacional de Productores de Coca: Pronunciamento," *Presencia*, November 15, 1985.
38. "El congreso extraordinario de la asemblea de derechos humanos de Bolivia demanda la vigencia de los derechos humanos conculcadas por los decretos 21060–21132," *Presencia*, February 2, 1986.
39. *Narcotráfico y Política II*, pp. 131–135.
    Interviews with U.S. and Bolivian agricultural experts in La Paz and Cochabamba, May 15–19, 1986.
40. "Carta abierta de Roberto Suarez al presidente Ronald Reagan," in *Coca, Cocaína*, p. 433.
41. *Coca, Cocaína*, pp. 273–281.

Presidency of the Republic, "Régimen legal de control de sustancias peligrosos," Annex to Supreme Decree 20811, p. 3.
42. "Bolivia: Riding High," p. 7.
    Narcotráfico y Política II, p. 74.
43. "Project Agreement Between the Government of the United States of America and the Government of the Republic of Bolivia," p. 8.
44. *Narcotráfico y Política II*, pp. 109–113.
45. Ibid., p. 110.
    "Congress to Review Secret Drug Accords with U.S.," Paris AFP, February 3, 1984.
46. "Peasant Farmers Riot," *Hoy*, La Paz, March 29, 1984.
    "Campesinos del Chapare no aceptan erradicar los cultivos de coca," *Presencia*, May 27, 1984.
47. *Narcotráfico y Política II*, p. 160.
48. "El gobierno declara zona militar a la región del Chapare trópical," *Presencia*, August 1, 1984.
49. "Jefe militar dispone que se levante bloqueo de caminos," *Presencia*, August 2, 1984.
    "Coca Producers Declare State of Emergency," *La Paz Cadena Panamericana*, August 1, 1984.
50. *Narcotráfico y Política II*, pp. 168, 181.
51. Ibid., pp. 181–185.
52. "Hunger Strike Lifted," Paris AFP, November 2, 1984.
53. *INCSR*, 1987, p. 69.
    INCSR, 1988, p. 72.
    "Second Day in Siege," Madrid EFE, July 2, 1987.
    "Bolivia's U.S.-Aided Attack on Cocaine an Uphill Struggle," *Los Angeles Times*, May 13, 1988.
54. "Second Day in Siege," see note 53.
55. Peter McFarren, "Workers Strike to Protest the Killing of Six Coca Leaf Farmers," The Associated Press, International News, June 30, 1988.
    "Coca Violence," *Latin American Newsletters*, July 28, 1988, p. 5.
    Alberto Zuazo, "Workers' Protests: Peasant Deaths Blamed on U.S. Agents," United Press International, July 1, 1988.
56. "Campesinos del Chapare aceptan reducción de cultivos de coca," *Presencia*, November 9, 1985.
57. "President, Peasants Sign Coca Eradication Pact," *La Paz Cadena Panamericana*, November 9, 1985.
    "Colonizadores apoyan plan de reducción de cultivos de coca," *Presencia*, March 21, 1986.
58. "A los campesinos no nos asusta la amenaza de los gringos," *Opinión*, Cochabamba, March 6, 1986.
59. "Colonizadores de Carrasco trópical no aceptan reducir cultivos de coca," *Presencia*, December 4, 1985.
    "Colonizadores contra quema de coca," *Aquí*, La Paz, December 7, 1985.
60. "Piden la cabeza de Eudoro Barrientos productores que rechazan la reducción," *Los Tiempos*, Cochabamba, November 30, 1986.
    "Un 80% de productores de coca está en contra de la reducción," *Opinión*, Cochabamba, November 28, 1985.
61. "Asociación Nacional de Productores de Coca: Pronunciamiento," see note 37.

"Colonizadores de Carrasco trópical no aceptan reducir cultivos de coca,"
see note 59.

"Minister Says Peasants Should Accept Coca Plan," Paris AFP, November
16, 1985.

62. *INCSR*, 1987, p. 70.

Shirley Christian, "Bolivia Hoping U.S. Drug Forces Will Extend Stay," *The
New York Times*, August 22, 1986, p. B4.

63. *Mid-Year Update, INCSR*, September 1987, p. 10.

64. "Residents Protest Presence of U.S. Troops, Leopards," Paris AFP, October
11, 1986.

65. "MNR Leader Scores President, Founds Party," Paris AFP, July 31, 1986.

"Criticism from Various Sources," Madrid EFE, July 17, 1986.

"Congress Split Over Presence of U.S. Troops," Paris AFP, August 5, 1986.

66. "Plan trienal de la lucha contra el narcotráfico," La Paz, December 1986, p.
11.

"Triennial Program," pp. 12, 14.

(These are two different versions of the same plan.)

67. "Triennial Plan," pp. 13, 14, 16.

68. "Peasant Leaders: Official Statements," La Paz, *La Red Panamericana*, May
26, 1987.

"Coca Plantation Defense Committee Formed," Madrid EFE, April 24, 1987.

69. "Acuerdo entre el gobierno," pp. 1–5.

70. *INCSR*, 1988, p. 69.

"Convenio de reducción de cocales no solo comprende la indemnización,"
Presencia, November 8, 1987.

71. "Productores de coca decidieron suspender programa de reducción," *Presencia*, December 16, 1987.

72. "Productores de coca levantaron ocupación y liberaron a rehenes," *Los
Tiempos*, June 10, 1988.

"Productores de coca iniciaron bloqueo general de carreteras," *Opinión*, June
7, 1988.

"Campesinos se movilizan en defensa de sus cocales," *Opinión*, May 25,
1988.

73. "Matan la coca—y a los campesinos," *Aquí*, La Paz, July 2, 1988, p. 16.

Interviews with U.S. narcotics experts in La Paz, October 11, 1988.

74. "Ley de sustancias controladas y ones disposiciónes transitorias," *Presencia*,
July 18, 1988.

75. "111 encuentro nacional de productores de coca," *Hoy*, August 20, 1988.

76. Peter McFarren, "New Eradication Program Winning Over Coca Farmers,"
Associated Press, Business News, December 31, 1987, p. 8.

Interviews with U.S. narcotics experts in La Paz, October 2, 1987.

77. Interviews with AID officials in Washington, D.C., August 16, 1988.

78. Telephone interview with U.S. expert on Bolivian rural development, Washington, D.C., July 24, 1988.

79. Peter Kerr, "Bolivia, with U.S. Aid, Battles Cocaine at the Root," *The New
York Times*, April 17, 1988.

80. Interview with U.S. narcotics experts in La Paz, October 11, 1988.

81. Raul Gonzalez, "Coca and Subversion in the Huallaga," *Quehacer*, Lima,
September–October 1987, pp. 58–72.

82. Comité Regional de Productores de Coca de la Provincia de Leoncio Prado,
"Letter to Senator Andres Quintana Gurt," February 18, 1986.

"Las razones del frente de defensa de Leoncio Prado" ("Las razones"), *Pura Selva*, Tingo María, July 1987, p. 18.
83. "Debemos tratar el problema de la coca," *Pura Selva*, April 1986, pp. 6–8.
84. Interviews with Catholic priests in Tingo María, February 17–18, 1986.
Tito Jaime Fernandez, "Letter to Attorney General of Leoncio Prado," November 11, 1982.
85. Interviews with representatives of ENACO, February 18–19, 1986.
86. Interviews with representatives of ENACO and CORAH in Tingo María, February 17–19, 1986.
87. "Pliego de reclamos," Frente de Defensa de los Intereses del Pueblo de la Provincia de Tocache, Tocache, April 24, 1986.
DIPOD, Guardia Civil, "Intelligence Note," June 10, 1985, p. 3.
88. "Coca and Subversion in the Huallaga," pp. 58–72.
89. "Counterinsurgency and Anti-Narcotics Measures Become Intertwined in the Upper Huallaga Valley" ("Counterinsurgency and Anti-Narcotics"), *The Andean Report*, June 1987, p. 102.
90. "Pliego de Reclamos," see note 87.
91. "La Conexión," September 7, 1987, p. 36.
92. "Crack Secret Police Outfit to Combat the Shining Path's New Offensive," *The Andean Report*, March 1987, p. 39.
93. Interview with Ambassador Alexander Watson in Lima, October 16, 1987.
94. "Pliego de Reclamos," see note 87.
95. "Las Razones," p. 18.
96. Ciro Gallegos, "Referencias," unpublished memorandum, Tingo María, February 1986, pp. 2–4.
97. Interview in Tingo María, October 14, 1987.
98. "Overproduction of Coca at Root of Shining Path New Prominence in the Region," *The Andean Report*, June 1987, p. 107.
Interviews with ENACO representatives in Tingo María, October 14, 1987.
"U.S. AID Project Wins Few Friends and Fails to Match the Drug Industry's Complete Package," *The Andean Report*, December 1985, p. 244.
99. "Derrotaremos al ejército a la policía y a los mercenarios y asesores Yanquis," *El Diario*, Lima, September 17, 1987.
100. "Coca y catástrofe," *Caretas*, March 7, 1988, p. 69.
Monte Hayes, "Drug Traffickers Kill Five Policemen and a District Attorney," Associated Press, International News, April 25, 1986.
101. *INCSR*, 1988, p. 109.
102. "Mixed Signals," p. 248.
103. Ibid., p. 243.
104. "15,000 Tocache Coca Growers Well Organized," *El Comercio*, November 16, 1985, p. A-13.
105. "Pliego de Reclamos," see note 87.
"Narcos pretenden paralizar Tocache con terror y chantaje," *La República*, Lima, May 12, 1986.
106. "Coca and Subversion," pp. 58–72.
107. Ibid.
"Hablan los líderes guerrilleros del PCP-SL de la Selva," *El Diario*, September 15, 1987.
108. "Marginal 70 km," pp. 31–35.
109. Bases Huallaga, "Paro de 72 horas," August 1988.

110. Raul Barrionuevo, "Mafia corrompe y agita a autoridades y campesinos," *Ojo*, May 5, 1986.
111. Marlise Simons, "Peruvian Rebels Halt Drive Against Cocaine," *The New York Times*, August 13, 1984, p. A4.
    Jackson Diehl, "Model Anti-Drug Drive Fails in Peru," *The Washington Post*, December 29, 1984.
112. "Counterinsurgency and Anti-Narcotics," p. 107.
113. "Narcos pretenden paralizar,"see note 105.
114. Interviews with U.S. narcotics officials in Lima, October 15–17, 1987.
115. "FF. AA. asume control en zona de emergencia," *Extra*, Lima, November 11, 1987.
116. *INCSR*, 1988, p. 108.
117. Joel Brinkley, "Bolivians Deny Asking GIs for Aid in Raids," *The New York Times*, July 20, 1986, p. 21.
118. *INCSR*, 1988, p. 108.
119. Ibid., p. 91.
120. Frederico Nier-Fischer, "Health: Double Dealing Denounced in Anti-Drug Campaigning," Inter Press Service, Vienna, February 19, 1988.
121. "To Spike or Not to Spike," *The Economist*, June 27, 1988, p. 23.
    See also Chapter 5 discussion of spraying.

3

The Cocaine Mafia

*Virtue, honor, truth, and the law have all van-
ished from our life.*

—Al Capone, 1931

Structure and Organization

The cocaine mafia is the organizational embodiment of the downstream
phases of the cocaine industry: refining, smuggling, and distribution. Like
the coca lobby, it is a potent political force in South American countries.
The source of the cocaine mafia's power, however, is not so much
numerical strength (for example, masses of peasants who can blockade
highways), but rather superior financial and logistical resources, sophisticated weaponry, and extensive protection networks. In Colombia and
Bolivia, mafia organizations have penetrated deeply into key decisionmaking structures (such as legislatures and the military) and have virtually
substituted for state power in parts of the country.

South American cocaine mafias fall into the category of what Professor
Mark Moore calls "large, durable criminal organizations."[1] U.S. law
enforcement officials believe that Colombian syndicates are vertically
integrated "from the clandestine laboratories of Colombia to the stateside
distribution."[2] According to a 1986 U.S. indictment against nine Colombian drug traffickers, the operations of Jorge Ochoa's "family" extends
"from the purchase of raw materials through and including cocaine production, transportation, distribution, and sale."[3] However, these organizations seem to be more amorphous than criminal organizations in the
United States or Western Europe. Their boundaries are fluid, the cast of
characters changes continually, and the links in the chain are bound
together in an intricate system of contracts and subcontracts.

In Colombia, the cocaine trade is dominated by two coalitions of crime
families; the larger one is centered in Medellín and the other in Cali. The

99

capos of these organizations typically reside or maintain residences in Medellín or Cali. Five major export syndicates exercise informal leadership over these coalitions: the Medellín export syndicates are headed by Pablo Escobar, Jorge Luis Ochoa, and José Gonzalo Rodríguez Gacha; the Cali syndicates are run by Gilberto Rodríguez Orejuela and José Santa Cruz Londoño. These five major exporters produce and market their own cocaine, but they also market cocaine supplied by other Medellín or Cali families. The major syndicates apparently export a large share, perhaps 70–80 percent, of the cocaine manufactured in Colombia. They also handle some percentage of Bolivian and Peruvian cocaine exports.

Apparently no effective cocaine cartel is operating in Colombia; that is, the leading organizations seemingly cannot restrict production or maintain prices. (The U.S. wholesale price of cocaine dropped from $55,000–$60,000 per kilo in 1980 to $10,000–$15,000 per kilo in 1988.)[4] Competition, especially intercity competition, clearly operates in the system. For example, Medellín and Cali coalitions (often called, confusingly, cartels) are currently fighting for control of the lucrative New York City market. Also, the Medellín and Cali groups probably do not account for much more than 60–70 percent of the total world market; most of the balance is in the hands of Colombian independents or Peruvian and Bolivian traffickers. Yet, if the Colombian mafia does not constitute a cartel in the strict economic sense, it is capable of coordinated action. Mafia leaders form joint business ventures, pool cocaine shipments, cooperate in insurance schemes, issue joint communiqués, and even jointly plan assassinations.

The sheer size of mafia operations requires the explicit coordination of many transactions as well as a system of information gathering and record keeping. Cocaine syndicates are too big and too complex to escape detection, and they are too vulnerable to penetration by law enforcement agents. Hence, they have to make large cash payments to the authorities to protect their laboratories and smuggling routes and to keep their chief executives out of jail. Their system of protection also includes a far-flung intelligence network that extends to enforcement agencies (and superordinate bureaucracies) and even, perhaps, to U.S. embassies operating in drug-producing countries. Mafia syndicates also have a capacity for violence. Such violence or the threat of it is used to discipline employees, to enforce contracts with business associates, and to exterminate rival traffickers. In Colombia, violence is also a means of influencing judicial outcomes—the *"plomo o plata"* alternative—and of shaping the government's overall policy on drug control. The parade in recent years of mafia-sponsored hits against uncooperative judges, public officials, and newspapermen has no counterpart elsewhere in Latin America or in the United States.

State Department officials like to talk about narco-terrorism, but drug violence should be distinguished from terrorist violence. To the stray judge, policeman, or cabinet minister who gets in the line of fire, this may seem like a distinction without a difference. Still, terrorists who are interested in destabilizing the existing government target the civilian population more broadly than drug traffickers; the latter do not randomly kill civilians, but rather single combatants—enemies of the narcotics industry. Bombing public buildings, hijacking airplanes, destroying railway links, blowing up oil pipelines and refineries, and attacking military bases are acts of revolutionaries, not drug dealers. Foreign and Colombian businessmen are not afraid of being kidnapped by the cocaine mafia; however, the threat of kidnapping by the M-19, the FARC, and the National Liberation Army (ELN) is real and ever-present.

In some recent cases, traffickers have kidnapped political figures to convey an anti-extradition message. One such case was the abduction of Andres Pastrana, a conservative candidate for mayor of Bogotá (who was later elected) by a paramilitary group called "The Extraditables." Pastrana was snatched from Conservative Party headquarters in Bogotá, transported to Medellín by helicopter, and held for 1 week on a farm outside the city. He was rescued by police acting on an anonymous tip—possibly from the traffickers themselves. In a wrathful communiqué sent to the Colombian government the day before Pastrana's return, the group denounced the "surrender of Colombians to North American imperialism" and declared "total war" against the Colombian "traitors" who favored extradition.[5] The second case was the abduction on January 25, 1988, of pro-extradition Attorney General Carlos Mauro Hoyas while he was traveling to Medellín's José María Cordoba airport. Mauro was fatally shot during the abduction. A communiqué from The Extraditables after the incident said that Mauro was "executed because of treason to the fatherland." However, U.S. narcotics experts in Bogotá believe that Mauro's death was "probably an accident"—the result of a bungled political kidnapping.[6]

Such instances, however, are the exception rather than the rule. In contrast, political kidnappings by guerrillas are "the bread of each day" in Colombia. For example, nine mayors of small towns in the departments of Cesar, North Santander, and Bolivar were kidnapped by the ELN and other subversive groups in January–February 1988.[7] Most of these operations in effect were involuntary escorted tours into guerrillas' jungle hideouts; following several days of indoctrination, the "guests" were presented with a list of guerrilla demands, told to communicate those demands to the higher authorities, and then released.

Finally, South American cocaine traffickers are intensely political; they want not just protection (in the traditional sense of immunity from prosecution) but also legitimacy. They work hard at image building, trying (with some success) to pass themselves off as patriotic, progressive, and public-spirited citizens. They seem intensely status conscious: "We reject with indignation," said a communiqué of The Extraditables, "declarations by the national newspapers that it is 'the mafia' that is holding Señor Pastrana." (Mafia evidently is considered a term of disrespect: Call us *narcotraficantes*, they seemed to be saying, but not mafia.)[8] Cocaine traffickers wage a sophisticated and relentless propaganda campaign against drug enforcement measures, characterizing such measures as just another form of U.S. meddling in Latin American affairs. Extradition, Carlos Lehder once said, is an "anti-Latin invention."[9] Traffickers' charitable and public works projects, which reach thousands of peasant villagers and poor slum dwellers whom governments cannot reach, have earned them a dedicated popular following in these societies. Cocaine dealers attempt to purchase political power, contributing massive sums to presidential and congressional political campaigns and even offering governments huge cash loans to bail them out of financial difficulties. Finally, individual cocaine capos have themselves entered the political arena: Carlos Lehder, for example, founded a new political movement in his native department of Quindío; Pablo Escobar was elected to the Colombian Congress as an alternate deputy from Antioquia.

The mafia's power is extraordinary. Enrique Parejo, Colombia's Minister of Justice under Belisario Betancur, remarked, "At one time or another, in one way or another, all state organizations have suffered the corruption of the narcotics traffickers."[10] Betancur himself recently called the mafia "an organization stronger than the state." The mafia constitutes a challenge of sorts to traditional political elites and has earned their antipathy. Yet, the mafia's enormous web of protective relationships greatly complicates the task of law enforcement officials. In Parejo's words, "Here in Colombia, we see well-known traffickers walking around as if they owned the place."[11] As of 1988, no major traffickers were being held in jail anywhere in Colombia. A few leading traffickers—Jorge Ochoa, Gilberto Orejuela, and Evaristo Porras—were arrested in 1986 and 1987, but then released by criminal court judges. Major capos, in other words, operate in a kind of twilight zone: They are wanted men, sort of, but a protected species nonetheless.

Definitions

Organizational scope.   Mafia syndicates tend to concentrate on downstream activities—on refining, transporting, and distributing coca prod-

products. Most are not engaged in coca cultivation (Gonzalo Rodríguez Gacha's organization in Colombia may be an exception), although traffickers sometimes provide financing and even seeds and fertilizer to growers. Organizations differ greatly in the sophistication of their refining operations and in their capacity to move cocaine into major consumer markets. Here, a rough comparison can be drawn between Colombian syndicates on the one hand and Peruvian and Bolivian organizations on the other. The former buy coca paste and cocaine base—mainly from Peru and Bolivia, convert these intermediates to cocaine hydrochloride (CHCL), and ship the finished drug to distributors. Colombians dominate the coca trade; according to the National Narcotics Intelligence Committee, 75 percent of the refined cocaine entering the United States in 1985–1986 was of Colombian origin.[12]

In contrast, mafia organizations in Peru and Bolivia are mainly in the business of supplying crude cocaine to Colombian middlemen, who capture the value added in further refining and in delivery of the product to overseas markets. Peru's trade is especially poorly integrated. The vast majority of cocaine leaves Peru in the form of cocaine base and is often carried out in Colombian airplanes that fly the routes between the Upper Huallaga Valley and the Amazon Basin. Bolivia's cocaine exports apparently include a larger percentage of CHCL. (In 1985–1986, Bolivian-refined cocaine accounted for an estimated 15 percent of the U.S. market, but cocaine of Peruvian origin accounted for only 5 percent.) Both Bolivia and Peru have every economic incentive to integrate forward and may succeed in doing so—up to a point. Yet, Colombia will continue to dominate smuggling and distribution, at least for North American markets. Colombia's geographic location, its extensive transportation links with the United States, and a large Colombian immigrant population in United States cities give Colombian traffickers an enormous commercial advantage over their Bolivian and Peruvian counterparts.

Organizational assets—physical assets. Large mafia organizations own or control an array of physical assets used in running the cocaine business. The most important of these are laboratories, means of transportation, and means of communication. Laboratories constitute the core of syndicate operations. They may produce intermediate products, such as cocaine paste or cocaine base (purified paste), or they may produce cocaine hydrochloride—the finished cocaine consumed by most end users. The larger and better integrated the trafficking organization, the more sophisticated its processing capability. Transport also is essential to mafia organizations; boats, planes, and helicopters are used to ship products from remote jungle laboratories to customers and also to supply the laboratories with raw materials and chemicals. Traffickers also build and maintain the literally thousands of clandestine airstrips in Colombia,

Bolivia, and Peru. In addition, traffickers rely on sophisticated communications systems to maintain secure communications within their organizations and to monitor law enforcement surveillance. Such systems include state-of-the-art radio equipment, sometimes outfitted with scramblers (to prevent interception of messages), and digital encryption devices. In Colombia, as U.S. Army General Paul Gorman (Ret.) notes, the government communications system "is regularly intercepted, indeed used, by the *narcotraficantes.*" Furthermore, says Gorman, "The *narcotraficantes* can track the movement of Colombian armed forces and aircraft and ships better than their respective commanders, know more surely where they are and where they are going."[13]

Two other assets are also critical to the functioning of cocaine syndicates: weapons and money. Both factors carry political as well as business connotations. For example, weapons provide security for installations but also convey an image of power. Money is plowed into direct operating expenses—equipment, raw materials, salaries, and the like—but also is used to buy protection, fund political campaigns, and even create political movements.

Traffickers' weapons characteristically include high-quality firepower, often automatic weapons such as Ingrams, Uzis, and Urus. Cocaine trafficking organizations in Colombia, Bolivia, and Peru are better armed than the antinarcotics police—at least, the police believe that to be the case. Such weapons are used for guarding laboratories, airstrips, and other facilities against both police and predatory guerrilla groups. Personal escorts of leading drug capos also carry weapons.

Bluffing is also part of the drug traffickers' arsenals. For example, a major Bolivian trafficker, Roberto Suarez, bragged to reporters in 1983 that he had 12 Brazilian-made combat aircraft, some armed with rockets and missiles. Suarez even said in an interview that he "could practically destroy the Bolivian air force in 1 minute."[14] After being jailed in July 1988, Suarez admitted that his claims were false, but his saber-rattling made the Bolivian government nervous at the time—which was the intent in any case. As a member of Bolivia's labor confederation (COB) said, "Public opinion does not believe that Suarez acquired sophisticated weapons only to defend himself against the DEA. Undoubtedly, this public display hides very well-defined political objectives."[15]

The financial resources available to drug trafficking organizations are seemingly enormous. Colombia's major cocaine capos reported in 1984 that their business earned "an annual income close to $2 billion," but the earnings are probably far higher today. The personal fortune of one of Colombia's most important capos, Pablo Escobar, is estimated at $3 billion and Gonzalo Rodríguez Gacha's at $1.3 billion.[16] Some drug money ends up in banks for investment overseas, but a significant sum is spent domestically on overhead; for example, on running laboratories, maintaining fleets of planes and helicopters, and carving out airstrips in the jungle. Traffickers also buy protection from law enforcement officials and maintain networks of informants in key government ministries.

In many respects, South American cocaine mafias behave very much like U.S. criminal organizations. However, the South Americans apparently have penetrated much further into the political realm. They have poured millions of dollars into national electoral campaigns, built grassroots political organizations, run for political office, and even offered to pay off part of their countries' foreign debts. For South American drug lords, money is not just operating capital or a means of acquiring luxury; it is also a powerful tool for influencing political processes and outcomes.

Organizational assets—human factors. The structure of mafia organizations also can be defined in terms of their human assets. There are several main categories of people: a core element comprising syndicate leaders and key lieutenants—the latter often blood relatives—operators of cocaine laboratories, and professionals such as lawyers, bankers, and financial managers. According to Ramón Milian Rodríguez, a former money launderer for the Medellín syndicates, all the members of the Medellín syndicates' financial management team have advanced degrees in their individual specialties.[17] Traffickers also maintain private security forces that (in Colombia) have acquired the dimensions of private armies; one reason is that traffickers, who have invested in landed estates in the countryside, seek to protect their properties against predatory guerrilla groups (see the discussion in Chapter 4). Finally, large exporting syndicates have their own boats, planes, and pilots to smuggle cocaine to overseas markets, and they sometimes hire specialized transport-courier companies as well to move their products.

In addition to the above characteristics, the most important component of cocaine organizations is the system of protection and intelligence. Protection, as defined here, means general immunity for criminal operations—traffickers pay people in authority to leave them alone. The mafia pays the police (or military) not to raid laboratories, not to make arrests, and to block investigations. It pays district attorneys (or their Latin American equivalents) not to prosecute, judges not to convict, and penal officials to release those traffickers who, in spite of everything, do manage to land in jail.

There is a limit, however, to the mafia's ability to penetrate and to corrupt enforcement agencies; it cannot buy immunity for all of its activities. The mafia consequently needs an intelligence network to supplement the protection network and to provide advance warning of planned antidrug operations such as raids on laboratories, customs searches, and arrests. The network includes informants strategically placed in police organizations, the military, and key government ministries such as Justice, Interior, or Foreign Relations. Sometimes cocaine traffickers themselves occupy positions of trust and responsibility within the law enforcement bureaucracy. In Peru, a trafficker named Reynaldo Rodríguez Lopez simultaneously was an adviser to the Director of the Peruvian Investigations Police (PIP) and maintained an office at PIP headquarters. Rodríguez, whose arrest in mid-1985 resulted largely from a DEA investigation, had some important associates. His drug ring allegedly included several PIP generals as well as the private secretary, Luis López Vergara, of Fernando Belaunde Terry's Minister of Interior, Luis Percovich Roca.[18]

The United States also is a target of mafia intelligence gathering. Cocaine syndicates reputedly have informants inside U.S. embassies in drug-producing countries. U.S. narcotics experts in Bogotá have speculated that the cocaine mafia might have access to some of the U.S. embassy's cable traffic. According to an article in Colombia's *Semana* magazine, the mafia pays its own agents three times as much to inform against DEA as DEA pays Colombians to inform against the mafia. Colombian syndicates also are said to maintain a list of DEA agents and their code names—a list that is circulated to counterpart organizations in other South American countries.[19]

This intelligence capability functions within a broader system of social relationships created by the mafia. Cocaine traffickers earn friends and supporters within the society by spending money within the society. In some cases, traffickers have acquired a kind of Robin Hood image by donating vast sums to local development projects or by simply giving money and gifts to the poor. The standing that some major capos hold in their communities enables them to co-opt the local populace into their early-warning systems. As a result, within major mafia strongholds, such as the Beni Region in Bolivia and the city of Medellín in Colombia, the "fat fish" of the cocaine trade can operate with relative impunity. With the notable exception of Carlos Lehder, who was arrested near Medellín in February 1987 (and who may well have been betrayed by his colleagues in the cocaine cartel), no major Colombian cocaine trafficker has ever been brought to justice.

Industry Tendencies

Specialization—cocaine versus marijuana. Cocaine trafficking is a highly specialized business; the organizations that handle cocaine do not overlap much with those that handle South America's other major drug export, marijuana. In Colombia—the largest producer of both drugs—the cocaine and marijuana businesses display distinct hierarchies, assets, employees, and methods of operation. They have different regional bases: The main centers of refined cocaine production appear to be in Antioquia, Cordoba, and the Middle Magdalena Valley. Coca grows predominantly in the southern departments (comissariats) of Meta, Guaviare, Vaupes, and Caqueta. The centers of the marijuana industry are in the Sierra Nevada de Santa Marta and the Serranía de Perija mountains in the northeastern part of the country. (The Sierra Nevada de Santa Marta also contains some coca cultivation.) Trafficking patterns are also different: The vast majority of cocaine smuggled into the United States is shipped by air (the majority by general aviation aircraft). Most Colombian marijuana, on the other hand, enters the United States by sea, often in stages. "Mother ships" may carry the cargo most of the way, then discharge it to smaller, faster craft that make the final run into the United States, particularly along the Florida coast.

Cocaine traffickers regard marijuana as not particularly lucrative; moreover, they hold marijuana dealers in low esteem, seeing them as uncouth peasants with little intelligence or entrepreneurial talent. In a 1984 memorandum, a group of Colombian cocaine capos stated that marijuana "was not an organized or important business in Colombia."[20] Part of the problem with marijuana, in the view of the cocaine mafia, is that the higher value-added stages of the trade traditionally have been in the hands of Cuban-Americans and other North Americans. In the case of cocaine, however, Colombians have been able to control the movement of the product through at least the upper levels of the distribution system.

What convergence there is between the two industries may occur after the drugs leave South America and before they reach U.S. shores. In one well-documented case, a major Colombian trafficker, Carlos Lehder, managed a huge cocaine and marijuana smuggling operation from a Bahamas island that he controlled, Norman's Key, between 1978 and 1980. Lehder describes his own role on the island as that of an "intermediary" for Colombian cocaine and marijuana syndicates.[21] (The U.S. prosecutor in Miami, Robert Merkle, has said that Lehder was to the transportation of drugs what Henry Ford was to automobiles.) Lehder bought out or expelled the legitimate local residents and turned the island into a "well-fortified refueling and storage base." He ran Norman's Key "with military discipline, deploying radar, German and Colombian armed guards, and attack Doberman Pinschers to protect airstrips and caves hiding large cocaine caches." Planeloads of cocaine and marijuana would arrive from Colombia and fly to rural airstrips in south Florida—especially on Saturdays, when the air traffic between Florida and the Bahamas was especially heavy. Lehder received a cut of each drug shipment—in the case of cocaine, his share was 1 kilo out of every 4 kilos passing through the island—and smuggled the drugs to the United States in his own fleet of aircraft. According to testimony at his trial, he earned $250 million to $300 million just from the cocaine part of the operation.[22]

Intraindustry specialization. Another question concerns specialization within the cocaine industry itself. In Colombia, the Medellín-Cali network imports raw materials, coca paste, and cocaine base from Peru and Bolivia; processes these products; and exports refined cocaine to international markets. However, a second cocaine industry in Colombia centers around the 20,000 tons or so of coca leaf that are grown domestically. Colombian leaf, which has an alkaloid content one-half to one-third of that grown in Peru and Bolivia, is relatively expensive to process into good-quality cocaine. Small peasant entrepreneurs process the leaf into cocaine base; some of this enters the Medellín-Cali refining system, and some is sold to independent cocaine refiners. Colombian guerrillas—notably the Fuerzas Armadas Revolucionarias de Colombia (FARC)—protect or control many of the base laboratories. The FARC also may have some CHCL processing capability, although the FARC's technique for marketing their products is not clearly understood. The main point to remember—and this is crucial for understanding the relation between drug traffickers and guerrillas discussed at length in Chapter 4—is that the Medellín-Cali networks do not depend significantly on domestically produced coca and coca products. If Colombia stopped growing coca tomorrow, there would be no appreciable effect on the supply systems of the major syndicates.

The cocaine mafia in Colombia has made every effort to disassociate itself publicly from the bazuco trade. It is not difficult to see why. Bazuco consumption is one of Colombia's *major* public health problems—an estimated 200,000 to 600,000 people regularly use the drug. Civic and professional groups have increasingly labored to raise public concern and governmental response. In a memorandum presented to Colombia's Attorney General in 1984, Colombia's top 100 cocaine traffickers denied any association with the bazuco trade. The memorandum read in part:

> Colombia participates in the drug trade as a processor of Peruvian and Bolivian coca and as a transporter to countries where it [the refined drug] is consumed. . . . [We who control the cocaine business are not involved, nor have we been involved, in the coca trade within Colombia, much less in the distribution of coca in the form of bazuco."][23]

Obviously, these claims are self-serving and a political tactic of sorts. Bazuco consumption is one of the Colombian government's main

arguments for convincing itself and the Colombian people of the importance of the war against drugs. Yet, the claims have been corroborated by
others. Two prominent Colombian writers on narcotics argue, "Bazuco is
not a market of the major capos but rather one dominated by the small
trafficker."[24] DEA officials interviewed in Bogotá and Washington generally agree with this assessment. Also indicative is that mafia organizations
have not made an issue in their public statements of sporadic U.S.-
Colombian efforts to spray Colombia's coca plantations. This reaction
suggests that domestically-grown coca and its products are not major
factors in mafia operations. In other words, the image may fit the reality:
The cocaine mafia—which tries very hard to characterize its activities as
beneficial to Colombians, with any ill effects falling on foreign shores—
may find it expedient to leave the bazuco business to lesser traffickers.

   Cooperation and conflict. The structure of the cocaine business differs
from one country to the next. In Colombia, the bulk of the business
apparently is controlled by coalitions of crime families based in Medellín
and Cali, respectively Colombia's second and third largest cities. (There
reportedly are 20 such families in Medellín.)[25] The Medellín-Cali networks
buy crude cocaine (paste or base) in Peru and Bolivia, refine it in laboratories in Colombia, export CHCL to the United States (and other international markets), and sell cocaine within the United States as wholesalers
and possibly as distributors. In addition, some trafficking organizations
are based in Leticia, in the departments of Armenia and Pereira, and on
Colombia's north coast, but these are closely linked to the Medellín-Cali
axis.

   In Bolivia and Peru, in contrast, refining and marketing structures are
relatively poorly developed. The Bolivian Senate's Ad Hoc Commission
on Narcotics estimates that "not more than 12 to 15 families" are engaged
in drug trafficking in Bolivia; however, the State Department has identified
25 organizations that each buy paste—often on credit from farmers—and
process it within their own organizations to produce cocaine base, CHCL,
or both.[26] Virtually all of the base is sold to Colombian buyers. Although
Bolivia produces some 15 percent of the world's CHCL, that product, too,
is marketed largely to Colombian buyers. In Peru, the DEA estimates that
12 organizations in the Upper Huallaga Valley supply coca paste or cocaine
base to Colombian refiners. Colombian traffickers, who maintain an extensive presence in the Valley, provide leadership, technical expertise, and
armed protection for many of these organizations. A few Peruvian traffickers (such as Reynaldo Rodríguez) produce cocaine hydrochloride and
manage to market it in the United States; however, for practical purposes,
Peru's cocaine industry is a supplier of raw materials and hence an
appendage of Colombia's trafficking syndicates.[27]

As already noted, large Colombian syndicates seemingly do not constitute a cartel in the sense of being able to control production and prices. Yet, there are tendencies toward cooperation. Like mature criminal syndicates in the United States, Colombian syndicates apparently have staked out territories, such as distribution markets in major U.S. cities. Moreover, they actively help each other in certain respects. If one family does not have enough cocaine on hand to meet delivery obligations to a customer, it can obtain the necessary product from other families. Composite shipments—loads of cocaine belonging to several families—are increasingly common. Families take turns insuring each others' shipments of cocaine. If the cocaine is confiscated en route, the insurer pays the owner his initial investment in product plus his transportation costs. If the shipment reaches its destination, the insurer gets a percentage of the take—usually between 30 percent and 50 percent of the price paid by the foreign wholesaler.[28]

There is also evidence that Colombia's vertically integrated organizations occasionally pool their strengths and form joint ventures. The DEA gave the President's Commission on Organized Crime a chart detailing a temporary cooperative venture, based in Medellín, between the Escobar and Ochoa families. That chart is reproduced in Figure 3.1. As diagrammed, the two families "combined and divided trafficking responsibilities typically completed by a single organization." Roughly, Escobar's group assumed responsibility for production and marketing and Ochoa's for enforcement and finance. Normally, however, both organizations are capable of handling all these operations independently.[29] Medellín and Cali families have also collaborated: In mid-1984, Gilberto Rodríguez Orejuela and Jorge Luis Ochoa journeyed to Spain, apparently to set up a distribution network to serve the growing Western European market. (That effort was temporarily aborted when Ochoa and Rodríguez were arrested in Madrid and extradited to Colombia.)[30]

Moreover, cocaine syndicates share intelligence about enemy operations. They circulate lists of names and descriptions of DEA agents both to each other and—in a gesture of transnational cooperation—to criminal organizations overseas. Major assassinations, like that of Rodrigo Lara Bonilla (a former Colombian Minister of Justice), conceivably were jointly planned and financed by several trafficking organizations.[31] The establishment in 1981 of the anticommunist vigilante organization Muerte a Los Secuestradores (Death to Kidnappers) was the product of a summit meeting of 223 cocaine traffickers (see the discussion in Chapter 4). Finally, in a rather extraordinary show of unity, 100 leading Colombian cocaine capos issued a joint manifesto to the nation's Attorney General in 1984. The document was the product of a Colombian government crackdown on drug

FIGURE 3.1
A Cocaine Collaboration:
The OCHOA/ESCOBAR Joint Venture

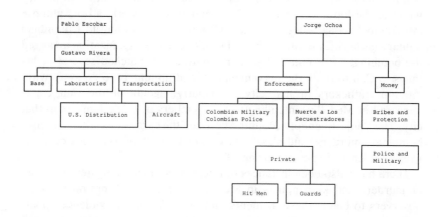

Source: President's Commission on Organized Crime, *America's Habit: Drug Abuse, Drug Trafficking, and Organized Crime,* March 1986, p. 102.

traffickers that began after the assassination of Justice Minister Lara Bonilla in April 1984. The authors proposed to *dismantle* their cocaine operations in Colombia in return for "reinstatement in Colombian society" and for implied guarantees against extradition to the United States.[32]

Yet, evidence of conflict abounds. There currently is open warfare between the two epicenters of the cocaine trade, Medellín and Cali. The dispute stems in part from Medellín's attempt to intrude on Cali's sales territory in New York City. However, differences in operating style also contribute to the conflict. The Medellín group has relied heavily on violence—from assassination of leading government officials to massacres of peasants who collaborate with guerrillas—to promote its political and social objectives. The Cali group is less confrontational; as the Army Commander of the Medellín-based IV Brigade noted, it "has not traditionally been violent and has succeeded to the extent that this is possible in legalizing its operations."[33]

When the dispute began is not clear. The conflict can, perhaps, be traced to the capture of Jorge Ochoa on the Palmira-Buga highway near Cali in November 1987. (Ochoa was later freed from a Bogotá prison on December 30 of that year.) There is speculation that conceivably the Cali cartel provided the information that led to Ochoa's arrest. In January 1988, a car bomb attack on a Pablo Escobar residence in Medellín, "Monaco," wrecked the top floors of the building and gave the world a brief glimpse into Pablo Escobar's life style (see Chapter 1). According to Colombian military authorities in Medellín, Gilberto Orejuela's organization arranged the bombing. In response, Escobar reportedly dispatched several of his thugs to Cali to track the movements of, and ultimately to do away with, the top traffickers in that city.[34] Similarly, agents of the Cali cartel appeared in Medellín, intending to kill members of crime families in that city. The "adjustment of accounts" between the cartels has taken its toll— bombings, murders, and shootouts between bands of assassins cost the lives of at least 150 people during 1988.[35]

There have also been instances of intercity conflict. A mysterious spate of murders and kidnappings in Medellín in early 1986 prompted some observers to blame these incidents on the DEA, but the violence apparently was triggered by the breakdown in the insurance system described above. Specifically, the Ochoa clan had guaranteed a large collective shipment of cocaine that was seized by U.S. Customs in January. The Ochoas then failed to pay the resulting claims. The conflict seemingly involved primarily the Ochoa and Escobar families. In any event, a summit meeting of mafia chiefs later that year apparently settled the dispute.[36]

Still, cooperation (at least intracity cooperation) is the norm among Colombian organizations. The fact that mafia syndicates have shared risk, pooled information, developed joint marketing enterprises, and issued a joint proposal to close down most of the cocaine industry suggests a rather impressive system.

The mafia organizations and the coca lobby constitute what might be called the cocaine constituency in South American countries. These organizations—especially those based in Colombia—integrate a range of activities, are multinational in scope, and command substantial technical, financial, and human resources. In Colombia, the cocaine mafia exhibits a tendency toward oligopoly; the industry is relatively concentrated, and the actors cooperate on both strategic and operational matters. In general, the mafia's structure, capabilities, and methods of operation convey the impression of strength and resiliency.

However, the cocaine mafias in Colombia, Bolivia, and, to a minor extent, Peru are not merely criminal organizations. They have gone beyond routine forms of corruption (such as payoffs to police and local officials) to intervene directly in the political process. The mafia's political goals, its ideologies, and its tactics of political participation will be explored in the following sections.

Ideology

General Comments

South American drug barons over time have developed something in the nature of a political and social philosophy to give an aura of legitimacy to their drug trafficking activities. They pose as defenders of national values, as civic leaders, and as fighters for progress. Drug barons strive to convey the message that drug control is "anti-Latin," a violation of national sovereignty, and a threat to the freedom of individuals. They argue openly that drug dealers are essential to economic stability and to the public welfare. They are critical of particular administrations and even certain aspects of regime types, but not necessarily of the political status quo; some capos want to work within the system, and some wish to change it.

The main sources of mafia political thought, such as it is, are Bolivia's Roberto Suarez and Colombia's Pablo Escobar and Carlos Lehder. The three have impeccable criminal credentials. Escobar and Suarez are under indictment in the United States for conspiring to import cocaine, and Lehder was arrested and extradited to the United States in February 1987. (He was convicted in a Jacksonville court in March 1988 on 11 counts of drug smuggling and sentenced to life imprisonment plus 135 years.) Suarez, who had largely retired from the drug business by the end of 1985—he was reported in financial difficulty and in poor health—was arrested in the Beni in July 1988 and could serve up to 12 years in jail in Bolivia on drug charges. The United States is still seeking Escobar's extradition, although successive decisions by Colombia's Supreme Court and State Council have temporarily halted the extradition process in that country. Escobar is also thought to have been the "intellectual author" of at least three high-profile assassinations: those of Rodrigo Lara Bonilla, Jaime Ramírez Gómez, and Guillermo Cano—respectively, a Colombian Justice Minister, a former chief of the Anti-Narcotics Division of the National Police, and the editor of a leading Bogotá newspaper, *El Espectador*. It would be a mistake, however, to view Escobar, Lehder, and Suarez as merely common criminals. All are political personalities who have disseminated their views exclusively through articles, open letters to the press, and interviews. And they do have a following in their respective societies, not only among *narcotraficantes*, but also among broader publicists who share their anti-Yankee feelings and their professed concern for the poor and downtrodden.

Nationalism

Drug capos are first and foremost nationalists. Their nationalism may be linked to a specific aspect of U.S. drug control policy. For example, in Colombia, the U.S.-Colombian extradition treaty has been a prime target of the cocaine establishment. Carlos Lehder wrote in the Medellín newspaper *El Colombiano* in 1982, "From any point of view, the extradition of nationals has no reason for existing, and even less reason exists for making a pact with a country which does not even have borders with the U.S. and where customs have not one iota of affinity with ours."[37] A writer in *Medellín Cívico*, a newspaper controlled by Pablo Escobar, observed in a 1984 article, "The nation's face has been disfigured by the imperialist boot of the treaty."[38] In Bolivia, Roberto Suarez said in a December 1985 letter to two national deputies that the 1983 U.S.-Bolivia accords for coca reduction violated the nation's constitution as well as the "fundamental rights of countless Bolivians."[39]

The cocaine mafia also may target specific U.S. institutions and individuals associated with drug control. The Colombian mafia tends to pick on the U.S. DEA, accusing it of committing espionage against Colombians, controlling Colombia's borders, restricting private air travel within the country, and even committing murder. An article in the weekly magazine *Semana*—an article that U.S. officials in Bogotá think was paid for by the mafia—claims that the DEA hired Cuban or Puerto Rican hitmen to kidnap and kill some traffickers in Medellín in early 1986.[40] (*El Espectador*, in a more credible account, attributed the murders to a dispute among mafia families over the payment of insurance claims for a lost cocaine shipment. See the discussion in the above section, "Cooperation and Conflict.") In Bolivia, Roberto Suarez apparently has conceived a particular hatred for Edwin Corr, Washington's Ambassador to La Paz during the Siles administration. A 1984 letter to Siles Zuazo accused Corr of "humiliating and trampling on Bolivian national sovereignty." The same letter also accused Corr of extortion, saying, "This aspiring policeman extorted from me sums worth millions, which were carried away by special commissioners and by other servants of the North American Embassy."[41]

A particularly virulent and extreme form of drug-based nationalism was expounded by Colombia's Carlos Lehder. Lehder used the drug enforcement issue as a springboard from which to develop an all-encompassing attack against Colombia's "monarchical oligarchy," which he sees as hopelessly dependent on "North American Imperialism." This dependence, in Lehder's view, touched every aspect of Latin American life and culture, but is epitomized by the Colombian government's willingness to extradite Colombians to the United States.[42]

To create a new Colombia, free of U.S. influence, Lehder has advocated a broad popular alliance among groups as politically diverse as the M-19 guerrillas and the nationalist elements of the Colombian military. The struggle is to be financed by the cocaine and marijuana trade—what Lehder called "a revolutionary weapon against North American imperialism"— and spearheaded by an anti-imperialist army. Lehder has talked at different times about a 500,000-man force to be created with the help of the Colombian army and about a Latin American "NATO" encompassing all South American countries.[43]

Lehder's ideology was a curious amalgam of extremism that borrowed from both the left and the right. The Latin Nationalist Movement (MLN), a political party founded by Lehder, opposed "communism, imperialism, neo-colonialism, and Zionism" and also holds that "we are Catholic, Apostolic, and Roman."[44] Lehder and his followers espoused a Latinized version of Hitler's master race theory. Admiration for Hitler, "the greatest warrior of all time," was coupled with a belief in Latin superiority. As one of Lehder's lieutenants put it, "In 50 years, the Latin race will be the dominant one; the Europeans are finished."[45] Lehder spoke warmly of right-wing military figures such as General Landazabal Reyes, a former Minister of Defense dismissed by Betancur in early 1984, apparently for his opposition to Betancur's efforts to reconcile with the nation's major guerrilla groups. And Lehder wants the "nationalist sector" of the Colombian army to play a role in his anti-imperialist revolution.[46]

At the same time, Lehder played to the extreme left. He talked in interviews about starting a "dialogue" with the leaders of the M-19 movement.[47] Confidential Colombian police reports say that M-19 guerrillas served intermittently as part of Lehder's personal guard force. Lehder reportedly was dallying with Quintin Lamé, an Indian-based revolutionary movement in southern Colombia. In a major political turnabout, Lehder's fascist political party supported the communist (Unión Patriótica) candidate for president, Jaime Pardo Leal, in the May 1986 presidential election. In an interview, one of Lehder's chief political lieutenants said that the MLN backed Pardo because the communists oppose the extradition treaty. Politics, it is said, makes strange bedfellows, and Lehder's extreme anti-Americanism made him willing to welcome allies of many political stripes. The DEA official's description of Lehder as the Qaddafy of international cocaine traffickers is probably as accurate a summary as any of the man and his world view. In general, Lehder's political antics embarrassed other more conservative members of the cocaine cartel, and this may have been part of his undoing.

To some extent, "Latin nationalism" is an elaborate projection of its architect's personal problems. Lehder has many. He has the distinction of being the first Colombian whose extradition was approved by the Colombian Superior Court and by the government (under Betancur). Also, Lehder once spent 2 years in a U.S. jail in Danbury, Connecticut, for possession of 200 pounds of marijuana. Probably for these reasons, he feels especially bitter toward both the Colombian government and the United States. In addition, Lehder comes from mixed parentage: His father is a German engineer and his mother a Colombian schoolteacher. He mounted an aggressive defense of Latin culture and values, possibly to overcompensate for his divided heritage. All of these factors contributed to, if they do not fully explain, the virulence of Lehder's political messages.

Populism

Drug capos try to make the case that the narcotics industry is good for progress and employment. Escobar said once that drug dollars kept Colombia from suffering "a grave crisis similar to that of other Latin American societies." He also said that drug money created new employment for the Colombian people. In a similar vein, Carlos Lehder once remarked, "If it were not for these hot dollars, Colombia would be in worse shape than Argentina."[48]

Also, leading cocaine traffickers—such as Carlos Lehder, Roberto Suarez, Pablo Escobar, and Gonzalo Rodríguez Gacha—have won the hearts and minds of local populaces by their personal largesse; all have financed a vast array of social services in their native towns and regions, for example, housing projects, sports stadiums, schools, roads, and sanitation facilities. Such narco-welfare activities are the stuff of folklore (see the section later in this chapter, "Building a Legend") and have enormously complicated the task of drug enforcement in the Andean countries. "The people love him for what he has done," said a Colombian official about Pablo Escobar's public works activities in Antioquia.[49] The Robin Hood image of Escobar and his criminal colleagues represents an important part of their protection shield; it raises the political costs to governments of arresting these outlaws and (especially) of extraditing them to the United States.

Obviously, Carlos Lehder's brand of populism extended far beyond philanthropy to advocacy of radical political reforms. Lehder described his Latin Nationalist Party, which he formed in 1982, as a "product of the absence of popular power." Said Lehder about the Colombian political system: "Bipartisanism has placed the people on the margin of major national decisions." Lehder called for the creation of a new Colombian political body, a congress of between 3,000 and 4,000 people in which all "popular sectors" of Colombian society—"men, women, peasants, priests, and soldiers"—would be able to voice opinions. It must be stressed, however, that Lehder is not typical of the Colombian trafficking establishment, most of which prefers to work within the Colombian system.[50]

Support for the System

Is the cocaine mafia a conservative or revolutionary force in Latin American societies? Does it represent a threat to democratic systems and values in the Hemisphere? In Colombia and Peru, these questions acquire special urgency because of the presence of Marxist revolutionary movements. Narco-ideologies do have a few anti-establishment overtones: They focus on Latin America's economic and political dependence on the United States, social inequalities, and the failure of governments to provide services to the poor. Yet, for all that, most cocaine traffickers—if not exactly pillars of society—are conservative if not atavistic in their political thinking. In this respect, they resemble stereotypical mafia figures in Sicily and in the United States. For example, America's king of crime, Al Capone, denounced "Bolshevism," praised the free enterprise system, and supported family values. (He once remarked that if America had a leader like Mussolini, "She could conquer the world.")[51] Many South American drug lords apparently are cut from the same mold.

In Colombia, the cocaine mafia, with the apparent exception of Carlos Lehder, has never sought radical changes in the Colombian political system. A memorandum from 100 major capos to Attorney General Jiménez Gómez in 1984 stated, "We have no connection, nor do we accept any such connection, with armed guerrillas. Our activities have never been intended to replace the democratic and republican form of government."[52] Pablo Escobar has expressed, in slightly different terms, his preference for the political status quo. Responding to efforts by U.S. Ambassador Lewis Tambs to link him to FARC guerrillas, Escobar said in *Medellín Cívico*, "I share with them [the guerrillas] a desire for a Colombia with more social equality for all, but I do not agree with their plans to obtain power by means of weapons, because to achieve power there exists a democratic system, faithfully watched over by our army, guardian of the constitution and of the laws of the Republic."[53]

The mafia's antidemocratic tendencies, such as they are, run more toward vigilantism than toward subversion. For example, in 1981, more than 200 cocaine traffickers founded Death to Kidnappers (MAS). Both Pablo Escobar and Carlos Lehder reportedly were associated with the creation of MAS. Designed originally to retaliate against guerrillas who kidnapped for money, MAS evolved into an instrument for the indiscriminate persecution of leftists, including labor organizers, peasants who collaborate with guerrillas, civil rights activists, and members of the Unión Patriótica (the civilian arm of the FARC). Some Colombian army officers also have been members of MAS; in fact, the organization seemingly served as a communication channel of sorts between the mafia and the military.

Furthermore, Colombia's cocaine dealers have acquired huge tracts of land in the countryside—an estimated one million acres between 1983 and 1988.[54] Some of these areas were traditionally strongholds of guerrilla groups such as the FARC and the Ejército de Liberación Popular (EPL). The acquisition of rural property by leading drug dealers apparently has raised their political consciousness; as one Colombian government official put it, "As soon as they become landowners in guerrilla zones, they view communism as a threat and an enemy. Suddenly, they see themselves as pillars of the establishment."[55]

The new mafia landed gentry not only have refused to pay taxes to guerrillas, but also have used their private armies to spearhead local self-defense and to destroy guerrillas' political support networks. In their *labor de limpieza* (clean-up work) they have received support from other groups: traditional landholders, conservative politicians, and right-wing elements of the Colombian army. Such alliances apparently have dislodged guerrillas from large sectors of the Middle Magdalena Valley—the Puerto Boyaca–Puerto Triunfo area, for example—and from parts of Cordoba, Magdalena, Santander, and Meta departments. A clandestine guerrilla radio station, Radio Patria Libre, referred to a "Narco-Military Republic of the Middle Magdalena Region" that "has control over the mayor's offices in nine municipalities and covers more than 20,000 square kilometers, equal in size to the Guajira department."[56] Significant social changes apparently are occurring in the Colombian countryside: Narco-control is replacing guerrilla control in some regions.

The narco-guerrilla thesis has become very difficult to sustain in the face of such developments. To be sure, the FARC still dominates the coca-growing region. Many of the FARC's 39 fronts maintain themselves by taxing and in some cases directly managing coca cultivation and cocaine processing facilities. Yet, most of Colombia's cocaine refining industry— the more lucrative part of the cocaine trade—is not controlled by the FARC, but rather is in the hands of powerful trafficking syndicates that have deployed manpower, weapons, and resources against communist guerrillas and that are hostile to the Colombian left in general.

In Peru, the situation is somewhat different. The cocaine industry in that country is immature and fragmented; traffickers have not developed a common anti-leftist agenda (as they have in Colombia), nor have they been able to establish close alliances with the propertied classes and with the military. One reason is that Peru's cocaine industry is relatively underdeveloped—it still accounts for only a small percentage of South American exports of cocaine hydrochloride. Peru has no major trafficking personalities comparable to Pablo Escobar or Gonzalo Rodríguez Gacha in Colombia or Roberto Suarez in Bolivia. The minimal leadership in the existing Peruvian cocaine industry is provided mainly by Colombian traffickers. The industry's shallow roots and fragmented structure and the dominant role played by foreigners may have allowed Sendero Luminoso to penetrate some trafficking organizations. Still, as the discussion in Chapter 4 will show, there is substantial evidence of narco-guerrilla conflict in Peru; the narco-guerrilla relationship seemingly depends on the balance of forces in a given region at a given time.

In Bolivia—where there is no revolutionary movement to speak of and where the narco-bourgeoisie traditionally has had rightist leanings—the critical question is: Does the cocaine mafia favor a return to military authority? In Bolivia, the mafia and the military are related, both historically and ideologically. The military regimes of the 1970s provided state bank loans that supported the development of the cocaine industry; money borrowed ostensibly to finance cotton farming and other agricultural ventures in Santa Cruz department apparently was diverted to building laboratories and other elements of a cocaine infrastructure. Narco-traffickers provided financial backing for García Meza's coup in June 1980, and there was a virtual symbiosis between drug trafficking and the state under García Meza's regime. The Bolivian writer Amado Canelas sees an ideological affinity between the mafia and the military, a common concern for "God, home, and country" and a common fear that democracy would undermine these values.[57]

Some leaders of the democratic Siles and Paz administrations see the mafia as having a vested interest in authoritarianism. A former vice president under Siles Zuazo, Jaime Paz Zamora, argued in 1983 that the mafia—far from being politically colorless—had a definite goal: to topple democracy and to restore the military dictatorship.[58] Some leading traffickers were clearly uncomfortable with the advent of democracy in 1982. For example, in a 1984 letter to Siles Zuazo, Roberto Suarez referred to the "fragile foundation" of democracy, its "rotten structure of power," and the "increasing panorama of political confusion and social malaise resulting from the ineffective party system and from anarcho-syndicalism."[59] Clearly, Suarez was no friend of democracy, although he did not openly advocate a return of the military dictatorship to Bolivia. Suarez represents the authoritarian, elitist wing of Bolivia's cocaine elite—he was a major financial backer of the 1980–1981 military regime of General Luis García Meza. Yet, his views may no longer be shared by most Bolivian traffickers, who by now are probably comfortable with democracy in Bolivia. By all indications, the cocaine industry has expanded enormously since the early 1980s, and there are now a significantly greater number of actors. (Interestingly, Suarez himself in various statements has bemoaned the democratization of the industry.) Still, the possibility of a cocaine-backed military coup should not be dismissed out of hand.

To return to the original question: Is the cocaine traffic a destabilizing political force? Unquestionably it is, in the sense that the violence and corruption associated with the drug trade erode public commitment to democratic institutions. Yet, most cocaine traffickers are not revolutionaries—they seek to penetrate and to manipulate established economic and political institutions. The rightward orientation of cocaine traffickers may itself be destabilizing—consider, for example, García Meza's antidemocratic coup in 1980. Yet, today even Bolivia's traffickers probably prefer to corrupt people in authority rather than to overthrow them. Mafia vigilantism in Colombia arguably reduces the chance of an accommodation between the government and leftist guerrillas. Yet, some observers—among them this writer—believe that the peace process initiated by the Betancur administration in 1984 has merely provided Colombia's revolutionary groups with the opportunity to strengthen their military forces.

Tactics

Cocaine traffickers use a combination of carrot and stick to influence drug enforcement policies in their countries. Like their counterparts elsewhere, South American mafias use coercive tactics against officials who are "uncooperative" or who publicly condemn their activities. Yet, traffickers prefer to use financial blandishments—bribes, donations, and charitable activities—to achieve their ends. Money is by far the mafia's most important political weapon; with it, the mafia buys protection from law enforcement officials, corrupts the political establishment, and builds a public following, especially among poorer classes. Violence is usually the last resort—that is, it is used against the policeman, judge, or politician who cannot be bought. Yet, mafia-sponsored violence against government and judicial representatives has been a common feature of the Colombian political scene. (The Medellín group of traffickers displays a particular penchant for bloodshed; the Cali group seems almost benign by comparison.) The behavior of Colombian traffickers reflects a violent national culture. Colombia's murder rate is six times that of the United States, itself one of the most violent societies in the world. Murder is the leading cause of death for males between the ages of 15 and 44 and the second leading cause of death among all age groups.[60]

Coercion

Mafia pressure tactics fall into basically two categories: blackmail and the threat or use of violence. In Colombia, the mafia has used money—especially campaign contributions—as a wedge for later blackmail or defamation of an official. The most famous case on record involved a Minister of Justice in the Betancur administration, Rodrigo Lara Bonilla, and a drug trafficker from Leticia named Evaristo Porras. Lara was elected to the Senate in 1982 and appointed to Betancur's cabinet in August 1983, and he was a prime mover in a 1983 congressional campaign against "hot money," that is, drug money, in Colombian politics. However, days after becoming Justice Minister, Lara was himself accused of being on the mafia payroll. His accuser was Jairo Ortega, an Antioquian congressman with close ties to Pablo Escobar, who presented as proof a check that Porras had made out to Lara's name for one million pesos (about $12,000 U.S.) as well as a tape of a supposed conversation between Lara and Porras in the Bogotá Hilton.

Lara's basic defense was that he had been set up: The check "never passed through my hands," he never had met Porras, and the check was part of a transaction between one of Lara's companies and one owned by Porras. However, Lara almost certainly was acquainted with Porras. Furthermore, a second tape of an alleged later telephone conversation between the Minister and Porras was published in the Bogotá daily *El Espacio* and suggests that Lara knowingly took Porras' check, probably to cover campaign debts, and showed bad judgment in "not registering the temperature of the money." The affair almost cost the Minister his job and did cost him the support of Luis Carlos Galan, the head of the New Liberal Party to which Lara belonged. However, Lara remained in Betancur's cabinet and continued as an active fighter against drugs until he was shot to death in April 1984.[61]

The drug mafia's repertoire also includes threats against government officials. Many such threats apparently are linked to extradition cases. Mafia authorship is not necessarily certain—extradition arouses strong antipathy among many Colombians who have nothing to do with the drug traffic. Yet, most of the more than 100 extradition requests by the United States to the Colombian government involve drug trafficking and related offenses, and the narcotics lobby is clearly at the forefront of national opposition to the treaty. In fact, it would be fair to say that extradition has been the number-one bone of contention between the mafia and the

Colombian government and will in all likelihood continue to be so in the future.

The assassination of Lara Bonilla triggered a chain of actions and countermeasures that sharply raised the level of mafia-government confrontation. The Colombian government began to honor the extradition treaty with the United States and to deliver accused Colombian traffickers to U.S. justice. The result was a spate of death threats directed especially against top Colombian law enforcers—such as Betancur's Minister of Justice, Enrique Parejo—and against justices of Colombia's Supreme Court, which until recently ruled on extradition cases. Some of the messages were anonymous and did not give a reason for the threatened violence. Parejo's office received many telephone calls that said simply, "We are preparing to kill you in a few days"—or words to that effect.[62] Other messages were specific, blunt, and terrifying. For example, a letter circulated by The Extraditables to several Colombian Supreme Court justices in December 1986 warned:

> We declare war against you. We declare war against all the members of your family. As you may suppose, we know exactly where they are—we will do away with your entire family. We have no compassion whatsoever—we are capable of anything, absolutely anything. We also have families. Botero [a pro-extradition Colombian Supreme Court judge murdered earlier that year] had a family, too, wife, sons, parents, and brothers. He was a miserable government patsy and an anti-nationalist, pro-Yankee traitor to his country.[63]

The mafia also decided to make life more difficult for U.S. officials. Traffickers are said to have bribed Colombian guards around the U.S. embassy to murder U.S. Ambassador Lewis Tambs. *Newsweek* magazine reported in February 1985 that drug traffickers had offered $350,000 to anyone who would kidnap Francis Mullen, then head of the DEA. The plan, according to *Newsweek* sources, was to exchange Mullen for six accused Colombian traffickers who were in custody in the United States and Spain.[64]

The cocaine mafia tries to dictate the national rules of the game on narcotics control. The traffickers' number-one political objective clearly is to force the Colombian government to scuttle the U.S.-Colombian extradition treaty (in this they have almost succeeded) and to adopt a policy of not extraditing Colombians to the United States. Moreover, the mafia seeks to paralyze the top echelons of the nation's criminal justice system and to discourage potential crusaders against the cocaine industry. Where national drug policy is concerned, violence rather than bribery has been the traffickers' main political weapon. There has been a veritable parade of mafia-sponsored hits against prominent Colombians in recent years, as the following tragic examples indicate.

In July 1986, Hernan Baquero Borda, a Supreme Court judge who helped draft the 1979 extradition treaty, was gunned down by motorcyclists in a Bogotá street. Also in July, Raul Echevarría, deputy director of the Cali daily *El Occidente*, was shot to death the day after he wrote an article advocating the death penalty for major traffickers.[65]

In October, a Medellín Superior Court judge, Gustavo Zuluaga Berna, was murdered and his wife wounded by unknown assassins in Medellín. Zuluaga had several months earlier issued an arrest warrant against Pablo Escobar and his cousin Gustavo Gaviria as the possible "intellectual authors" of the murder of two detectives of the Department of Administrative Security (DAS). (The policemen had participated in an arrest of Escobar and his cousin for possession of cocaine in June 1976.) The day after the arrest warrant was issued, four armed men intercepted Zuluaga's wife while she was driving her car near Medellín, forced her to get out, and then pushed the car over a cliff. "Next time, we'll make you stay with the car," they warned her as she walked back toward the city.[66]

In November 1986, Colonel Jaime Ramírez Gómez, a former head of Colombia's Anti-Narcotics Police (CONAN), was machine-gunned to death in his car outside of Bogotá. (He had been returning to the city from vacation; 28 bullet holes were found in his body.) Ramírez, at the time Colombia's and perhaps Latin America's most distinguished antidrug policeman, was clearly a major liability to the mafia. He was preparing to write a "black book" revealing the results of his many years of investigation into Colombia's drug syndicate. He allegedly had evidence linking Pablo Escobar to the assassination of Lara Bonilla. Ramírez and Lara were the primary architects of a well-publicized CONAN raid against a gigantic complex of cocaine laboratories at Yari in Caqueta department in March 1984, an operation that made a significant, if temporary, dent in the mafia's cocaine processing capability in Colombia. He was a prime mover in developing antinarcotics cooperation between Colombia and other countries in the region: Peru, Bolivia, Ecuador, and Venezuela. (Ramírez, for example, was instrumental in creating RIPOL, an international police communications network for the exchange of information on drug trafficking.) Finally, Ramírez was a leading proponent of extradition, calling it a "key factor in the war against drugs" in Colombia.[67]

In December, the mafia disposed of another leading crusader against drugs. Gunmen killed Guillermo Cano, the editor and co-owner of the Bogotá daily *El Espectador*. Cano's signature had appeared on a number of editorials advocating that Colombian drug traffickers be sent to the United States to stand trial. In early 1987, Enrique Parejo González, who had been Minister of Justice under Betancur, was shot and severely wounded by unidentified assailants in, of all places, Budapest. (Parejo was Colombia's Ambassador to Hungary at the time.) Parejo had been an outspoken supporter of extradition and in his capacity as Justice Minister had approved several U.S. extradition requests.

Finally, there were the kidnapping of Andres Pastrana, then a candidate for mayor of Bogotá (and now mayor of that city), and the kidnapping-murder of Attorney General Carlos Mauro Hoyas in January 1988. Both actions were carried out by the mafia paramilitary group The Extraditables, both culminated in the environs of Medellín, and both were political statements against extradition.

Cocaine traffickers also were widely believed to have financed the hit against Lara Bonilla—the architect of what some observers felt was Colombia's first serious effort to overcome the drug industry's influence. The man held in the shooting allegedly was paid $10,000 for the murder. The Bogotá judge in charge of the pretrial hearing was murdered, too. Yet, for what it is worth, the cocaine mafia has vigorously denied any involvement in Lara's death. (The mafia, on the other hand, has not denied killing judges and other public figures who are pro-extradition.) The denial is partly credible in the sense that the assassination was a disaster for the illicit Colombian drug industry, touching off a wave of antidrug hysteria in Colombia—"narco-McCarthyism," in the words of one Colombian columnist—and forcing many leading capos into exile or hiding.[68] The assassination also prompted the government to abandon its earlier opposition to the extradition treaty and to the spraying of illicit crops. These actions were highly desirable from the U.S. point of view, and some Colombians, especially those on the extreme left, have speculated that U.S. government agencies (the CIA or the DEA) might have been behind the assassination. Another theory has it that the assassination was the work of small-time drug traffickers in Colombia who hoped to increase their market share when the finger of suspicion pointed (as it inevitably would) to the major cocaine capos.

Some circumstantial evidence links Escobar to the crime—specifically, evidence of Escobar's past personal association with the four assassins (and also records of telephone calls made by one of the killers to a number listed in Escobar's name). Moreover, Escobar had reason to dislike Lara, who was the leading Colombian official responsible for the Yari operation—Escobar reportedly was one of the owners of the complex. Lara also had orchestrated the expulsion of Escobar, then an aspiring politician, from the New Liberal Party 2 years earlier. Evidently, Lara took exception to Escobar's criminal history as a cocaine smuggler. (Escobar subsequently joined the main wing of the Liberal Party and was elected to the

Colombian Congress as an alternate deputy from Antioquia.) Despite the evidence, in late 1986 a Bogotá Superior Court judge suspended an arrest warrant that had been issued against Escobar in connection with the slaying; it now seems unlikely that Escobar will ever go to jail for Lara's murder.[69]

One result of all this bloodshed has been the destruction of the confidence of Colombians in their political institutions. A national Colombian survey taken in March 1987 reported that nearly one-half of the population believed that the drug traffickers were too powerful to combat. In a 1988 interview, former president Belisario Betancur said, referring to the drug mafia, "We are up against an organization stronger than the state."[70] Moreover, the extradition process has been torpedoed. In June 1987, the Colombian Supreme Court nullified the legislation that enabled the government to implement the 1979 extradition treaty. The court based its ruling on the technical ground that the president (at the time, Julio Cesar Turbay Ayala) had not originally signed the enabling legislation (see discussion in Chapter 5). However, the mafia's record of murdering pro-extradition Colombians as well as the death threats against members of the court understandably contributed to the court's decision. In January 1988, the Colombian government issued warrants for the arrest "with the attempt to extradite" of Pablo Escobar and four other major traffickers; the government based the order not on the 1979 treaty but on a multinational convention that the United States and Colombia had signed in Montevideo in 1933. However, the Council of State, Colombia's supreme administrative tribunal, declared the warrants invalid in March 1988.

Aside from exercising a "veto by assassination" over national drug policy, the Colombian mafia is also progressively destroying the nation's judicial system. Judges trying drug trafficking cases in Colombia are offered the proverbial choice of *plomo o plata* (lead or silver)—death if they convict, a bribe if they set aside the charges. Not surprisingly, few judges opt to convict. In the past 2 years, criminal court judges released from jail or dropped charges against four major cocaine dealers: Gilberto Rodríguez Orejuela, José Santa Cruz Londoño, Evaristo Porras, and Jorge Luis Ochoa (the U.S. government has offered $500,000 for Ochoa's arrest and conviction). Ochoa was released twice within 16 months, and corrupt judges played a role in both occasions.[71] According to a Western diplomatic source, the Ochoa clan paid $3 million the second time to get Jorge out of jail and an additional $20 million to arrange every step of his escape route so that he would not be murdered or recaptured. Indeed, the Colombian criminal justice system has almost ceased to function in drug trafficking cases. Recently in Medellín, police arrested a middle-ranking trafficking chief implicated in the murder of Guillermo Cano (the editor of the Bogotá daily *El Espectador*). After several days in jail, he was released, because no judge in Medellín was willing to try the case.[72]

Curiously, the Colombian government's case against Ochoa involved not cocaine trafficking but rather the illegal importing of fighting bulls into Colombia. (There is a parallel here to the history of organized crime in the United States; the federal government ultimately convicted Al Capone in 1931 not of racketeering but rather of income tax evasion.) The magistrate in charge of the case, Cartagena customs judge Fabio Pastrana Hoyos, sentenced Ochoa to 20 months in prison in August 1986 and fined him $11,500. Unfortunately, the judge suspended the sentence, although he required Ochoa to appear before the court every 2 weeks for the remainder of the 20-month term.[73] (Pastrana subsequently was removed from his post; in early 1988 allegations surfaced that he had received hundreds of thousands of dollars in bribes from the Ochoa family.) Ochoa dropped out of sight and was re-arrested for violating parole in November 1987. He was re-released in December of that year, despite an apparent promise by the Colombian government to the United States that he would remain in jail pending a decision on extradition.[74]

A few months before the trial of Ochoa, a penal customs judge in Medellín, Carmencita Londoño de Rojas, had begun an investigation of Pablo Escobar on a similar charge: importing exotic animals and birds for his zoo at Puerto Triunfo. (The zoo is on one of the Escobar family estates, "Napoles," which is located about 90 km from Medellín.) In May 1986, the judge received a letter that, loosely translated, read as follows:

> We admire and esteem Señor Pablo Escobar, because we and our families are able to subsist thanks to him. For him, we are prepared to sacrifice our lives whenever necessary.
>
> It is disgraceful that you—showing no respect for law and propriety—want to put Pablo Escobar in jail for having brought progress to Colombia and for having contributed to our country's nature and wildlife. He has done all this selflessly, having only the interests of the Colombian people at heart.
>
> We guarantee that you will not find promotion (ascenso) in your professional career, but rather demotion (descenso) into the depths of the earth, which is all that you deserve.[75]

Judge Londoño was shot to death in her car in Medellín 7 days after receiving this letter.

Cocaine Trafficking and the State

The Colombian mafia has accomplices and informants in law enforcement institutions, in key government ministries (such as Justice, Defense, and Foreign Relations), in the diplomatic community in Bogotá, and in the national and local news media. The network extends well beyond Colombia and also includes political or military leaders in several Central American and Caribbean countries. Moreover, the network probably encompasses corrupt police, customs officials, and air traffic controllers in the United States, as well as some members of Latin American diplomatic missions overseas.[76] In Bolivia, there was a period, roughly from the mid-1970s to the early 1980s, when the cocaine traffickers and the state apparatus became almost indistinguishable from one another. The era of what one Bolivian writer calls "the cocaine superstate" ended with the introduction of a democratically elected government in 1982;[77] however, the cocaine industry, which accounts for as much as one-half of Bolivia's yearly inflow of foreign exchange, still exerts a tremendous if informal influence over official policy.

Cocaine traffickers, as already noted, buy protection from police, prosecutors, judges, and, where necessary, the military. *Time* magazine reported in February 1985 that at least 100 Colombian air force personnel and 200 national policemen had been discharged because of drug connections. Also, 400 judges reportedly were under investigation by the Colombian Attorney General's office for alleged complicity in the trade.[78] Documents captured during a Colombian army raid on traffickers' hideouts in Medellín in early 1987 provided solid evidence that traffickers had infiltrated the Ministries of Justice and Foreign Affairs. In April 1988, the intelligence chief of the Colombian army's Fourth Brigade, based in Medellín, was dismissed, because investigations verified that he had "contacts with drug traffickers."[79] Such extensive penetration of the state apparatus protects trafficking operations up to a point; at the very least, the mafia has acquired an excellent early-warning system—that is, a capacity to anticipate raids on laboratories, police dragnets, and other official forays against the cocaine industry.

On the rare occasions when leading traffickers are arrested, they can bribe their way out of custody on the spot. For example, a car carrying Pablo Escobar was stopped at a police checkpoint outside of Medellín in November 1986. Escobar managed to buy his freedom with a bribe of $250,000 to $350,000. (Police held Escobar's wife, who was traveling with him, for security until the money was actually delivered.)[80] When traffickers do, in spite of everything, land in jail, frightened or corrupt judges may release them from custody; as noted above, there have been several such releases between 1986 and 1988. Recently, in a particularly horrendous incident, one of Latin America's most notorious drug traffickers, Juan Ramón Matta Ballastreros, escaped from Modelo Prison in Bogotá by paying more than $2 million or $7 million (stories differ) to 18 guards.

Matta was given the key to his own cell and walked through seven unlocked jail doors to freedom. "God opened the doors for me," the trafficker reportedly commented after his escape.[81]

Cocaine traffickers sometimes try to sway official policy by capitalizing on governments' financial problems. For example, Roberto Suarez, in a meeting with President Siles' narcotics adviser in June 1983, offered to give the Bolivian government $2 billion in four $500-million installments to help pay off Bolivia's foreign debt. Suarez, according to accounts of the meeting, wanted the Siles government to acknowledge the independence of his cocaine trafficking enclave in the Beni.[82] (If genuine, the offer was possibly underwritten by Colombian trafficking syndicates—it is hard to believe that Suarez could have raised such a large sum in Bolivia.) In early 1984, a Peruvian trafficker by the name of Guillermo "Mosca Loca" ("Crazy Fly") Cárdenas—shortly before being murdered in jail—reportedly offered to pay off Peru's national debt in return for his freedom.[83] In May 1984, Colombian cocaine traffickers, in meetings with that country's attorney general, offered to repatriate an estimated $2 billion to Colombia in return for official amnesty. Roughly 2 years later, they offered informally to pay off Colombia's $13-billion national debt.[84] Finally—according to a Bolivian police official interviewed in May 1986—Bolivian traffickers at the end of 1985 helped the financially strapped government of Victor Paz Estenssoro to pay a traditional end-of-the-year bonus to government employees.

Under the García Meza regime in Bolivia, a virtual symbiosis occurred between the state and the cocaine mafia. Drug traffickers, as noted above, had borrowed money from Bolivia's State Bank during the military regimes of the 1970s. The money—ostensibly earmarked for cattle ranching or cotton farming ventures—had gone into building up the cocaine trade. In 1980, traffickers, fearing a restoration of democracy in Bolivia, helped finance García Meza's military coup. Also, they are reliably reported to have loaned the new government $100 million to help tide it over initial obstacles.[85]

During the García Meza administration, there were, in the words of U.S. Senator Dennis DeConcini, "multiple and pervasive linkages" between the junta and cocaine-smuggling organizations.[86] Indeed, it was hard to tell where the former left off and the latter began. Cocaine traffickers financed and manned right-wing paramilitary squads that were dedicated to repression and terrorism in the service of the state. García Meza's Interior Minister, Luis Arce Gómez—dubbed by CBS' "60 Minutes" the "Minister of Cocaine"—himself participated in the traffic; he was a partner in an air transport company that flew loads of cocaine paste out of Bolivia. He also reportedly was the owner of several laboratories in the Beni. At the same time, in his capacity as minister, he collected huge sums in protection money both from coca merchants and from cocaine exporters. Roberto Suarez, for example, once paid Arce $50 million to stop a government operation (apparently conducted to impress the United States) that was interrupting the supply of coca leaves to Santa Cruz department, then an important center for the manufacture of cocaine.[87]

Bolivia in the García Meza period was a kind of model worst-case of drug-related corruption—a "cocaine superstate." The cocaine superstate passed from the scene with the advent of democratic government in 1982, but because of Bolivia's frail government and its sinking economy, the cocaine mafia still wielded (and continues to wield) enormous influence in the country. In 1985, for example, Roberto Suarez allegedly conspired with two members of Hugo Banzer's center-right Acción Democrática Nacional (ADN)—a former general and an ADN congressmen—in an election plot. The plan was to bribe congressional representatives of the Movimiento Nacional Revolucionario (MNR), the party of current president Victor Paz Estenssoro, to cast their votes for Banzer in a runoff presidential election that year. Earlier popular elections failed to give either Paz or Banzer a majority of the popular vote, so the outcome was decided in the congress. Whether any money changed hands is not clear, but, in any case, Paz won the election and the presidency.[88]

In July 1988, the Bolivian government arrested the King of the Beni at a ranch, "El Sujo," 35 km from the Beni capital of Trinidad. The arrest was hailed in La Paz and Washington as a major coup against the Bolivian cocaine trade. Such a claim was exaggerated. First, Suarez had more or less disengaged himself from the cocaine trade after 1985. His apparent retirement was the result of several factors. The loss of 2 tons of cocaine shipped in 1984 and 1985, worth perhaps $80 million at U.S. wholesale prices, constituted a significant factor (some of the cocaine was seized in Panama and Miami, and the rest mysteriously disappeared en route to the United States). Another factor influencing Suarez was a dispute with Colombian buyers: Suarez apparently had incurred some huge losses in 1984, when Colombian buyers suddenly lowered the price of cocaine base below the level that Suarez paid to Bolivian producers. A third factor was Suarez's health: The trafficker had suffered several heart attacks and had developed an addiction to bazuko. At the end of 1985, the leadership of the Bolivian cocaine industry reportedly had passed to Suarez's nephew, Jorge Roca Suarez. The king became really nothing more than a legend, although his pioneering role in developing the Bolivian industry is established beyond a doubt.

The circumstances of Suarez's capture are obscure. Suarez claims that he gave himself up to the authorities, saying, "I knew what time they would come—I was ready with my things, dressed, and smoking a ciga-rette."[89] This is quite possible. The six UMOPAR policemen who raided "Sujo" encountered only two bodyguards and no perimeter defense sys-tem—Suarez typically surrounded his ranches with sentries and main-tained a waiting airplane to fly him to safety. Suarez claims that he gave himself up because the police were holding his family hostage at another ranch some 15 km away, a version of the event that the government denies. One mid-level Ministry of Interior official interviewed in October 1988, however, does believe that Suarez arranged his own arrest, possibly in return for guarantees against extradition to the United States. With the help of DEA, the Bolivian government had mounted a major effort to capture Suarez. One reason was that the trafficker in a 1988 television interview insulted the president of Bolivia as "a boss in the service of the U.S. government."[90] Conceivably, Suarez also calculated that he would be able to negotiate a reduced jail term (he had earlier been sentenced in absentia by a Bolivian court to a 12-year sentence). The true story of the Suarez arrest, however, may never be known.

The Politics of Cocaine

South American mafias seem to intrude more directly into their nations' politics than do criminal syndicates in the United States. They spend large sums on financing electoral campaigns (both national and local), building a favorable public image, and—in Colombia—mounting direct bids for polit-ical office. Such initiatives do not always increase the mafia's influence. In Colombia, for example, the mafia may have made a mistake by going too public. Yet, they represent an interesting commentary on mafia political strategies and on South American politics in general.

Funding political campaigns. Campaign contributions are one of the ways that drug mafias seek to extend their influence in the political realm. Such contributions do not in themselves ensure influence, but nevertheless constitute a hold of sorts over office holders. The more open the mafia's funding—or, at least, the more visible it is to the candidate—the greater the likelihood of compliance. An incumbent may feel gratitude toward his mafia backers. He may perceive mafia financing as essential to his future political plans, such as getting reelected. He may fear exposure and blackmail if he knowingly received contributions from traffickers. On the other hand, he may act completely contrary to his backers' expectations and, in fact, may take a principled stand against the drug industry. Lara Bonilla was, perhaps, a case in point. So the mafia takes what amounts to a calculated risk. The odds are, however, that its financial leverage will corrupt some politicians and—in numerous subtle ways—weaken a country's political will to fight against drug trafficking.

Drug money pervades Latin American politics, but the best documented cases are in Colombia. In that country, according to a November 28, 1983, *Wall Street Journal* article, an estimated $1 million in narcotics money supported candidates in the 1982 congressional campaigns.[91] The former Colombian Justice Minister Rodrigo Lara Bonilla himself may have accepted drug money to cover debts incurred in his 1982 senate race. More recently, Betancur's Minister of Justice Enrique Parejo denounced the influx of "hot money" into the 1986 congressional and local campaigns. Parejo claimed that some politicians were not honestly fighting the mafia, by which he meant that they were accepting contributions indiscriminately. Complaints of corruption received by his office, he said, most often implicated politicians in regions that are noted centers of cocaine or marijuana trafficking: Colombia's north coast, Antioquia, Caqueta, and the Amazon commissariats in the south of the country.[92]

Colombian capos have made some startling revelations (if they can be believed) about their support for the 1982 presidential campaign of Belisario Betancur and Alfonso López Michelsen. The mafia's own accounts of the election suggest that the donations may have totaled close to $3 million (U.S.) and that some capos may have given money to both sides. Pablo Escobar claimed that he donated 80 million pesos ($1.14 million U.S.) to López's campaign.[93] Escobar and Carlos Lehder say that they and several associates—Gonzalo Rodríguez Gacha, José Ocampo, and others—gave a joint donation of 26 million pesos ($370,000 U.S.) to support López's election. The money was reportedly given to López's campaign manager, Ernesto Samper Pizano, in a suite in the Intercontinental Hotel in Medellín.[94] Lehder also swore, in a letter written to the Bishop of Pereira (the capital of Risaralda) that Betancur "knowingly" received 110,000,000 pesos (about $1.6 million U.S.) in campaign funds from Escobar, Rodríguez Gacha, and other accused traffickers.[95]

Drug dollars are important to aspiring politicians in Colombia. Colombian law makes no provision for public financing of campaigns, and in some regions of the country—in cocaine and marijuana strongholds—drug income may be the leading source of private political funds. Money is a tool of influence, but in ways that are complex and—to the eye of the outsider—somewhat opaque. Mafia contributions do not necessarily bear a signature (like Evaristo Porras' check), but candidates may be generally aware that part of their funding comes from dubious sources.

This awareness can constrain their behavior, both as candidates and, later, as incumbents. However, it is extremely difficult to draw inferences. For example, observers of the Colombian scene point to the absence of public debate on drugs during national election campaigns. Hot money may partly account for this, but so does the fact that opinion polls show that drug trafficking ranks near the bottom of concerns of Colombian publics. Similarly, a politician's opposition to extradition might reflect a past or current financial nexus with the mafia, but also might be attributable to nationalist convictions. Assumptions about influence therefore must be made with caution. Yet, it is a safe bet that the mafia's use of money can win some converts to its cause.

Building a legend.   Cocaine traffickers represent what one Colombian sociologist has called a "new illegitimate bourgeoisie."[96] In a strictly economic sense, they are one of South America's great success stories—the continent's purest version of an indigenous capitalist class. Not surprisingly, traffickers portray themselves not as criminals but rather as successful entrepreneurs—paragons of capitalist virtue. As Pablo Escobar—the son of a vegetable farmer, a former car thief, and today one of the world's richest men—once remarked in response to a question about the origins of his fabulous wealth:

> Fortunes, large or small, always have a beginning. Most of the great millionaires of Colombia and of the world have begun with nothing. But it is precisely this which converts them into legends, myths, and an example for the people. To make money in a capitalist society is not a crime but rather a virtue.[97]

Such philosophical reflections on capitalism—considering the source—are almost ludicrous. At the same time, Escobar and his colleagues serve as role models for aspiring groups within their societies: After all, they stand for the expansion of economic opportunities. Their philosophy doubtless strikes a chord in societies where economic wealth has always been highly concentrated and where the state, a few leading families, and foreigners own a large share of the productive assets. The American political scientist Bruce Bagley compares Colombia's cocaine elite to an earlier nouveau riche group, the coffee oligarchy that emerged in that country in the late nineteenth and early twentieth centuries.[98] Both cocaine barons and coffee barons have sought to change the economic rules of the game to their advantage; in the case of the former, efforts at assimilation have been compounded by an ideology that is almost revolutionary in its glorification of the acquisitive spirit.

Yet, the mafia legend is based on more than just rags-to-riches entrepreneurship. Enlightened mafia chieftains such as Escobar, Lehder, and Suarez have made a conscious effort to purchase political support among the urban and rural poor. They have earned the gratitude of local residents—and sympathy for the cocaine industry—by delivering welfare and social services to poor communities that governments are unable to reach. Such narco-philanthropy represents a minuscule fraction of traffickers' total illicit earnings, but it is more than just hype; in any event, the political returns from this relatively small investment have been incalculably great. Even the church, which is by no means prodrug, has welcomed the proceeds of the industry. As the Bishop of Pereira put it in separate 1984 interviews, "I myself have received money from drug traffickers and distributed it to the poor—God's hands do not get dirty when they receive money from the mafia."[99]

Traffickers have dispensed their largesse in the form of money and gifts and also in the form of public works. To take some examples from the 1980s: The Bolivian trafficker Roberto Suarez donated sewing machines to poor women in his home town of Santa Ana de Yacuma. Evaristo Porras in Leticia wrote checks to needy citizens and arranged for the sick to get medical care at local hospitals.[100] The Escobar family estate, "Napoles," gave away 5,000 toys every Christmas to children of needy families in the Middle Magdalena Valley.[101] In Quindío, Carlos Lehder's Latin Nationalist Party used to distribute 500-peso notes (the equivalent of $3.50 to $4.00) to people who attended "patriotic Saturdays," as party rallies were called. (At one 1984 rally, the faithful discovered in their lunch boxes—free lunches were served at these events—a U.S. $5.00 bill wrapped in gold foil. With the money there was a message that read, "With this you are invited to the next gathering. Thanks. Brother Latin.") In a somewhat more altruistic spirit, Lehder also distributed cash and medical supplies to the inhabitants of Popayan after an earthquake there in March 1983.[102]

More important than their acts of charity are traffickers' contributions to the development of poor communities and regions. Lehder, for example, built a housing project for the poor, "San Julian," outside of Armenia, the capital city of Quindío. He also reportedly sponsored literacy campaigns in some of the rural areas of the department. Gonzalo Rodríguez Gacha restored the facade of the town hall in his native town of Pacho (in Cundinamarca, about 80 km from Bogotá); in addition, he built a large outdoor basketball court for the residents of the town. Roberto Suarez paved streets and restored churches in Santa Ana and supplied electric generators and water pumps to other small communities in the Beni. He developed a system for supplying medical services by air to villagers living in the remotest parts of the region. He reportedly provided scholarships to young Beni residents for technical or college education abroad. Finally, according to a foreign coca expert who regularly visits Bolivia, Roberto Suarez and other traffickers virtually reconstructed a town in northwestern Bolivia (San Buenaventura, in La Paz department), providing roads, a police station, a post office, and a school, as well as a hotel and a restaurant.[103]

Perhaps the archetype of mafia civic leaders is Pablo Escobar. According to various laudatory columns in *Medellín Cívico* (a newspaper founded by Escobar's uncle, Hernán Gaviria Berrio, and financed in part by the trafficker himself), Escobar is a "gospel of generosity" who is "dedicated to redeeming the forgotten class of Antioquia," from the slum dwellers of Medellín to the poor peasants of surrounding villages. His public works span almost every social sector: health, education, housing, recreation, and urban renewal. Escobar's civic efforts, proclaims *Medellín Cívico*, are nothing less than a "creative rebellion" against misery, social inequality, abandonment, and neglect.[104]

Escobar's showpiece project, called "Medellín Without Slums," was launched in 1982 to build 2,000 new housing units for poor families in that city. "Medellín Without Slums," said *Medellín Cívico*, would provide a new "life of noble dignity" for families that had been living in a "pestilential inferno of garbage." The project was later scaled back to 1,000 units, and only 450 to 500 dwellings were actually completed. Escobar's troubles with the law—especially his implication in the death of Lara Bonilla—prevented the full realization of his ambitious plan. Yet, "Medellín Without Slums" still is seen by many as a symbol of Escobar's civic leadership and of mafia public spiritedness in general.[105]

Escobar also seemed to have a special interest in sports facilities for the poor. He built, outfitted, and illuminated 80 sports arenas in Medellín and surrounding communities in Antioquia. In another famous project, Escobar and some relatives reportedly built an immense zoological park at "Napoles"—a family estate located near Puerto Triunfo, 180 km from Medellín. The zoo is open to the public, and entry is free of charge. Explained Escobar, "The fact is that the Napoles Zoo belongs not to us but to the Colombian people—and the people cannot pay to visit that which it owns." A nice touch at the zoo is the display at the front entrance of an old Piper Cub airplane, mounted on a concrete arch, that was reportedly used to fly some of the first shipments of Colombian cocaine to Florida.[106]

Escobar's civic action programs had a basic methodology: to send teams of activists into the barrios to determine, in consultation with residents, the works that would be of most benefit to the community. Escobar himself made the final selection. The results, if reports can be believed, were far-reaching. The following report is suggestive of both the scope of Escobar's programs and the populist fervor behind them.

Fifty thousand trees planted in fifty barrios of Medellín . . . schools built with plenty of space, with an eye to beauty and pedagogical function. Broken sewers repaired to protect residents from contaminated water and from epidemics, [sewers that were] a health hazard that the government has ignored for years. Basketball courts, skating rinks, multi-sport arenas . . . .thousands of bricks to expand the houses of poor families, to finish buildings, churches, and wings of schools. Illumination of barrios trapped in darkness because of indifferent bureaucrats or politicians who do not keep their promises . . . ."[107]

Escobar and his supporters constantly justified their civic campaigns in terms of the failings of the local bureaucracy and the general selfishness of the ruling oligarchy. Escobar's campaign, said *Medellín Cívico*, "frightened politicians and bureaucrats who had done nothing for the people."[108] Apparently Escobar did occasionally run afoul of the local authorities, who accused him of taking matters into his own hands. For example, the local Secretary of Education, Recreation, and Culture wrote Escobar that his efforts to refit a sports arena in the Santander section of Medellín reflected a "scorn for order and procedure" and told him to desist from further activity on the matter. Escobar wrote back that the project and others like it "filled a vacuum created by the indifference, the apathy, the negligence, and the irresponsibility of the municipal administration."[109] The media hype surrounding Escobar's campaign was at times intensely class-conscious. An enthusiastic supporter wrote:

> . . . there exist in Colombia two classes of bourgeoisie. That of the Lleras, Sampers, Ospinas, and Laras who earned their capital at the expense of the labor of millions and millions of Colombians, only to invest it in North America or Europe . . . and the other bourgeois class which invests in Colombia out of concern for the misery of the masses and their desperate struggle for survival. To this second class belongs Pablo Escobar . . . .[110]

The activities of Escobar and other capos clearly pose a challenge to their governments. The cocaine capos have created a base of support not only "above"—among law enforcement officials, bureaucrats, and politicians—but also "below"—among urban slum dwellers and residents of remote jungle towns. The extensive welfare and civic-action initiatives of cocaine capos convey a broader message that is not lost on Latin American leaders; namely, that the mafia may have become an important link between the formal structures of power and the people on the margins of society. Destroying this link will be difficult; even harder will be finding institutions to take its place.

Direct political participation. A distinctive feature of the Colombian cocaine mafia has been the open bid by some of its members for a share of political power. Pablo Escobar, for example, ran on the Liberal Party ticket for the Colombian House of Representatives in 1982. Escobar ran together with Jairo Ortega—Lara Bonilla's nemesis—for a parliamentary seat from Antioquia. Ortega and Escobar were elected, respectively, principal and alternate representatives for the seat. Escobar's campaign, not surprisingly, centered largely around his civic and social works in Antioquia; his sports stadiums and "Medellín Without Slums" campaign were prominent themes. Carlos Lehder, although a fugitive from justice, was a candidate for the Senate from Quindío in the March 1986 congressional elections. (He lost, overwhelmingly.) Lehder ran as a representative of his Latin Nationalist Party. In Leticia, Evaristo Porras sponsored in his own name a slate of Liberal Party candidates for the city's municipal council in the local elections of March 1986. During the 1988 mayoral elections, traffickers associated with Gonzalo Rodríguez Gacha reportedly gained control over five city governments in the northern coastal department of Magdalena.[111]

Colombia was also the home of Latin America's only mafia-organized political party, Carlos Lehder's Latin Nationalist Movement (MLN). MLN was founded in Quindío in early 1983 with money that Lehder had earned from drug smuggling activities in the Bahamas. As mentioned earlier, the party's ideology stressed a "pure nationalism" that was unaligned but opposed to "communism, imperialism, neo-colonialism, and Zionism." The major planks in the party's platform include nationalization of banks, transport, and the assets of multinationals; an end to "foreign intervention" in Colombian life; the abrogation of the extradition treaty; and the creation of a united Latin American army to safeguard Latin sovereignty, culture, and frontiers.[112] Of these, the anti-extradition plank was the most important; Lehder admitted on several occasions that the party would never have come into being had it not been for the 1979 treaty. There was even a line in the MLN party hymn that ran, "Don't destroy your Nation by surrendering your sons—let's struggle as brothers against extradition."[113]

Other points in Lehder's political program included legalization of marijuana for personal use and protection of Colombia's wildlife and natural resources. To highlight the MLN's ecological focus, the party had a green flag, the front of its headquarters in Armenia was painted green, and its newspaper, *Quindío Libre*, was printed on green paper.[114]

Lehder and his political lieutenants relied on a combination of modern mass communication and cold cash to build a popular following; indeed, the citizens of Quindío had never seen anything like the MLN's style of political campaigning. In Armenia, the MLN maintained a fleet of 20 yellow buses to take people to rallies, which were held outside of town in Lehder's Posada Alemana hotel complex. People who got on the buses would be handed banknotes, usually of 500 pesos. At rallies, political messages were introduced almost subliminally—Lehder's harangues against the Colombian "oligarchy" and against U.S. "imperialism" alternated with sets of loud disco music. Those attending such occasions were well-fed (an MLN lunch might consist of pieces of chicken, steak, and tongue), and at some rallies, the faithful might find money as well as food in their lunch boxes (see the section, "Building a Legend," earlier in this chapter). To reach people outside of the capital city, the party relied on helicopters equipped with loudspeaker systems; Lehder and his MLN colleagues would broadcast their messages to farmers and villagers from the air. Lehder's fleet of helicopters and private aircraft were also used to mass-distribute leaflets throughout the department and to carry *Quindío Libre* to major Colombian cities, especially to Medellín, Bogotá, and Cali.[115]

The political fortunes of Lehder's party looked promising for a while. MLN won 10,857 votes—about 12 percent of the electorate—in regional elections in Quindío in March 1984. This represented a significant achievement, because Lehder was actually a fugitive at the time. They won 2 out of 13 deputy seats to the departmental assembly, as well as a total of 11 seats on several city councils, including 2 in Armenia, the capital. These electoral successes did apparently convey some influence. For example, by shrewd politicking that exploited nationalist tendencies, the two MLN deputies managed to persuade the entire assembly to pass a resolution in November 1984 condemning the U.S.-Colombian extradition treaty. MLN's political clout, such as it was, derived in large part from its ability to exploit a serious local economic situation. Quindío's economic mainstay, coffee production, collapsed in 1984, the result of a failed harvest. Production fell more than 50 percent in that year, and continuing low prices in world markets aggravated the situation. Thousands of people were thrown out of work, and many became susceptible to MLN's appeal, which may have had more to do with money than with ideology.[116] The "Lehder phenomenon," said a former governor of Quindío, "is the most pathetic symbol of the appearance of money from narcotics trafficking in politics." He went on to say:

> They have millions and millions to spend. They have won over people, especially the unwary, with gifts and raffles. At the meetings held each week, which they called Patriotic Saturdays, they raffle off sewing machines, television sets, and other things, in addition to distributing goods and hundreds of 500-peso notes to those attending. The people are attracted by these things, especially the lower classes, the local people, the hungry, and the unemployed.
>
> . . . You know that Quindío is essentially a coffee-growing department, and that the coffee harvest mainly depends on the temporary employment of thousands of people. The last harvest was a failure; 50 percent was lost and thousands of

people were left hungry, even the little growers. This partly explains the emergence of a movement such as the one headed by Carlos Lehder.[117]

Other local politicians blamed the rise of MLN on the central government's failure to create new industry and to provide jobs. "We have been totally forgotten by the central government," said a Liberal senator from Quindío.[118] The political establishment was clearly alarmed. Fears were voiced that MLN, building on massive unemployment and wide popular discontent, would gain 20,000 supporters in the next election. The election of an MLN senator and an MLN representative to congress was seen as virtually certain. A conservative councilman from Armenia thought that MLN might take over the government of Quindío. None of this, as it turned out, came to pass. The party only received about 4,000 votes in the March 1986 elections, lost both deputies in the Quindío departmental assembly and six out of eight city council seats, and sent no representative to congress. The explanation was in large part related to the coffee industry. Better harvests and a near doubling of world coffee prices—from $1.20 per pound to $2.10 per pound in December 1985 (thanks to a massive drought earlier that year in Brazil)—helped Quindío's economy begin to rebound. Also, Lehder, in hiding following the government's approval in July 1983 of his extradition to the United States, could not tend very well to the affairs of his party. Reports surfaced of serious altercations between Lehder and some of his party lieutenants. The MLN's financial resources began to run dry, and there was less money to use for buying votes or otherwise influencing the populace. When this writer visited Armenia in April 1986, MLN no longer seemed to be a going concern: Its supporters were drifting back to the traditional Liberal or Conservative parties or toward the Unión Patriótica (unified Marxist party).[119]

There is widespread agreement among U.S. and Colombian observers that Colombia's cocaine capos overreached themselves in their eagerness to handle power directly. The traditional parties felt threatened and began to band together against the newcomers. Lehder's Latin Nationalist Movement—its fascist-populist message, its flagrant vote buying, and its obtrusive style of political communications—positively infuriated local politicians. Lehder's public admission that he had been involved in narcotics trafficking—"I myself have participated in the great Colombian bonanza," he said in an interview with Radio Caracol in June 1983—sealed his political fate.[120] In mid-1987, a conservative party leader in Armenia issued a public communiqué denouncing "the strange political movements that seem to be in vogue" and calling for an investigation into both the MLN's aims and its sources of funding. Copies of the declaration were sent to President Betancur, the Ministers of Government and Defense, the

Attorney General, the Governor of Quindío, and the Mayor of Armenia. The establishment, in other words, decided to mobilize against Lehder and his "strange political movement."[121]

Pablo Escobar's election to Congress and the populist rhetoric of his civic action campaign in Antioquia also worried politicians; Escobar was viewed as an anti-establishment figure (although not to the same extent that Lehder was). The publicity surrounding Escobar's and Lehder's political activities helped touch off a major national debate in the first half of 1983 about hot money in politics. Bad things began to happen. An old cocaine trafficking charge from 1976 against Escobar was reactivated. (The charge had been buried because of the disappearance of records of Escobar's arrest and because of the mysterious murders of two policemen who had participated in the arrest.) In August 1983, Lara Bonilla accused Escobar on ABC television of being one of Colombia's major drug capos. In October 1983, Carlos Lehder went into hiding—apparently the government had issued a provisional warrant for Lehder's arrest after receiving an extradition request from the United States in September. In May 1984, Betancur signed an order approving Lehder's extradition to the United States. In July, a judge of the Bogotá Superior Court accused Escobar of complicity in the slaying of Lara Bonilla. Also in July, the U.S. government requested Escobar's extradition for conspiring to introduce cocaine into the United States via Nicaragua. In September, the Colombian government issued a warrant for Escobar's arrest, not for drug trafficking or murder but for "contraband—one rhinocerous and 85 exotic birds"— which the trafficker had imported to stock his zoo at "Napoles." At the same time, the Colombian Congress lifted Escobar's parliamentary immunity—an action that for practical purposes marked the end of Escobar's political career.[122]

The mafia's direct bid for political power, in other words, backfired: The spotlight of public attention proved to be disastrous. The leaders of the cocaine industry are unlikely to make the same mistake again. For criminal organizations, power does not go hand in hand with success at the polls— power is best exercised covertly. Since 1983–1984, the cocaine industry has retreated from the political front lines. (Mafia figures, for example, no longer hand over large sums of money to politicians; the sources of campaign funds are carefully disguised.) However, the industry's influence in Colombian life has if anything increased, and the hold of individual capos—native Robin Hoods—on the popular imagination remains strong.

Negotiating with Governments

The South American cocaine mafia has been called variously an "empire without frontiers" and a "state within a state." In Bolivia and Colombia, governments on two recorded occasions have acknowledged the mafia's independent political clout by conducting quasi-official discussions with drug traffickers. In June 1983, Rafael Otazo Vargas, the head of President Siles Zuazo's Advisory Commission on Narcotics, held a meeting with Roberto Suarez at one of the latter's hideouts in the Beni. In May 1984, a former President of Colombia, Alfredo López Michelsen, and President Betancur's Attorney General, Carlos Jiménez Gómez, held separate meetings with Pablo Escobar, Jorge Ochoa, and other major Colombian capos in Panama. Jiménez "said that he happened to run into the drug trafficker during a visit to Panama to investigate a bank robbery"; López said that he was in the country to observe the May 6 presidential election. Few U.S. or Colombian observers believed these versions, however. It seems likely that the presidents of both countries authorized the discussions. According to two Colombian writers who closely follow the drug industry, President Betancur "not only had prior knowledge" of the Panama meetings but actually hoped that the participation of López and Jiménez would produce a national accord with the mafia. Furthermore, Jiménez had conducted a previous (and unreported) meeting with mafia leaders in Colombia in late 1983. Otazo says that he "interviewed Suarez with the complete knowledge and support of the chief executive"—that is, Siles Zuazo—and his version is accepted by most U.S. and Bolivian observers.[123]

Neither episode seems to have resulted in a government-mafia deal; yet, the discussions conferred an aura of legitimacy on the cocaine mafia and, as a result, caused major national scandals in Bolivia and Colombia. The Suarez-Otazo meeting was condemned in a resolution by the Bolivian Congress and, indeed, may have hastened the departure from office of the Siles government.[124] In Colombia, Minister of Justice Enrique Parejo and many members of congress denounced the talks. Two Colombian senators called for Jiménez Gómez to resign because of his participation in the Panama meetings.[125] Possibly the idea of giving official recognition to the drug mafia bothered opponents most. As one El Tiempo columnist cynically observed, congressmen said it was a "moral impossibility to have a dialogue with narcos," but saw nothing wrong when "the same narcos gave generously to their political campaigns."[126]

The Colombian Mafia's Proposal

Escobar, Ochoa, and other major capos who met with López and Jiménez in Panama claimed to represent "100 persons who constitute the dome (cúpula) of the cocaine organization" in Colombia—that is, the cocaine establishment. Significantly, the traffickers made clear to the Colombian leaders that they did not speak for Carlos Lehder. Yet, the proposal can be considered as representing the mainstream of Colombian mafia thinking at the time.[127]

When the Panama meetings took place, Colombia's cocaine traffickers were more or less on the run, attempting to avoid the consequences of the wave of national antidrug hysteria that followed the assassination of Colombia's Justice Minister Rodrigo Lara Bonilla. The government declared a state of siege and initiated a series of reprisals against the drug industry. Police, sometimes accompanied by soldiers, broke into the houses and offices of suspected traffickers. Airplanes, boats, and automobiles were seized on the presumption that their owners were engaged in drug dealing. The government decreed that narcotics cases would be judged by military tribunals rather than by (more lenient) civilian courts. Government officials were forbidden under pain of dismissal to maintain friendships with traffickers. Most important, the Betancur administration indicated that it would begin honoring the 1979 extradition treaty with the United States.[128] López Michelsen, who met with Ochoa and Escobar in Panama, said that the traffickers were "very frightened"—hence, receptive to the idea of coming to terms with the Colombian government.

The proposal that the capos presented to López and Jiménez reflected their status as fugitives. According to the version published in *El Tiempo* in July 1984, the traffickers requested what amounted to official amnesty— "reinstatement in Colombian society in the near future." They also wanted the extradition treaty revised so that they would have the right to be judged under Colombian law. The traffickers drew a parallel between their proposal and the peace agreement that the government had worked out with the guerrillas. The government, they said, offered the guerrillas the "opportunity to return to civil life with dignity," and they wanted the same deal.[129]

To support the case for amnesty, Colombia's capos tried to cast themselves in the most favorable possible light. They did not assassinate the Justice Minister, they claimed. Moreover, they supported the "democratic and republican form of government in Colombia" and had no connection with the guerrillas who were trying to overthrow that government by force. They made a point of criticizing the "inaccurate image of the drug trafficking guerrilla," which, they claimed, was "suspiciously and maliciously coined in the days after the assassination of Lara Bonilla." They also asserted that they were in the business of exporting cocaine, that their cocaine business did not rely on home-grown coca, and that they were not involved in selling bazuco to the Colombian masses. In other words, the capos were saying, they did not constitute a threat to the Colombian state or to Colombian society.

What the traffickers offered in return for amnesty was radical indeed.

The main feature was the dismantling of their cocaine infrastructure: the surrender to the government of laboratories, clandestine runways, and aircraft "used in the shipment of raw materials and of the finished product." The traffickers announced that they would get out of the business of producing, shipping, and distributing cocaine. They claimed that their organizations accounted for 70–80 percent of Colombian exports, that their organizations had taken years to develop, and that it would be "difficult to replace or duplicate" them in less than 10 years. In other words, acceptance of the traffickers' proposal would seemingly result in a significant, if temporary, decline in the availability of cocaine in world markets.[130]

To make the deal more attractive, the mafia included some additional inducements. They offered to repatriate their capital to Colombia. The proposal as recorded in El Tiempo did not indicate an amount; however, most Colombian observers estimated that traffickers' bank deposits abroad amounted to several billion dollars. In addition, traffickers proposed to help the Colombian government combat the remainder of that country's drug trade. They said they would cooperate in "campaigns to abolish consumption of bazuco and to rehabilitate addicts." They also indicated that they would help the government replace the coca and marijuana grown in Colombia with other crops. The cocaine mafia, in other words, would now be in the front lines of the war against drugs. Finally, in a gesture to Colombia's traditional political elites, the mafia promised to refrain from overt political activity. Past participation of "some members of our organizations in politics," they explained, had been prompted by a "desire to work against the extradition treaty signed with the United States."[131]

Public reaction to the news of the talks was largely unfavorable, at least on the surface. As El Tiempo commented, "The announcement of the contacts was received with stupor and later with indignation. The political parties, the economic interest groups, almost the entire country completely rejected the idea, which would legalize one of the most scabrous criminal activities." Some political leaders took the line that negotiating with criminals would undermine Colombia's legal and institutional order. Others were skeptical that the traffickers would keep their part of the bargain. Said Ernesto Samper Pizano, a Liberal senator from Bogotá, "To ask the drug traffickers to teach us how to end the drug traffic is like inviting bank robbers to a symposium on bank security."[132]

The U.S. response also was essentially negative. A few U.S. officials saw the traffickers' offer as a real opportunity to reduce world supplies of cocaine, at least temporarily. However, this view did not prevail. Officially, the United States, which had indictments against many of the proposal's sponsors, adopted the position that it could only deal with cocaine traffickers individually, that is, on a case-by-case basis and not with the mafia as a group. The United States, in other words, refused to recognize the mafia as a "political" entity. Hence, the United States rejected the entire thrust of the Panama meetings—the purported idea behind the meetings was negotiating a collective withdrawal by most of the mafia's chief executive officers from the drug trade.[133]

Not everyone condemned the meetings. Some (unnamed) businessmen supported the mafia's proposal on the grounds that massive repatriation of drug money could help solve Colombia's major economic problem—at the time, the country's growing fiscal deficit and its declining international reserves. A law professor at Bogotá's National University, Emilio Robledo Uribe, believed that traffickers could help fight the drug traffic. He argued, "The primary responsibility of Colombia's leaders is to deracinate the drug dealing business, and if the drug dealers offer to cooperate in such an effort, isn't it the duty of the government to listen to them?" Furthermore, said Uribe, "using drug traffickers' power in the service of the nation" is better than "forcing them into permanent opposition" by rejecting their overtures for a dialogue.[134]

For their part, López and Jiménez defended the talks and urged that the government accept the mafia's proposal as a starting point for serious negotiations. Both saw negotiations with traffickers as a logical extension of the peace process that was underway between the government and various guerrilla groups. López even believed that the government could strike a better deal with the mafia than with the guerrillas: "The difference between the [proposed] surrender of narco-traffickers and the surrender of guerrillas is that the former gave up everything while the latter hold on to their shotguns."[135] There also were some congressmen—albeit a small minority—who argued in favor of government-mafia negotiations. One conservative parliamentarian felt that, if anything, traffickers were more deserving of amnesty than guerrillas. Drug money, he said, was "invested in important enterprises" and "created jobs for thousands of Colombians." Guerrillas, in contrast, had contributed to "thousands of Colombian deaths and incalculable losses in production" over a 30-year period.[136]

Still, Colombia's political establishment seemed to overwhelmingly oppose striking a bargain with cocaine dealers, and, eventually, Betancur himself killed the initiative. The president issued a communiqué on July 19, 1984, that said in part, "There has not been, there is not now, nor will there ever be any kind of understanding between the government and the signers of the memorandum."[137] Thus, an extraordinary chapter in the history of mafia-government relations apparently ended, although individual Colombian officials may have continued to engage in low-key, sporadic, and highly informal discussions with drug traffickers.

The Otazo-Suarez Meeting

The meeting in June 1983 between President Siles' narcotics adviser, Rafael Otazo, and Roberto Suarez took place under circumstances different from those of the Panama meetings. At the time, Suarez was technically a fugitive from justice with warrants issued for his arrest. Yet, for all practical purposes, he was untouchable. Suarez controlled what amounted to an independent kingdom or fiefdom in the remote Beni region of the country. "The state is not present in those territories," he once remarked about the Beni.[138] Suarez apparently maintained his own private army and air force. Also, the "King of Cocaine," as Suarez was popularly called, could count on many loyal subjects: Cocaine dollars had brought wealth, employment, and social services to thousands of Beni residents. The Bolivian government simply did not have the economic, political, or military resources to dislodge him. Suarez' empire was for practical purposes a "state within a state" and also constituted a serious political challenge to the Siles regime.[139]

Suarez had no interest in forsaking his cocaine business in return for the right to live peacefully as an ordinary citizen. He sought conversations with the Bolivian government, but as part of a pattern of activity designed to pressure, and perhaps even to destabilize, the Bolivian government. Suarez had written to Siles in 1983 seeking what he called a "summit meeting" to "consider a solution to the political, economic, and social crisis confronting the country."[140] Suarez later made it clear that the democratic system of government, introduced in 1982, was at the root of the country's problems. Siles refused to meet with Suarez but—for reasons that are still unclear—authorized Otazo to arrange a meeting with the trafficker. On June 2, 1983, Otazo flew in a private plane from La Paz to one of Suarez's ranches in the Beni. He interviewed the cocaine king for several hours and returned to La Paz on the same day.

Suarez used the meeting with Otazo to convey an image of his political and economic power. He talked about his "magnificent communications and transportation system and first quality armament." He claimed that he had a "network of people in uniform and workers" in all of the country's main departments. He talked about the various public work projects that he was supporting in the Beni region: electrification, water control, medical support services, and so on. He expressed his distaste for democracy, which he associated with inefficient government and a deterioration of public order. Through Otazo, he challenged Siles to respond with a "clearly stated national and international policy" that would address "the fundamental problems of the country" and "defend the dignity of Bolivians." Finally, Suarez offered to loan the Bolivian government $2 billion, in four $500-million installments. (It ·is highly unlikely that Suarez himself had this sum in hand; if the offer was genuine, the money almost certainly would have come from Colombian traffickers.) Possibly, the proposal was just a grandstand play—a patronizing gesture by Suarez to the weak and financially troubled Siles government. On the other hand, Suarez's intention may have been obtaining official sanction for his independent kingdom in the Beni. In any event, according to Otazo, the Siles government did not accept the money.[141]

After the interview, Suarez continued to pressure the Siles government. In July, he gave an interview to reporters in which he bragged about his military power. According to accounts of the interview, the cocaine king boasted of having a Libyan-trained private army equipped with modern automatic weapons. He also claimed to own three jets "of the Harrier type" and a dozen Brazilian-made combat aircraft, some armed with missiles. In addition, Suarez told reporters of his ambition to overthrow the Siles regime and to become the next leader of Bolivia. The Bolivian government's reaction to these statements was understandably negative. Mario Rueda Peña, the Information Minister, issued a communiqué that accused Suarez of having "the intention to destabilize democracy" in Bolivia.[142]

News of the Suarez-Otazo meeting did not break for more than a year. In August 1984, the news was leaked to the media from "various official levels," and the result—as in Colombia—was a major national scandal. The difference was that there was almost no overt public support in Bolivia for the meeting. Both houses of Bolivia's Congress voted to "condemn the scandal, which compromises national dignity by involving the government in negotiations with drug traffickers." Another resolution asserted that Siles should be called to account for "his immorality and the lack of capacity of his government." Furthermore, a Bolivian congressional commission summoned Siles to testify under oath about the case. Siles refused, and there were pressures in Congress to declare the president "in contempt and in defiance of the law."[143]

The government, seeking a scapegoat, fired Otazo from his job as narcotics adviser. Spokesmen for Siles also claimed that the president had "not instructed" Otazo to meet with Suarez. Few Bolivians believed this version of the incident, however. Otazo presented a detailed and generally credible account of the affair to congress, indicating that he had, in fact, acted on a direct order from the president. Otazo also reported that during the interview, Roberto Suarez had fingered a former Siles Minister of the Interior, Mario Roncal, as a major drug trafficker—which did not help the image of the Siles administration. Clearly, the administration was in hot water. American columnist Georgie Anne Geyer called the affair a

"Bolivian Watergate" and said that "narcocracy" and "coca dollars" had soiled the president and his closest followers.[144] Siles, like Nixon, departed office well before the end of his term. The catastrophic state of the Bolivian economy (which had a 10,000-percent rate of inflation in 1985) was probably the major reason for his departure, but the revelations about the Siles-Otazo meeting certainly helped to discredit Siles politically.

Commentary

As the episodes recounted above demonstrate, government discussions with narcotics traffickers aroused strong political resistance in Bolivia and Colombia. Congressional leaders, and to some extent the public, view cocaine dealers as political pariahs and blanch at the thought of any official dealings with them. The same congressmen, however, may welcome financial support from traffickers for their political campaigns. There seemingly is a world of difference in Latin American societies between accepting the drug traffickers as a kind of necessary social evil and granting them political legitimacy. The United States, for its part, has more or less rejected out of hand the idea of a bargain with the mafia. "We do not negotiate with criminals" apparently is the predominant reaction of U.S. officials to the idea.

Yet, the idea of negotiating with the mafia was not totally without redeeming features. The Colombian capos' offer, on the face of it, had merit—if one accepts its two most important assumptions: that the traffickers who authorized the proposal controlled 70–80 percent of the cocaine market in Colombia and that their cocaine infrastructure had taken 10 years to build. Amnesty for Colombia's cocaine establishment seems a small price to pay for reducing world supplies of cocaine—and U.S. consumption of the drug. Moreover, the Colombian economy clearly would have benefited (especially at the time the proposal was made) from the repatriation of narco-dollars held abroad. The fundamental issue is whether the traffickers would or could keep their word. For example, international commissions would have to be established to supervise the dismantling of laboratories and other elements of the traffickers' infrastructure. The government would have to be in a position to impose severe sanctions on traffickers should they decide to reinvolve themselves in the cocaine business.

Also, the Colombian and U.S. governments would have to be willing to accept the political costs involved in negotiation. Such costs would be considerable—one can imagine the screams of outrage from the Colombian political establishment, the U.S. Congress, and world leaders in general. One notes in this connection that the Reagan Administration paid a high political price for negotiating with General Manuel Noriega in Panama. The Administration tried to persuade Noriega—indicted by a federal court in Miami on drug smuggling and money laundering charges—to step down as head of the Panamanian defense forces. The negative political fallout from the Noriega affair prompted both candidates for U.S. President in 1988 to assure the American public that they will never under any circumstances negotiate with drug dealers.

Ironically, the idea of negotiation is gaining popularity in Colombia today. According to a poll commissioned by the Medellín newspaper *El Mundo* in August 1988, 55.1 percent of Medellín residents support the idea of a government-trafficker dialogue.[145] The current mayor of Medellín, Juan Gómez Martínez, says, "It is necessary to engage in dialogue with the Medellín cartel."[146] However, some of the more prominent advocates of this course—for example, a head of Colombia's State Council and an acting Colombian Attorney General—seem to see discussions with traffickers as a prelude to legalizing (and taxing) cocaine rather than a means of shutting down the industry.[147] These new pleadings for negotiations reflect more than anything the increasing powerlessness of the Colombian government vis-à-vis the cocaine industry. In 1984, the government had the trafficking establishment on the run—100 of the country's leading cocaine operators sued for peace from exile in Panama. A functioning extradition treaty existed at that time between the United States and Colombia. That was the time—if there ever was a time—for the United States and Colombia to seek a negotiated solution to the cocaine trafficking problem.

Notes

1. Mark Moore, "Drug Policy and Organized Crime," in *America's Habit: Drug Abuse, Drug Trafficking, and Organized Crime (America's Habit)* (Washington, D.C.: U.S. Government Printing Office, 1986), p. 23.
2. Select Committee on Narcotics, Abuse, and Control, *South America Study Mission, August 9–23, 1977* (Washington, D.C.: U.S. Government Printing Office, 1977), p. 9.
3. Thomas Ricks, "Indictment of 9 Alleged Gang Members Portrays How Cocaine Industry Works," *Wall Street Journal*, November 19, 1986.
4. The Colombian cartels are less successful in maintaining cocaine prices than OPEC is in maintaining oil prices.
5. "Comunicado de los Extraditables," *El Tiempo*, January 25, 1988.
6. "Colombia's Chief Prosecutor Murdered," *Los Angeles Times*, January 26, 1988.
   Interviews with U.S. narcotics experts in Bogotá, May 1988.
7. "Secuestro y terrorismo," *El Espectador*, February 16, 1988.
8. "Comunicado de los Extraditables," p. 40.
9. "Extradition Treaty Viewed as Anti-Latin Invention" ("Anti-Latin Invention"), *El Colombiano*, Medellín, May 24, 1982.

10. "Colombia's Parejo: Narcotics Traffickers 'Winning,' " Bogotá Television Service, April 4, 1986.
11. Ibid.
    "Where Cocaine is King," *Newsweek*, February 29, 1988, p. 10.
12. NNICC, *The NNICC Report 1985–1986 (NNICC Report 1985–1986)* (Washington, D.C., June 1987), p. 36.
13. Committee on Foreign Relations, U.S. Senate, *Drugs, Law Enforcement, and Foreign Policy: Panama* (Washington, D.C.: U.S. Government Printing Office, 1988), Hearings before the Subcommittee on Terrorism, Narcotics, and International Communications, Part 2, p. 33.
14. R. W. Lee, "The Latin American Drug Connection," *Foreign Policy*, No. 61 (Winter 1985–1986), p. 154.
15. "Siles rechaza entrevista pedida por Roberto Suarez," *Presencia*, La Paz, July 5, 1983, p. 1.
16. David Henry, "Pablo Escobar Gaviria," *Fortune*, October 5, 1987, p. 153.
    "Vivo a salto de mate y no puedo entrar a las ciudades," *Meridiano*, La Paz, July 4, 1983.
17. Committee on Foreign Relations, U.S. Senate, *Drugs, Law Enforcement, and Foreign Policy: The Cartel, Haiti, and Central America* (Washington, D.C.: U.S. Government Printing Office, 1988), Hearings before the Subcommittee on Terrorism, Narcotics, and International Operation, p. 177.
18. "El asunto del auto," *Caretas*, August 12, 1985, pp. 12–13.
    "Caso gigante," *Caretas*, July 30, 1985, pp. 40, 42.
    "Police Generals Ousted," *Facts on File: World News Digest*, December 31, 1985, p. 996 G-1.
19. "¿Quién está matando a la mafia?" ("Quién Está Matando"), *Semana*, April 1, 1986, p. 32.
    Interviews with U.S. narcotics experts in Bogotá, March–April 1986.
20. "Text of Drug Traffickers' Terms for Ending Activities," ("Text of Drug Traffickers' Terms"), *El Tiempo*, July 7, 1984.
21. "Lehder cuenta como se hizo millionario con bonanza de la droga" ("Lehder Cuenta Como"), *El Espectador*, June 29, 1983.
22. Michael Isikoff, "Drug Cartel Founder Convicted; Carlos Lehder Sent Tons of Cocaine into the United States," *The Washington Post*, May 20, 1988.
    Michael Satchell, "A Narcotraficante's Worst Nightmare," *U.S. News & World Report*, January 11, 1988, p. 30.
    Ruth Marcus, "Assault on Cartel Fails to Halt Drugs," *The Washington Post*, February 14, 1988.
23. "Text of Drug Traffickers' Terms," see note 20.
24. Mario Arango Jaramillo and Jorge Child, *Narcotráfico Imperio de la Cocaína* (Medellín: Editorial Percepción, 1984), pp. 203–204.
25. "The Medellín Cartel: World's Deadliest Criminals," A Miami Herald Special Report, *Miami Herald*, February 1987.
26. "Senate Estimates Drug Traffic Yields $3 Billion," La Paz, *La Red Panamericana*, July 11, 1986.
    State Department, *International Narcotics Control Strategy Report (INCSR)* (Washington, D.C., 1988), p. 71.
27. Peru reputedly accounts for only five percent of the refined cocaine consumed in the United States. See *NNICC Report 1985–1986*, p. 36.
28. "Guerra en la mafia," *El Espectador*, March 29, 1986.

29. "America's Habit," p. 103.
30. Alan Riding, "Gangs in Colombia Feud Over Cocaine" ("Gangs in Colombia"), *The New York Times*, August 23, 1988.
31. Fabio Castillo, *Los Jinetes de la Cocaína (Los Jinetes)* (Bogotá: Editorial Documentos Periodistas, 1987), p. 207.
32. "Text of Drug Traffickers' Terms," see note 20.
33. "Gangs in Colombia," see note 30.
34. "Pablo Escobar dirige complot para acabar con cartel de Cali," *El Tiempo*, March 31, 1988.
35. "Ojo por ojo," *Semana*, August 29, 1988, pp. 26–28.
    Alan Riding, "Massacres Are Jolting Colombia," *The New York Times*, December 15, 1988.
36. "Guerra en la mafia," see note 28.
37. "Anti-Latin Invention," see note 9.
38. "Estamos con la patria," *Medellín Cívico*, March 1981, p. 6.
39. "Letter to National Deputies Mario Velardo Dorado and Franklin Anaya," *Hoy*, November 6, 1985.
40. "Quién Está Matando," pp. 28–32.
    See also note 28.
41. "Carta abierta de Roberto Suarez," *Los Tiempos*, Cochabamba, October 19, 1984, p. 9.
42. Mario Arango Jaramillo and Jorge Child Velez, *Los Condenados de la Coca (Los Condenados)* (Medellín: Editorial J. M. Arango, 1985), pp. 141–147.
43. Ibid.
    Movimiento Latino Nacional, *Bases Ideológicas*, Armenia, 1983, p. 19.
44. *Bases Ideologicas*, pp. 7, 9.
45. George Stern, "Cocaine Kingpin Flees Colombia," *Miami Herald*, September 18, 1983.
46. *Los Condenados*, pp. 143–144.
47. Ibid., p. 140.
48. John Corry, "Cocaine in Colombia: Dad-Daughter Sleuths," *The New York Times*, August 19, 1983.
    "Belisario no entregará a ningún colombiano" ("Belisario no entregará"), *Quindío Libre*, October 1, 1983.
49. Bernd Debussmann, "Robin Hood Image of Latin Drug Kings Worries Authorities" ("Robin Hood Image"), Reuters International News, July 15, 1986.
50. *Los Condenados*, p. 144.
    "La patria acorralada," *Quindío Libre*, October 1, 1983.
    "Belisario no entregará," see note 48.
51. "Al Capone: How I'd Run This Country," *Star*, August 24, 1987, p. 24.
52. "Text of Drug Traffickers' Terms," see note 20.
53. "Escobar Gaviria refuta a Tambs," *Medellín Cívico*, March 1984.
54. "El Narco-Agro," *Semana*, December 5, 1988, p. 37.
55. Alan Riding, "Colombian Drug Lords Buy Land, Gain Acceptance," *The New York Times*, December 21, 1988.
56. "Military Drug Trafficking Link Alleged," Radio Patria Libre (clandestine), November 15, 1988.
57. Amado Canelas Orellana et al., *Bolivia: Coca, Cocaína (Coca, Cocaína)* (La Paz: Los Amigos del Libro, 1984), pp. 140–141.
58. "Bolivia es más interesada que EE. UU. en combatir narcotráfico," *El Diario*, La Paz, April 13, 1983.

59. "Carta abierta de Roberto Suarez," see note 41.
60. Bruce Bagley, "Colombia and the War on Drugs" ("Colombia and the War"), *Foreign Affairs*, Fall 1988, pp. 71–72.
61. "Se prendió la mecha," *Semana*, No. 69 (August 23-29, 1983), pp. 22–28.
    "Soy victima de una celada," *El Tiempo*, August 18, 1983.
    "Nubes que el viento aparte," *Semana*, September 20-26, 1983, p. 26.
    "El pulso de la nación," *Semana*, August 30-September 5, 1983, pp. 22–25.
62. "Los narcotraficantes amenazan a ministros," *El Siglo*, Bogotá, November 24, 1984.
63. "Comienza a destaparse 'olla mágica,' " *El Espectador,* March 3, 1988.
64. "The Evil Empire," *Newsweek*, February 25, 1985, p. 14.
65. Richard B. Craig, "Illicit Drug Traffic: Implications for South American Source Countries" ("Illicit Drug Traffic"), *Journal of Interamerican Studies and World Affairs*, Summer 1987, p. 29.
66. *Los Jinetes*, pp. 61–63.
67. "Ramirez Gomez iba a escribir el libro negro de la coca," *El Tiempo*, November 19, 1986.
    "Urga grupo especializado en captura de narcotraficantes," *El Espectador*, November 14, 1986.
68. *Los Condenados*, pp. 84–94.
69. *Los Jinetes*, pp. 199–215.
70. "Where Cocaine Is King," p. 10.
71. *INCSR*, 1988, p. 88.
    "Estupor por subornos de la mafia," *El Tiempo*, January 10, 1988.
    R. W. Lee, "Drugs," in Richard Feinberg and Gregg Goldstein (eds), *The U.S. Economy and Developing Countries* (Overseas Development Council, February 1988), p. 3.
72. "Libre capo porque ningún juez quiso procesarlo," *El Tiempo*, January 10, 1988.
73. Fabio Rincon, *Ochoa* (Bogotá: Vea, 1987), p. 25.
    Tom Wells, "Search Yields Results But Not the Main Target," Associated Press, International News, August 26, 1986.
74. "Si compromiso existía," *El Tiempo*, February 5, 1988.
75. "Los jueces y la mafia," *El Espectador*, June 4, 1987.
76. See, e.g.: "Colombia and the War," p. 83.
    Los Jinetes, pp. 114–115.
77. *Coca, Cocaína*, p. 138.
78. "Fighting the Cocaine Wars," *Time*, February 25, 1985, p. 30.
79. "4th Brigade Intelligence Officer Linked to Drug Traffickers," *El Tiempo*, April 13, 1988.
80. "El dossier de Medellín," *Semana*, January 27, 1987, p. 25.
81. *Los Jinetes*, p. 71.
82. Guillermo Zavala, "Rafael Otazo Manifestó: Soy un cultor de la verdad y no he cometido ningún delito" ("Rafael Otozo Manifestó"), *El Diario*, October 21, 1984.
83. Perfecto Conde, "Cocaína y poder político," *La República*, Lima, September 15, 1985.
84. Alan Riding, "Cocaine Billionaires," *The New York Times Magazine*, March 8, 1987, p. 32.
85. *Coca, Cocaína*, pp. 127, 129–131, 153.

Kevin Healy, "The Boom Within the Crisis" in Deborah Pacini and Christine Franquemont (eds), *Coca and Cocaine* (Petersborough, New Hampshire: Transcript Printing Company, 1986), pp. 104–106.

Christopher Mitchell, "The New Authoritarianism in Bolivia," *Current History*, February 1981, p. 76.

86. IEPALA, *Narcotráfico y política, militarismo y mafia en Bolivia (Narcotráfico y Política)* (Madrid: Graficas Margaritas, 1982), p. 30.

87. Ibid., pp. 61, 81, 87.

88. "Declaramos anti la Comisión de Constitución de Deputadas," *Ultima Hora*, La Paz, June 1, 1988.

89. "Rey de la cocaína Roberto Suarez dice que se entrego para solucionar problemas de narcotráfico Boliviano," *Los Tiempos*, Cochabamba, September 25, 1988, p. 10.

90. "Drug Boss Arrested by Bolivians," *Miami Herald*, July 22, 1988, pp. 1A, 6A.

91. R. W. Lee, "The Latin American Drug Connection," *Foreign Policy*, No. 61 (Winter 1985–1986), p. 149.

92. "Parejo on Politicians Financed by Drug Money," Madrid EFE, January 18, 1986.

93. "La mafia colombiana," *El Nacional*, Barranquilla, January 12, 1985.

94. "La suite Medellín: opus magnus del dinero caliente," *Guión*, July 29, 1983, pp. 20–25.

95. *Los Condenados*, p. 107.

96. Alvaro Camacho Guizado, *Droga, Corrupción, y Poder* (Cali, Colombia: Universidad del Valle, 1981), p. 98.

97. *Los Condenados*, pp. 128–129.

98. Bruce Bagley, "The Colombian Connection: The Impact of Drug Traffic on Colombia," in *Coca and Cocaine*, pp. 97–98.

99. "Colombian Bishop Says He Took Money from Drug Traffickers," Reuters, North American Service, July 17, 1984.

100. "El hombre que puede hacer caer a Siles" ("El Hombre que Puede Hacer"), *Los Tiempos*, Cochabamba, September 30, 1984.
"Robin Hood Image," see note 49.

101. *Los Condenados*, p. 128.

102. Jorge Eliecer Orozco, *Lehder . . . El Hombre* (Bogotá: Plaza y Janes, 1987), pp. 57–60, 162, 185.

103. Ibid., p. 120.
"Robin Hood Image," see note 49.
"El Hombre que Puede Hacer," see note 100.
Author's field trip to Pacho on March 5, 1988.

104. "Pablo es La Paz," *Medellín Cívico*, March 1984, p. 7.
Edgar Escobar, "Pablo amigo, Pablo pueblo," *Medellín Cívico*, March 1984, p. 4.
"Aquí viven," *Medellín Cívico*, March 1984, p. 1.

105. "En la mitad del camino," *Medellín Cívico*, March 1984, p. 3.
Los Condenados, p. 127.

106. "Del pueblo colombiano," *Medellín Cívico*, March 1984, p. 23.
"Medellín: epicentro de la mafia," *El Nacional*, January 16, 1985.

107. "En la mitad del camino," p. 3.

108. "El pueblo fué superior a los pequeños dirijentes," *Medellín Cívico*, March 1984, p. 10.

109. "Una lección de educación cívica de Pablo Escobar a la Secretaria de Educación," *Medellín Cívico*, March 1984, pp. 16–17.
110. "Pablo es la paz," p. 7.
111. Michael Isikoff and Eugene Robinson, "Colombia's Drug Kings Becoming Entrenched," *The Washington Post*, January 8, 1989.
112. *Bases Ideologicas*, pp. 5–19.
113. *Lehder . . . El Hombre*, p. 183.
114. Ibid., pp. 164–165.
115. Ibid., pp. 141, 162, 181–186.
116. Ibid., pp. 191, 222–223.
117. Pedro Claver Tellez, "Quindío: The Devil's Workshop," *Cromos*, March 11, 1985, pp. 14–19.
118. Ibid.
119. Interviews with MLN leaders in Armenia, April 20–21, 1986.
120. "Lehder Cuenta Como," p. 12A.
121. *Lehder . . . El Hombre*, pp. 150–151.
122. *Los Condenados*, pp. 129–133.
    "Esta es Colombia, Pablo," *Semana,* October 1983, p. 28.
123. *Los Condenados*, p. 95.
    "Rafael Otazo Manifestó," see note 82.
    Interview with a former president of Colombia, October 23, 1987.
    "Secret Drug Talks Hamper Amnesty," *Latin American Weekly Report*, July 20, 1984, p. 3.
124. Again, the lesson is that *direct* political participation by the mafia evokes extremely negative reactions from established groups.
125. "Jiménez Gómez Criticized" and "Political Parties Reject Dialogue," *El Tiempo*, July 6, 1984.
126. Lucy Nieto de Samper, "Narco-político," *El Tiempo*, July 23, 1984.
127. German Santamaria, "El país tiene que hacerse cargo de la magnitud del problema de la droga" ("El País Tiene que Hacerse Cargo"), *El Tiempo*, July 29, 1984.
128. *Los Condenados*, pp. 87-94.
129. "Text of Drug Traffickers' Terms," see note 20.
130. Ibid.
131. Ibid.
132. "Political Parties Reject Dialogue," p. 8A.
    Guillermo Perez, "Repudio a contacto en Panamá," *El Tiempo*, July 8, 1984.
133. "El País Tiene que Hacerse Cargo," p. 8A.
134. *Narcotráfico Imperio de la Cocaína*, p. 13.
    Emilio Robledo Uribe, "El diálogo con los narcotraficantes," *El Tiempo*, October 2, 1984.
135. "El País Tiene que Hacerse Cargo," p. 8A.
    "Attorney General Talks with Drug Traffickers," Bogotá, Emisorias Caracol, August 3, 1984.
136. "Political Parties Reject Dialogue," p. 8A.
137. "Betancur Will Not Hold Dialogue with Traffickers," *El Siglo*, July 20, 1984.
138. "Roberto Suarez se confiesa," *Correo*, La Paz, June 28, 1983.
139. "Bolivia's Cocaine 'Godfather' Untouched by Crackdown," *Miami Herald*, June 27, 1983.
    "Un 'rey' destronado," *Guión*, August 19, 1983, p. 55.

"Oro blanco—suicidio inconsciente," *Guión*, August 26, 1983, p. 46.
140. "The Latin American Drug Connection," p. 154.
141. "Rafael Otazo Manifestó," see note 82.
142. "Siles rechaza entrevista pedida por Roberto Suarez," *Presencia*, July 5, 1983.
   "Vivo a salto de mate," *Meridiano*, La Paz, July 4, 1983.
143. "Congreso condenó el gobierno por negociaciones con narcotráfico," *Hoy*, October 25, 1984.
   "Presidente se excusa de declarar ante Comisión," *Los Tiempos*, Cochabamba, December 12, 1984.
144. "Se reitera que Siles no instruyó a Otazo que converse con Suarez," *Presencia*, September 19, 1984.
   Georgie Anne Geyer, "El watergate Boliviano," *El Diario*, October 11, 1984.
145. "Piden dialogo entre gobierno y guerrilla," *El Mundo*, Medellín, August 17, 1988.
146. Jorge Matiz, "Proposed Dialogue with Drug Traffickers Is Based on Conviction, Not Fear," *Cromos*, Bogotá, April 12, 1988, pp. 18, 19.
147. See, e.g., "Lo único que hacemos es el oso," *El Tiempo*, February 22, 1988.
   "Illicit Drug Traffic," p. 24.

4

The Narco-Guerrilla Connection

*If coca, marijuana, gold, coal, emeralds, or what-
ever we have can provide us a foothold [piedra de
apoyo] from which to expel imperialism from Colombia or Latin America, then that commodity is
welcome.*

—Carlos Lehder, 1985

The Political Context

Colombia and Peru are major national producers of illicit drugs. Unlike Bolivia, both countries confront sizable left-wing guerrilla movements. Rural insurgency and drug production or smuggling facilities may be collocated: Both thrive in rugged areas where the central government is weak and where a nationally integrated economic infrastructure is absent. The question is: Do drug traffickers and guerrillas simply coexist in these areas, or do they actively collaborate?

Many reports suggest collaboration. In Colombia and Peru, guerrillas reportedly finance their revolutionary activities by taxing the drug trade. The guerrillas also allegedly protect traffickers, plantations, laboratories, and airstrips against raids by government forces. One Colombian guerrilla group, the Fuerzas Armadas Revolucionarias Colombianas (FARC), is accused of owning its own coca plantations and processing laboratories— of being in the business, so to speak. Drug traffickers purportedly finance guerrilla ventures that serve their interests. Some U.S. and Colombian officials allege that traffickers backed the raid by the 19th of April Movement (M-19) on the Colombian Palace of Justice in November 1985—an operation that cost the lives of nearly half of Colombia's Supreme Court Justices. Other reports posit a different kind of link, alleging that guerrilla groups (especially in Peru) cultivate ties with coca farmers and others whose livelihoods are threatened by drug eradication programs.

Interpretation of the narco-guerrilla connection, such as it is, depends less on hard evidence—which seems to be in chronic short supply—than on the vagaries of politics and the motives of different institutional actors. Reagan Administration officials, especially in the early years of the Administration, aggressively promoted the notion of a drugs-insurgency nexus— an "unholy alliance," as some officials put it. The alliance theory reflected a general tendency of the Administration to fit many North-South issues into the framework of East-West conflict and the struggle against communism. Yet, the theory also served a propagandistic purpose, namely, advancing the threat perceptions of South American governments and publics to alert them to the evils of the drug trade.

In South America, the narco-guerrilla thesis (whatever its intrinsic validity) serves a variety of political and institutional purposes: for example, to discredit the left, to undermine the government's peace incentives for guerrillas, to disguise the connection of cocaine traffickers with established groups (such as the military), and to extract more foreign aid from the United States. (Narco-guerrillas make a better argument for expanded drug assistance programs than do just plain narcos.) In Colombia, the narco-guerrilla stereotype clearly constitutes a drug-fighting tool, a way to counter the powerful cocaine mafia, which itself is trying to shape public opinion. Affixing a Marxist label to the mafia interferes with its efforts to build a patriotic and public-spirited image.

Cocaine dealers, as might be expected, disavow any connection to the revolutionary left. As Pablo Escobar said, "You can accuse me of being a narcotics dealer, but to say that I'm in league with the guerrillas, well, that really hurts my personal dignity."[1] Spokesmen for Colombia's FARC and Peru's Sendero Luminoso deny financing their revolutionary activities from the drug trade. The political secretary of the FARC, Jacobo Arenas, brands the narco-guerrilla theory as part of a CIA-led "world-wide campaign against the revolutionary movement, against democracy, against the social progress of peoples."[2] The FARC's top military leader, Manuel Marulanda, notes, "Guerrillas and the narcotics traffic have nothing to do with one another. We are something very different."[3] A leader of Colombia's M-19 movement says about narcotics traffickers, "We have not had any relationship with them. We have repeatedly said that we are not interested in any relation—there has never been an official meeting between drug traffickers and the M-19 to discuss anything."[4]

At the same time, top political leaders such as Belisario Betancur and Virgilio Barco in Colombia have displayed relatively little interest in the narco-guerrilla connection. "The fight against narcotics will not stop," Betancur said in 1984, "but there is no analogy between this fight and the response to the armed groups."[5] In Colombia, presidents have had a personal stake in negotiating an end to civil strife—in promoting a dialogue with guerrillas and incorporating them into legitimate political life. The narco-guerrilla thesis makes for bad peace politics. Indeed, as a close political adviser to President Barco noted, the thesis creates some embarrassing and potentially unmanageable dilemmas for governments.

Is it possible to make peace with narco-guerrillas? Is it possible to give amnesty and pardons to drug traffickers? Is it possible, on the other hand, to extradite guerrillas? Can we leave to the Drug Enforcement Agency the treatment of the guerrilla problem in Colombia?[6]

In Peru, Fernando Belaunde Terry, who was president from 1980 to 1985, was a strong proponent of the narco-guerrilla thesis. The drug traffic, Terry believed, replaced international assistance from communist countries as a source of financing for revolutionary movements in Peru and other Latin American countries. Belaunde's successor, Alan García, for a long time seemed to reject the thesis, possibly because—like Colombia's leaders—he was committed to an eventual accommodation with guerrillas. However, in late November 1988, during a televised speech in Lima, García said that the "alliance between drug traffickers and subversives is the paramount threat to Peruvian democracy."

What, then, is the reality of the relationship? The weight of evidence suggests that although there are linkages between the cocaine industry and revolutionary organizations, these linkages do not add up to an alliance. Indeed, cocaine traffickers and guerrillas are usually competitors and sometimes mortal enemies. The complex interactions between the two groups can be summarized as follows.

First, most narcotics traffickers are not natural revolutionaries. They seek to buy into, to manipulate, and sometimes to coerce the political system, but not to change it in any fundamental way. Some of the mafia's actions—for example, the murders of prominent antidrug crusaders in Colombia—are destabilizing. However, the aim of mafia violence is creating a secure environment for business operations, not upsetting the political status quo. Given their limited objectives, drug traffickers do not typically engage in terrorism; they do not, for example, target public buildings, military bases, industrial property, or the civilian population at large.

Second, the relationship between traffickers and the revolutionary left is characterized by hostility as well as cooperation. In general, the stronger and more developed the trafficking organization, the less likely it is to collaborate with guerrillas. Narco-guerrilla conflict apparently centers on issues such as territorial control, relations with the coca-growing peasantry, and the distribution of economic benefits from the drug trade. In Colombia, conflict has been intensified by the cocaine mafia's purchase of large landed estates in areas that traditionally were guerrilla strongholds.

Third, some insurgent groups finance their activities in part by taxing the cocaine industry. However, the financial nexus is far stronger in the upstream phases of the industry (cultivation and low-level processing) than in the more lucrative downstream phases (refining and exporting). Most cocaine hydrochloride laboratories in Colombia are not "protected" by guerrillas. They are located in areas where drug traffickers have a preponderance of power (such as the Middle Magdalena Valley) or in regions where the guerrilla presence is virtually nonexistent (such as the Amazon jungle regions). Moreover, the connection seems to be more fully developed in Colombia than in Peru—unlike Colombia's rural-based guerrilla groups, Sendero Luminoso does not have a clear financial strategy vis-à-vis the cocaine trade.

Fourth, guerrilla organizations in Colombia and Peru have built a base of political (as opposed to merely financial) support among the coca-growing peasantry. Guerrillas play on class divisions between coca growers and cocaine operators and on peasants' hostility toward U.S.-financed eradication campaigns.

Some points of similarity do exist between cocaine traffickers and Marxist insurgent groups: They both rely on violence to promote their objectives, they both often share the same territory, they both use the same clandestine methods of operation, and they both operate outside the law. Extant trafficker-guerrilla ties, however, are basically low-level, opportunistic, and intermittent; they do not constitute a pattern of strategic cooperation. (Colombia's Carlos Lehder represents one possible exception to this rule—his case will be described in detail below.) In general, the narco-guerrilla stereotype is a misleading one, obscuring a more fundamental and more insidious reality: the increasing penetration by South American cocaine traffickers into established economic and political institutions.

The Relationship

The Setting

Narcotics traffickers and subversives are not natural friends. They do not share a common political and ideological agenda. They pursue basically different goals. Guerrillas attempt to overthrow the government and to transform society; traffickers, on the other hand, seek above all to be left alone, aspiring to a kind of quasi-legality within the political status quo. Drug dealers, especially the larger operators, do hold some anti-establishment views: They are strongly anti-U.S., and they favor a more egalitarian structure. Traffickers' populism, however, is a function of their drive for legitimacy and social acceptance and forms part of their protection strategy (as indicated in Chapter 3). Furthermore, traffickers are socially part of the big bourgeoisie. As landowners, ranchers, and owners of industrial property (including cocaine laboratories), dealers are far more closely aligned with the traditional power structure than with the revolutionary left—indeed, they are inclined to perceive the latter as a mortal threat.

In both Colombia and Peru, guerrilla organizations have successfully cultivated ties with coca growers, capitalizing, among other things, on the growers' fears of eradication. (Unfortunately, U.S. antidrug policies have produced a political bonanza for guerrillas, especially in Peru's Upper Huallaga Valley.) Guerrillas also play on peasants' resentment against drug dealers, who pay the lowest possible price for their coca leaves and coca paste. On an ideological level, groups such as Colombia's FARC and Peru's Sendero Luminoso distinguish between coca cultivation ("a social problem") and narcotics trafficking ("a product of social decay"). FARC and Sendero cast the peasants as the victims of both government oppression and exploitation by unscrupulous drug barons.[7]

The narco-guerrilla link, however, apparently deteriorates in the downstream phases of the cocaine industry. Cocaine dealers and guerrillas compete bitterly for territory and resources and for control over the coca-growing peasantry. Guerrillas increase the industry's business overhead; traffickers must either pay protection money (war taxes) to guerrillas or make large outlays to guard their laboratories, drug shipments, and clandestine airfields. The Colombian mafia—which invests much of its newfound wealth in farms, ranches, and landed estates in Colombia's relatively unprotected hinterland—is vulnerable to extortion by FARC guerrillas, because its class interests and those of Colombia's traditional rural elite are identical. In addition, in many rural areas, guerrillas try to drive a wedge between local cocaine dealers and cultivators of coca leaves. For example, in the "red" or liberated zones established by Sendero in the Upper Huallaga Valley, the guerrillas are mobilizing peasants to demand higher prices for their leaves and paste.[8] The generally depressed world prices for cocaine in 1987 and 1988—less than two-thirds of the price prevailing in 1985—already were putting great pressure on traffickers' profit margins. Sendero's pro-peasant line thus aggravates an already difficult situation for Peru's cocaine industry.

Patterns of Conflict

The conflicting social and economic interests cited above provoked confrontations. In Colombia, drug traffickers spearheaded efforts to organize ranchers and farmers to resist attacks by local guerrilla forces. Indeed, traffickers played the role of white knights. For years, guerrillas routinely extorted protection money from local landowners. Those who did not pay saw their farms burned down and their family members kidnapped. But when the big capos arrived and became the neighbors of the traditional landed gentry, the neighborhood actually improved, at least temporarily. The narcos created local self-defense associations. They brought in paramilitary squads that formed the nucleus of private armies. They received the enthusiastic backing of local farmers, cattlemen, and military commanders. For example, Gonzalo Rodríguez Gacha organized such a self-defense league of local landowners near Acacias in northwestern Meta department. His efforts apparently succeeded in driving off the FARC. In parts of the Middle Magdalena Valley, tripartite alliances of ranchers, cocaine dealers, and military men have expelled guerrilla forces and eliminated their peasant supporters. These countermeasures, however, are not always successful. A Medellín businessman who owns a farm near the Gulf of Uraba in Antioquia recently admitted in an interview that he and other landowners once paid dues to the local chapter of Muerte a Los Secuestradores (MAS), a mafia-backed vigilante organization. The FARC subsequently gathered strength in the area, and the MAS group collapsed. Now the businessman pays dues to the FARC.

Breaking the pattern of guerrilla extortion may be a worthy cause. Yet, the human rights consequences of such rural vigilantism have been horrendous. The white knights apparently have massacred scores of peasants who collaborated or sympathized with guerrillas. The events of March–April 1988 in the Uraba region of Antioquia provide a grisly example. On March 4, a group of 30 men armed with automatic weapons walked into a banana plantation shouting, "Long live peace, down with the Unión Patriótica and the Popular Front." (These are the civilian arms, respectively, of the FARC and of another guerrilla group, the Popular Liberation Army, or EPL). The gunmen awakened sleeping banana workers, lined up 17 of them against a wall, and shot them immediately. They then went to a second farm and killed three more peasants. Most of the workers apparently were members of the Popular Front. The same group of assassins killed nine more Uraba peasants the following month.[9] Preliminary allegations about these incidents suggest a rather vast conspiracy:

- The hitmen were recruited from Puerto Boyaca in the Middle Magdalena Valley, and Pablo Escobar and Gonzalo Rodríguez Gacha paid their salaries.
- Escobar and Rodríguez Gacha were acting on behalf of a shadowy group known as the Association of Peasants and Cattlemen of the Middle Magdalena, which owned banana plantations and other agricultural interests in the Uraba region.
- The killers were trained on estates belonging to a retired drug trafficker, Fidel Castaño, an associate of Pablo Escobar.
- The mayor of Puerto Boyaca helped to recruit the assassins and to coordinate their travel to Uraba.
- Local military commanders in Uraba drew up lists of suspected subversives and led the killers to their targets.[10]

There was another such massacre in April. A group of 10 men armed to the teeth machine-gunned to death 36 peasants during an Easter festival at a hacienda, "La Florida," near the Cordoba village of La Mejor Esquina, killing 15 percent of the village in the attack. The celebration, in fact, was held at a hacienda belonging to an alleged drug trafficker, Cesar Cura, who "paid 120,000 pesos for the orchestra and helped with other organizational aspects of the fiesta." In other words, the entire affair seemingly was a cruel trap. The Mejor Esquina killers, like their Uraba counterparts, may have been trained on Fidel Castaño's ranches. The reasons for the slayings are somewhat obscure, but the campesinos of Mejor Esquina, like many of the Uraba victims, apparently were members of the EPL-dominated Popular Front.[11]

The dirty war has extended to Colombia's towns and cities. Right-wing vigilante groups, many financed by drug money, have been carrying out an extermination campaign against members of the extreme left: labor organizers, university professors, amnestied guerrillas, human rights activists, and left-wing political leaders. Approximately one-third of the Unión Patriótica (UP) mayoralty candidates were massacred (many by drug traffickers) in the 6 months preceding the March 1988 elections. According to Colombia's Justice Minister, Rodríguez Gacha paid 30 million pesos (about $120,000) to henchmen to arrange the assassination on October 11, 1987, of Colombia's foremost leftist leader, Jaime Pardo Leal, the head of the UP. After the murder, Rodríguez reportedly hosted a reception for the killers—the three men hired to do the job—at one of his estates in his home town of Pacho.[12]

The slaying was the culmination of a long-standing vendetta between Rodríguez Gacha and the FARC. In early 1985, for example, the FARC tried to levy a vacuña (head tax) on 600 head of cattle that Rodríguez maintained at a ranch in San Martín (in the northwestern part of Meta department). Rodríguez imported a paramilitary squad from Puerto Boy-aca in the Middle Magdalena Valley. The hit squad ambushed and killed 10 guerrillas who came to collect the tax. Some observers, such as Fabio Castillo, trace the beginning of hostilities to late 1983, when the FARC successfully invaded one of Rodríguez Gacha's properties in the Llanos and made off with quantities of coca leaves, weapons, and cash (see the discussion later in this chapter).

Such carnage is in part a retaliation for the FARC's attacks on laborato-ries and other *narcotraficante* property. The mafia is not equipped to conduct search-and-destroy missions against guerrillas, so an alternative retaliation strategy is employed. Bogotá columnist "Ayatollah" recently remarked, "It is easier to assassinate members of the UP, born of the entrails of the FARC, than to enter into an armed confrontation with a guerrilla force which is more skillful, better prepared and which knows the territory very well."[13] The mafia also harbors a second strategic objective: Traffickers simply do not want communist leadership in the towns near their ranches and cocaine trafficking operations.

Vigilantism—which can be defined as establishment violence—is cer-tainly not a new phenomenon in Colombia, but it received a tremendous stimulus from the rise of the cocaine trafficking elite. Take, for example, the history of the paramilitary group MAS. In November 1981, M-19 guerrillas broke into the University of Antioquia in Medellín, grabbed Marta Nieves Ochoa (Jorge Ochoa's sister), and demanded $1 million in ransom. The Ochoa clan responded by calling a summit meeting of Colombia's leading cocaine dealers. The meeting, which reportedly was held in Medellín's Intercontinental Hotel and was attended by 223 drug lords, resulted in the formation of MAS. The founders pledged to contrib-ute a total of $4.5 million to the new organization. They subsequently issued a communiqué that was broadly distributed in Colombia, "handed out at busy city intersections and dropped from helicopters into crowded soccer stadiums."[14] The contents were a classic statement of vigilantes' principles, reading in part:

> At an emergency meeting, held only a few days ago, 223 mafia bosses met exclusively to discuss the issue of kidnapping. The mafia is aware that several kidnappings have taken and will be taking place throughout the nation;
>
> Kidnappings have been carried out both by common criminals and subversive elements, with the latter trying to finance their activities by targeting people like us, whose hard-earned money has brought progress and employment to this country, and much-needed schools, hospitals, etc.;
>
> At said meeting, the 223 mafia bosses, representing every region of the country, agreed to finance this endeavor through personal contributions of 2 million pesos

each [approximately $20,000] . . . In our effort to fight the practice of kidnapping, these resources will be used to pay for rewards, execution of perpetrators, and equipment;

At said meeting, we also agreed to create an operative group called MAS which will be under the direct control of the mafia; . . . .

Kidnappers will be executed in public; they will be hanged from trees in public places or shot by firing squads. They will be duly marked with a small cross which is the symbol of our organization—MAS; . . . .

A 20 million peso reward [approximately $200,000] has been created for those who, personally and directly, provide us with information on kidnappings . . . .[15]

MAS began a series of reprisals—taking some M-19 leaders hostage, turning others over to the Colombian army, and executing as many as 100 people associated with the organization. Some of the victims were hanged from trees as the MAS communique had promised. In one of its more colorful acts, MAS chained a young woman to the gates of the Medellín newspaper *El Colombiano,* with a sign identifying her as an M-19 militant and the wife of one of Marta Ochoa's kidnappers.[16]

Much of the M-19's organization was destroyed as a result of those reprisals, and the guerrillas had no choice but to sue for peace. In February 1982, the M-19 returned the Ochoa girl (no ransom was paid). There are reports that representatives of the organization and of the Medellín mafia met later that year and concluded a truce agreement. Yet, this was hardly the end of MAS, which grew and prospered, attracting establishment groups that had particular reason to despise guerrillas—again, members of the rural elite, right-wing businessmen, law enforcement officers, and elements of the military. In the middle sector of the Magdalena River Valley—where cocaine dealers had begun to purchase farms and ranches—MAS, the military, and local landholders formed a "triangle of terror" to hunt down guerrillas and their sympathizers.[17] In 1983, Colombia's Attorney General indicted 59 military men, including 11 officers, for being MAS members. MAS evolved into more than an anti-kidnapping organization, targeting political activists such as university professors, union organizers, students, civil rights workers, amnestied guerrillas, and left-wing party leaders. MAS spawned numerous clone organizations that operate nationally or regionally—for example, the Colombian Anti-Communist Alliance (AAC); the Colombian Anti-Communist Youth (JACOC); the American Anti-Communist Alliance (AAA); Death to Kidnappers and Communists (MASCO), which is based on the north coast; and Death to the Revolutionaries of Uraba (MRU).[18]

What about the supposed ties between the M-19 and the Medellín syndicates? There are some indications that mafia vigilantism in the 1980s was directed more against other revolutionary groups (the FARC and the EPL) than against the M-19. The M-19 apparently desisted from kidnapping family members of cocaine capos. Yet, the agreement did not involve collaboration (see the discussion of the Palace of Justice incident later in this chapter). A raid in September 1988 by troops of the Fourth Army brigade on an M-19 headquarters in Medellín discovered documentary evidence of a guerrilla plot to kidnap for ransom four close relatives of Pablo Escobar and two lawyers working for Escobar's organization. The agreement, such as it was, has apparently ceased to exist.[19]

In Peru, drug dealers and guerrillas apparently do not compete strategically, as they do in Colombia. Peru has not yet developed a self-conscious narco-bourgeois class comparable to those in Colombia and Bolivia. Peru's cocaine traffickers are mostly small-timers, heavily dependent on Colombian traffickers for leadership and weapons and extremely competitive with each other. Peru's cocaine traffickers have not developed a coordinated anticommunist strategy. Still, the Upper Huallaga Valley is the site of many bloody confrontations between cocaine trafficking gangs and Sendero Luminoso guerrillas. In the last half of 1987, clashes were recorded in or near the Valley towns of Sion, Uchiza, and Paraíso. The October 10 Paraíso shootout was an ambush staged by Sendero against one of the Valley's leading cocaine dealers, known as Machis, in retaliation for his efforts to organize the residents of Uchiza district against the guerrillas. (Machis was rescued from the encirclement by units of the Peruvian antinarcotics police flown in by U.S.-piloted helicopters; he is now in jail.)[20] According to an article in Bogotá's *El Tiempo,* Colombian crime syndicates in early 1988 dispatched 300 heavily armed traffickers to the Upper Huallaga Valley to help Peruvian traffickers protect cocaine shipments and supply routes against Sendero attacks.[21]

Given this pattern of conflict, it is not surprising that the Colombian sociologist Alfredo Molano suggests that drug dealers "can develop certain forms of cooperation and a tacit alliance with the state."[22] From the state's perspective, after all, guerrillas pose a greater strategic threat (or at least a more obvious threat) than the cocaine industry. For example, military factions in Colombia have been linked to cocaine traffickers through common membership in right-wing vigilante squads such as MAS. Colombian military units occasionally protect cocaine laboratories against FARC extortion attempts. In a November 1983 incident, for example, a Colombian Special Forces team from Villavicencio helped a cocaine trafficker move an entire laboratory complex from an area controlled by the First FARC Front to a safer location near the Brazilian border. The operation, which involved 5 officers and 43 noncoms, required 26 days.[23] During a

1984–1985 state of emergency in the Upper Huallaga Valley, Peruvian military commanders relied heavily on local cocaine dealers for information on the whereabouts, strengths, and weaponry of Sendero forces.

Areas of Convergence

Narco-guerrilla confrontation is not an across-the-board phenomenon. Cocaine dealers and Marxist guerrillas share certain perspectives: Both are ultra-nationalistic and (for different reasons) violently hostile to "Yankee imperialism." In Colombia, all of the major guerrilla groups and the cocaine mafia hold virtually identical opinions on the extradition treaty—that is, traffickers should not be tried in the United States by U.S. judges and under U.S. law. As an emerging social class—a "new illegitimate bourgeoisie"—cocaine dealers exhibit values, habits, and political views very different from those of the Colombian oligarchy. Pablo Escobar, for example, espouses the cause of slum dwellers and of "marginal people" in general. The Escobar family newspaper, *Medellín Cívico,* professes strong support for the Liberal party, but has a decidedly populist orientation. Recent articles in the newspaper criticized "the fabulous profits" of industrialists, claimed that "we are good friends of the working class," and advocated "employment for all, education for all, health for all, and bread for all."[24]

The nationalist-populist fervor of Colombian narcotics traffickers reached its most extreme form in the bizarre political philosophy of Carlos Lehder, who founded a fascist political movement, the Movimiento Latino Nacional (MLN), in his native department of Quindío. The MLN's raison d'etre was campaigning against the extradition treaty, but the party also supported a radical political program that called for replacing Colombia's traditional political parties with mass popular organizations. Although a fascist, Lehder maintained ties with several Colombian revolutionary organizations, and his party supported the extreme leftist (UP) candidate in the 1986 presidential elections. Lehder never backed the 1984 initiative of 100 top cocaine traffickers to negotiate with the Colombian government. He did not sign the manifesto that read in part, "We have no connection with, nor do we accept any such connection with armed guerrillas. Our activities have never been designed to replace the democratic and republican form of government."[25] Lehder's radicalism almost certainly put him at odds with Colombia's cocaine establishment. Indeed, many Colombian observers believe that the Medellín syndicates viewed Lehder as an embarrassment, were eager to cultivate a pro-establishment image, and consequently betrayed the trafficker to authorities.[26] Lehder now is in jail in the United States, probably forever.

The Colombian Pattern

Extortion and Protection

Clear signs—in Colombia at least—indicate that rural-based guerrilla organizations levy war taxes on the cocaine industry. The linkage is clearest in the case of the FARC—the "oldest and longest-standing guerrilla organization in all of Latin America."[27] The FARC exercises intermittent political and military control over some important coca-growing zones in the southern and eastern Llanos region. In these zones, coca farmers and leaf processors reportedly pay a tax of 10–15 percent on their outputs. The FARC also taxes the wages of laborers in the coca fields at a rate of 7–10 percent.[28]

However, the FARC's ability to shake down the Medellín-Cali syndicates is problematic. There is little evidence on this point; however, two general observations can be made. First, the cocaine syndicates (unlike the minor mafia of independent processors and refiners) hire well-armed security forces to guard their laboratories, supply routes, and cocaine shipments. Furthermore, they have the financial resources to purchase additional protection against guerrillas from local Colombian army units. The big cocaine operators can insulate their cocaine operations (at least in part) against guerrilla extortion attempts. Much depends on the local balance of forces at any given time: In southern Antioquia, a mafia stronghold, cocaine traffickers are less likely to pay taxes than in southern Caqueta, a region predominantly controlled by the FARC. Second, deteriorating market conditions in the cocaine industry—the U.S. wholesale price of cocaine dropped from $55,000 per kilo in 1980 to $15,000 per kilo in mid-1988—create strong incentives for cocaine traffickers not to pay protection money to guerrillas. No doubt the declining size of the "cocaine pie" has constituted an important factor in the recent open hostilities between cocaine operators and guerrillas in both Colombia and Peru.

Some of the reports of war taxes paid by cocaine operators to guerrillas are extremely suspect. For example, Colombian authorities reported that a large cocaine hydrochloride laboratory discovered in Vichada department in September 1988 paid 70 million pesos a month in protection money to the FARC. At prevailing rates of exchange, this would amount to $2.8 million a year. The economics of the alleged relationship are absurd. According to Colombia's Minister of Defense, General Rafael Samudo, Colombia's military expenditures per soldier amount to $1,300 per year. Drug traffickers paying double this rate could maintain a 500-man army for less than half the sum allegedly paid to the FARC. Such a force would be more than sufficient to protect the laboratory against any conceivable

FARC pressure or, for that matter, against forays by the antinarcotics police, whose total force numbers only 1,800 men.[29]

Whatever financial ties might bond cocaine traffickers and insurgents must be evaluated from the perspective of Colombia's overall security situation. The predominant political and military forces in many outlying regions of the country are guerrilla organizations, which have developed a financial strategy of exploiting all production assets in the areas that they control. Guerrilla targets, in addition to the cocaine industry, include cattle ranchers, farmers, merchants, hacienda owners, oil companies, and construction companies.

A recent incident in the intendency of Arauca illustrates the universality of the shakedown pattern. A German construction company, Mannesmann-Anlagenbau, was hired in 1984 to build a 170-mile pipeline from the Cravo Norte oil field to a terminal station at Rio Zulia (in north Santander department). The area along the pipeline route was more or less out of the hands of the central government, controlled by a particularly vicious antigovernment group called the National Liberation Army (ELN). Not long after Mannesmann started work on the pipeline, ELN kidnapped four of its employees and exchanged them for a $4-million ransom paid by the company. In addition, ELN reportedly orchestrated a number of work stoppages and even threatened to blow up the pipeline. In mid-1985, the commandant of the Colombian armed forces and the president of the Colombian Farmers Association accused Mannesmann of signing a pact with the guerrillas at the end of 1984 to pay a monthly war tax of $200,000 in return for an end to the harassment. Occidental Petroleum, the operator of the Cravo Norte field, was implicated initially in the payoffs, but, as the scandal developed, Mannesmann became the principal focus of attention.[30]

The Mannesmann affair created a political storm in Colombia. Some of the Colombian and foreign reactions are worth noting. Mannesmann, although denying the charge, removed its general manager from the country. The president of the company later visited Colombia and met with Betancur to smooth relations. The Colombian government issued a stern official warning to foreign companies against making payoffs to guerrilla groups. Armand Hammer, Occidental's chairman, made the extraordinary admission that his company was providing jobs to the guerrillas—presumably this meant employing them in the oil fields.[31] There were the predictable jingoistic statements that multinational oil firms were abetting subversion in Colombia and contributing to "the demoralization and deterioration of our fundamental institutions." At a meeting of the Democratic International Union in Washington in August 1985, former Colombian President Miguel Pastrano Borrero said that two factors contributed to the rise of terrorism in his country: the alliance with drug trafficking and financial support from transnational enterprises.[32]

Relationships between foreign multinationals and guerrillas persist to the present day. Interviews with representatives of several foreign oil companies in Colombia focused on security-management issues. The representatives deny making cash payments to the guerrillas à la Mannesmann. Yet, they admit that establishing a modus vivendi with a hostile environment means making compromises, including giving guerrillas or suspected guerrillas jobs, food, medicines, medical care, and valuable equipment such as radios, flashlights, and generators.

Obviously, then, drug traffickers and guerrillas are not engaged in an exclusive relationship. The point seems obvious, but it must be stressed, because the term narco-guerrilla carries certain ideological connotations— that is, it suggests a common anti-establishment posture. The inference is not warranted. If there are narco-guerrillas, then there must also be petro-guerrillas, rancho-guerrillas, and *ganadero*-guerrillas: The FARC and other insurgent movements fill their coffers from many sources. Indeed, the case can be made that cocaine traffickers, especially the large and powerful mafia organizations, are the best equipped of all the groups operating in Colombia's rural hinterland to resist guerrillas' extortion demands.

To the extent that the cocaine industry does pay taxes to guerrillas, what does it receive in return? One benefit is simply the right to operate in guerrilla-held areas. Moreover, some U.S. and Colombian observers agree that a mutually advantageous relationship has developed in which the FARC provides a substantive protective shield for trafficking operations. According to one theory, FARC contingents act as sentinels or watchmen for drug traffickers, alerting them to the impending arrival of government forces. If offered or provided, such services would benefit primarily the smaller cocaine operators—the minor mafia of independent processors and refiners. Large mafia organizations have little need for guerrilla sentinels; they maintain their own early warning system, relying on networks of official informants to provide tip-offs on planned raids or police sweeps. The FARC supplies short-term tactical intelligence, but the trafficking syndicates, which are well-supplied with manpower and well-equipped with aircraft and sophisticated communications, can fulfill this function as well.

Allegations have been made that the FARC actively defends traffickers' laboratories, plantations, and airstrips. That may happen in some cases, but U.S. and Colombian officials have been too ready to assume the existence of a FARC shield. Occasional reports surface that unidentified people wearing green fatigues fire on police on antidrug missions, but a mafia security force also could wear general military uniforms. Aerial photographs of laboratory sites sometimes show evidence of a guard contingent—hammocks, tents, shower stalls, and so on—but how is one to know whether the guards are guerrillas or traffickers' hired guns? Police and military forces operating in remote areas where both guerrillas and traffickers are active sometimes are fired upon—quite possibly by FARC and other guerrilla groups. Such incidents, however, may reflect general guerrilla-government hostility rather than a conscious strategy of insurgents to set up a defense perimeter around laboratories or cultivating areas.

U.S. and Colombian narcotics authorities occasionally assert that drug traffickers have a policy of supplying arms to guerrillas. The basic channels used to smuggle drugs and those used to smuggle arms clearly overlap to some extent. In a case from the early 1980s, a Colombian smuggler allegedly provided weapons from Cuba to M-19 guerrillas.[33] However, evidence of a sustained connection is absent. In fact, mafia organizations have good reasons for not funneling arms to guerrillas—why would the mafia enhance the guerrillas' power to extort? A Colombian police colonel interviewed in April 1986 indicated that where guerrilla and mafia organizations use the same transportation networks, the latter are not owned and operated by the cocaine syndicates, but rather by independent contractors. This is a technical distinction, perhaps, but an important one. Moreover, as Professor Bruce Bagley notes, most of the guerrilla organizations report that they can buy the arms they need on the black market or even from the military itself. "The link between guerrillas and arms trafficking," Bagley concludes, "has been overstated for political purposes."[34]

Finally, a few reports contend that the FARC has actually moved beyond taxing and protecting the cocaine traffic, that individual fronts cultivate their own coca and even operate their own processing laboratories.[35] Such a prospect is not beyond the realm of possibility—revolutionary organizations in other parts of the world have developed their own production and sales capabilities. (The Burmese Communist party is an outstanding example.) However, the FARC is, formally at least, part of the current peace process in Colombia. The FARC signed a truce agreement with the government and, via its civilian arm, the Unión Patriótica, is actually participating in national and local elections. For the FARC to be involved directly in cultivating coca or in manufacturing and selling cocaine runs counter to its political strategy (although not to its financial strategy). Politically speaking, the FARC is much better off claiming noninvolvement in the trade, while at the same time taxing its proceeds.

In sum, the narco-FARC connection, such as it is, can be characterized as limited, opportunistic, and tenuous. On the narco side of the equation, cooperation represents a cost of doing business that, because of worsening market conditions for cocaine, has become more burdensome over time. The big mafiosi, in fact, actively resist paying off the guerrillas. The FARC shakes down the narcotics industry as a way of raising money for the revolution; however, this apparently is a temporary expedient rather than a long-term strategy.

Indeed, the FARC seems to actively support the cause of drug control, especially with respect to coca cultivation. In the commissariat of Guaviare, for example, the Seventh FARC Front "has promised to cooperate with the government in the rehabilitation of the Guaviare and in curtailing coca cultivation." The quid pro quo for such cooperation is government aid for "substituting coca with food crops."[36] Similarly, in the Caguan region of Caqueta department, the FARC has worked with local community groups—as well as with Colombian government organizations such as the National Institute of Natural Renewable Resources (INDERENA, under the Ministry of Agriculture) and the Institute for Colombian Agricultural Reform (INCORA, also under the Ministry of Agriculture)—to put together an ambitious $25-million regional development plan. The basic thrust of the plan is providing Caguan peasants with a package of incentives for getting out of the coca-growing business. The package includes technical assistance for growing new crops; projects for developing roads, river transport, and telecommunication networks; new sewage and potable water systems; and legalization of peasant land holdings. According to a report from Caguan, "Representatives of both peasants and guerrilla chiefs have accepted the elimination of coca growing and its replacement by healthier economic activities."[37] Such accounts hardly suggest a pronarcotics stance. Although the FARC serves as an advocate for the coca growers vis-à-vis the Colombian government, the ultimate FARC cause apparently is phasing out the coca trade.

Yari, La Uribe, and the Palace of Justice Massacre

It is hard today to find evidence of interactions, other than hostile interactions, among Colombia's top mafiosi and the country's guerrilla groups. However, the relationship must be examined in its historical perspective; conceivably, cocaine traffickers and guerrillas were on better terms in the early and mid-1980s than they now appear to be. The nature and scope of past mafia-guerrilla cooperation will be discussed in some detail below.

In March–April 1984, Colombian police and U.S. narcotics officials conducted a series of raids on what was described as a cocaine industrial complex at Yari (named after the nearby Yari River) in the southeastern part of Caqueta department. Raids in early March discovered 6 airstrip-laboratory clusters (a total of 14 laboratories) stretched over an area of roughly 3,000 square kilometers. At the largest site, a cluster called Tranquilandia, police discovered a phenomenal 14 tons of cocaine, about 20 percent of the estimated exports of the drug from all South American countries in 1983. Tranquilandia apparently was also the administrative center for the Yari operation. A search of that site yielded maps and documents showing that the six sites formed a more or less unified enterprise. The controlling interest was held by several leading Medellín traffickers—Pablo Escobar, the Ochoa family, and Gonzalo Rodríguez Gacha. There were also indications, albeit less clear, that Carlos Lehder played a role in managing the complex.[38]

During the assault on Tranquilandia, the national police were fired upon from the jungle by snipers "in fatigue-type jungle uniforms."[39] Police returned the fire, secured the area, and arrested 40 individuals later identified as members of the laboratory complex. (All of these people were subsequently released by a Caqueta judge.) The snipers, who melted away into the jungle after firing a few shots, were never positively identified.

A second set of raids in April discovered a seventh airstrip with three associated laboratories. The new cluster, designated La Loma, was in the Serranía de Chiribiquete, a hilly area somewhat to the north and west of the other Yari sites. (The closest of these was Pascualandia, about 35 km to the southeast; Tranquilandia was 75 km to the southwest.) Near La Loma, the authorities found clear evidence of a FARC presence: sewing machines, uniforms with yellow triangle patches (the insignia of the Seventh FARC Front), and some literature describing the movement's strategy and goals. Colombian sources estimate that the FARC contingent was relatively small, possibly 15 to 20 men in all.[40]

U.S. and Colombian officials opted to interpret the hostile fire at Tranquilandia and the small FARC camp at La Loma as evidence of a narco-FARC connection in the operation of the Yari laboratories. Guerrillas, they said, were providing perimeter security to the complex. Assertions were made (based on no visible evidence) that the FARC was taxing cocaine processed at Yari at a rate of 10–20 percent. The Medellín cocaine kings and the FARC, it seemed, had joined forces. Yet, problems plague this interpretation. Pilots' maps discovered at Tranquilandia—the nerve center of the complex—did not indicate the existence of a seventh site; that is, La Loma could have been a completely different enterprise with no connection to the Medellín traffickers.[41] Furthermore, La Loma was most likely a case of local coexistence or cooperation. The FARC's presence there did not mean that the FARC was protecting or taxing all the cocaine laboratories at Yari. The true story of Yari will probably never be told; however, recent journalistic accounts and the author's conversations with State Department officials suggest that the original reports of the FARC's involvement in Tranquilandia were incorrect.[42]

In the early 1980s, actual negotiations took place between the FARC and a major mafia leader, Gonzalo Rodríguez Gacha. In his book, *Los Jinetes de la Cocaína (The Cocaine Jockeys),* Fabio Castillo says that Rodríguez Gacha once held discussions with a member of the FARC secretariat, Jacobo Arenas, about the construction of a mafia airstrip in the FARC's central base area at La Uribe (a mountainous stronghold in Caqueta department). Cocaine laboratories might have been part of the deal, although Castillo's account does not mention such a provision. The FARC stronghold, in one of Colombia's most rugged and isolated regions, presumably would have offered the traffickers some real protection against government raids. The La Uribe deal was apparently one of two demands pressed by Rodríguez. Perhaps the only major mafia figure to own coca plantations as well as laboratories, Rodríguez also wanted the FARC to provide armed protection for his cultivations of coca. In return for these concessions, the trafficker—who was already paying the FARC taxes on his lands—was willing to continue or even increase these payments.[43]

The idea of a cocaine-running operation in the middle of their central headquarters horrified the FARC, and the discussions were dropped. Indeed, Rodríguez Gacha's offer seemed more like a provocation or challenge to the FARC (reflecting dissatisfaction with what appeared to be a one-sided relationship) than a serious effort to establish an accommodation with the guerrillas. In any event, there was no accommodation. Shortly after the collapse of the talks, the FARC raided one of Rodríguez's plantations in Guaviare, making off with 180 kilos of coca, 15 pistols and rifles, and $500,000 (U.S.) in cash. This apparently marked the beginning of a vendetta between Rodríguez and the FARC—each side killing the other's supporters—that culminated in the murder in October 1987 of Colombia's top civilian communist leader, Jaime Pardo Leal.[44]

Finally, there is the attack by the M-19 on the Colombian Palace of Justice in Bogotá on November 6, 1985. More than 100 people, 11 Colombian Supreme Court Justices among them, died in the attack and in the ensuing counterattack by the army. The guerrillas who carried out the raid also perished. Some judicial archives, including files on extradition cases (which were merely photocopies of U.S. extradition requests) and testimony on alleged human rights abuses by the Colombian military were incinerated. To this day, it is not clear what happened inside the building. Much of the evidence (including eyewitness accounts) suggests that the judges were killed when the army stormed the building the next day. A single enormous cannon shell that the army fired through the top story of the building killed an estimated 50 people. Similarly, the destruction of the court records may have been an accident—the result of the fires started by the army shelling.[45]

The Palace raid, however, was described in Bogotá and in Washington as evidence of a narco-guerrilla entente. Betancur's Minister of Justice, Enrique Parejo, suggested that the aim was to implement a vendetta against Colombian Supreme Court magistrates who had come out in favor of the extradition treaty. Said Parejo:

> It must be said that there is one thing that must be obvious after this Palace of Justice incident—the alliance between the guerrillas and the drug traffickers. The judges who were the main targets of the attack on the Palace of Justice were precisely those who had been threatened because of their position on the Extradition Treaty . . . .It could have been a coincidence, but I don't think so. There is good evidence that behind the guerrilla action was an action to defend the dark interests of the drug traffickers.[46]

Such an interpretation was enthusiastically supported by ideologists within the Reagan Administration. In January 1987, for example, Assistant Secretary of State (for Latin American Affairs) Eliot Abrams was quoted as saying that the Medellín syndicates paid $5 million to have the extradition files destroyed and the justice hearing the extradition cases murdered.[47] Abrams told the House Foreign Affairs Committee on March 9, 1988:

> In Colombia . . . the combination of guerrillas and drug traffickers is obvious and direct. And the best example is the attack on the Supreme Court . . . where the guerrillas went into the Supreme Court building, the M-19, but the targets were justices and files that had to do with extradition, so there was a direct link there.[48]

There was also speculation in late 1985 and early 1986 that the Nicaraguan Sandinistas had played a role in the M-19's takeover of the Palace. A few rifles and submachine guns traceable to Nicaragua (either to the Sandinistas or to the preceding Somoza regime) were in fact found in the ruins of the Palace. A report published in *El Tiempo* on December 20, 1985, quoted an unnamed official source as saying that a group of Sandinista commandos arrived in Bogotá the day before the occupation and that their commanders coordinated the operation and gave instructions to the guerrillas. Some U.S. and Colombian officials apparently believed that the raid was the product of a tripartite Sandinista, M-19, and drug trafficker alliance. However, CIA and DEA officials were openly skeptical of at least the connection between the Sandinistas and the M-19.[49]

Many opinion leaders in Colombia, including some of Betancur's personal advisers, questioned such explanations. A special investigative committee of justice set up by the surviving members of the court concluded in June 1986 that neither the Medellín syndicates nor the Sandinista government had any connection to the raid. A separate inquiry conducted by Betancur's Attorney General, Carlos Jiménez Gómez, also concluded that the M-19 had acted alone (the Jiménez report was issued in June).[50] The theory of a linkage between the M-19 and the traffickers is especially difficult to sustain. The pattern of events tended to contradict the theory— the bloodbath resulting from the army's recapture of the Palace, the burning of court documents other than extradition files, and the fact that these files themselves were mainly photocopies (that is, their destruction would have served no useful purpose). The M-19's own statements immediately after the incident do not even mention the extradition issue. Such statements describe the takeover of the Palace as a protest against the supposed failure of the Colombian government to respect a peace agreement signed with the guerrillas in 1984. Declared one M-19 spokesman, Rudolfo Restredo, "The main objective was to return to the peace process and engage in dialogue again."[51] "The central idea," said a member of the M-19's national board of directors who called himself Commandante Alonso, "was to publicly denounce the government before the country. We didn't think there was going to be an intense fight." Alonso denied that the raid was financed by drug money, although he referred rather mysteriously to "friends" of the M-19 among the traffickers.[52]

Furthermore, it is difficult to believe that this high-profile terrorist venture was backed by Colombia's politically conservative cocaine establishment. Such support would only reinforce the official narco-guerrilla thesis, and the cocaine mafia, in its unceasing quest for political legitimacy, would have no desire to be linked to the revolutionary left. Furthermore, assassination by proxy is not the mafia's style. As a threatening message sent by The Extraditables to several Colombian Supreme Court justices in December 1986 declared, "You say that we were involved in the events of the Palace of Justice. Yet we need neither allies nor mercenaries. We have sufficient capacity ourselves and we have demonstrated this on many occasions."[53] Relying on the M-19 to kill judges would defeat one of the mafia's main objectives, which is to demonstrate its independent power vis-à-vis the state. Finally, mafia executions of judges and other public officials are carefully planned, highly individualized acts of vengeance (or warning). The instruments of death—gunmen riding on motorcycles—are virtually always the same. The cocaine mafia also engages in collective violence—witness the bloodbaths at Uraba and La Mejor Esquina—but the victims are peasants, not people with political and social stature.

It is most unlikely that the Medellín cocaine establishment had anything to do with the Palace of Justice massacre. However, some Colombian observers—although acknowledging the point—suggest that Carlos Lehder might have played a role in the affair. Lehder was the one major Colombian drug dealer who fit the description of a friend of the M-19. To reiterate an earlier point, Carlos Lehder's revolutionary politics set him apart from the other Colombian capos. He did not seek negotiation or accommodation with the Colombian government. He did not accept Colombia's two-party system: Rather, he wanted to overthrow the oligarchy and establish a radically different political order in Colombia. Lehder was ideologically ambidextrous. Although the leader of a fascist political party and an admirer of Hitler, he openly sought a dialogue with the extreme leftist M-19. The M-19 apparently fit into Lehder's paranoid vision; it was "nationalist," "revolutionary," and "against the extradition of Colombians to the United States."[54] Lehder's hatred of the Colombian government (which had already approved his extradition) and of the United States could have led him to form an association with the Movement.

If Lehder did not have a working relationship with the M-19, he at least might have had advance knowledge of the Palace of Justice raid. Although making a political statement against extradition was not the M-19's main concern, there still could have been a basis for an agreement with Lehder. The M-19 needed a financial boost, and Lehder saw in the M-19's plans an opportunity to promote his own political agenda. Paying the raiders to destroy extradition documents and to eliminate pro-extradition judges would have been in character for Lehder—hostility toward the extradition treaty, after all, lay at the heart of the trafficker's paranoid political vision. Such conclusions, however, are purely speculative: There is no credible evidence that the M-19 received support from Lehder—or any outside support, for that matter—in staging the occupation of the Palace.

The Peruvian Pattern

What Connection?

U.S. and Peruvian officials have never been able to define a precise link between Sendero Luminoso and the drug trade. Sendero is extremely elusive, and relatively little is known about its structure or operating strategy. Some sources interviewed in Lima and Tingo María doubt that Sendero has developed and implemented a financial strategy of shaking down the cocaine trade. The reasoning goes that Sendero would have the wherewithal to purchase sophisticated weapons if it were exploiting the trade. Yet, Sendero so far has made no display of expensive weaponry: Its armament (much of it captured from the police or the military) comprises revolvers, outdated rifles and shotguns, a few machine guns, and dynamite.

The converse is also true: The poor quality of Sendero's arsenal puts it at a disadvantage vis-à-vis drug operators. In Peru's Upper Huallaga Valley, traffickers and even coca growers (especially in the Tocache area) are armed with the latest automatic weapons—Ingrams, Uzis, and Urus. They rely on sophisticated booby traps and warning systems to protect their laboratories and plantations. The balance of military force in the Valley seems to favor the traffickers (who are closely linked to multinational Colombian organizations) over the guerrillas.

On the other hand, Sendero may prevail in individual confrontations— witness the October 1987 shootout at Paraíso described above. Furthermore, as already noted, Sendero has developed strong political ties with peasants in some parts of the Upper Huallaga Valley, and the movement's base of mass support may compensate somewhat for its lack of weaponry. According to some reports, cocaine dealers pay Sendero a tax on some shipments of cocaine that leave the Valley. In fact, traffickers may pay protection money to local police and military garrisons and to Sendero guerrillas for the same shipment (see the discussion on corruption in Chapter 5). A few traffickers may actively collaborate with guerrillas. One Peruvian trafficker named *Vampiro* (because he lacks all his front teeth except for two upper incisors) reportedly allowed his house to be used as a command post by Sendero Luminoso guerrillas when Sendero briefly occupied the Upper Huallaga Valley town of Tocache in April 1987. Still, the narco-guerrilla relationship apparently is primarily competitive, with each side trying to stake out territories (red and white zones, to use Sendero's terminology) where it can exercise predominant control.

Sendero's current strategy in the Huallaga appears to be oriented toward developing ties with peasants rather than drug traffickers. As noted earlier in this chapter, Sendero plays on peasants' fears of U.S.-backed eradication campaigns. Sendero also helps peasants resist exploitation by the cocaine dealers, who purchase their leaves and paste; there are even accounts of guerrillas executing traffickers who cheat the peasants.[55] A few reports contend that Sendero collects taxes from coca growers, "using the funds to pay for medicine and civic projects needed by the villagers themselves."[56] However, the movement's ability or disposition to tax the cocaine trade, as opposed to coca cultivation, are less certain.

The García administration seems to have converted recently to the theory of an alliance between drug traffickers and subversives. One wonders whether the conversion is based on solid evidence or on political factors. The administration is teetering on the brink of collapse; possibly

García is trying to present a tough anticommunist image to shore up his waning political fortunes.

Alan García's predecessor, Fernando Belaunde Terry, and Belaunde's Interior Minister, Luis Percovich Roca, were among South America's foremost proponents of the alliance theory (Belaunde called the supposed relationship "narco-terrorism"). The Belaunde administration held as political gospel that cocaine dealers provided Sendero Luminoso with money and arms, and in return Sendero protected drug shipments and distracted the armed forces and the police so that traffickers could operate freely.[57] More than a little irony inhered in these allegations. For example, the Peruvian military, which controlled the Upper Huallaga Valley during a 1984-1985 state of emergency, was enriching itself from the cocaine trade and collaborating with cocaine dealers in antiguerrilla operations. In addition, drug-related corruption had spread to the very top of the Peruvian government. The notorious cocaine trafficker Reynaldo Rodríguez (referred to in Chapter 3) was the center of a drug ring that apparently extended to several PIP generals and (very ironically) to a personal adviser to Percovich Roca. The narco-guerrilla, it can be hypothesized, was in part a projection of the Belaunde regime's own internal rot.

The Impact of Drug Control Programs

Many U.S. and Peruvian observers believe that rebel activities were prompted not so much by the cocaine trade itself, but rather by attempts to control it. In testimony before two U.S. Senate subcommittees in May 1985, then Deputy Assistant Secretary for Narcotics Matters (and now Ambassador to Paraguay) Clyde B. Taylor admitted that there was "substantial reason" to believe that Sendero had launched a recruitment drive aimed at coca growers in the Upper Huallaga Valley. U.S.-sponsored anti-coca policies, in Taylor's view, alienated farmers and made them susceptible to guerrilla appeals:

> Many see coca eradication efforts as a threat to their survival. When [Sendero] recruiters announce that they have come to protect the livelihood of growers against government interference, they find ready listeners. Paradoxically, the U.S.-funded eradication efforts may be making the remaining growers more desperate and more susceptible to the blandishments of terrorist recruiters.[58]

Taylor's testimony in a sense proved to be prophetic. He presented it on August 2, 1984, and about 3 weeks later, the Peruvian army moved into the Upper Huallaga Valley in response to an increasing pattern of Sendero violence. Since the late summer of 1983, the guerrillas had dynamited 10 out of 13 police stations in the region, killed 19 policemen, attacked a number of public buildings, laid siege to the PEAH compound, and—via death threat—forced the retirement of teachers and government officials in 14 different Valley communities. Sendero also had recruited nearly 2,000 Valley residents, doubtless playing on general anti-government and anti-U.S. sentiment.[59] During the state of emergency, which lasted until December 1985, the army in effect adopted Taylor's thesis of a correlation between rebel activities and narcotics control programs. The army kept CORAH out of zones where guerrillas had established a presence and virtually deactivated UMOPAR. The army commander of the zone, Julio Carbajal, publicly assured residents of the coca-producing Monzón district, "We guarantee that you will be able to continue with your normal economic activities."[60] The army left in December 1985, and, since that time, Sendero has reestablished a presence in the Valley—apparently infiltrating first those coca-producing areas that were hardest hit by CORAH eradication teams.

The Peruvian case emphasizes an apparent dilemma in narcotics control policy. Drug control measures can, in theory, dry up an important source of financial support for subversive movements. On the other hand, in regions that are more or less dedicated to the cocaine industry, such measures (especially those directed against peasant farmers) can precipitate widespread social and economic dislocation. Guerrilla movements may be waiting in the wings to pick up the pieces. Antidrug campaigns, in other words, can transform such movements into a lethal threat. Cato Institute policy analyst Ted Galen Carpenter notes, "It is a supreme irony of America's international narcotics policy that its implementation erodes popular support for 'friendly' regimes that Washington otherwise seeks to protect from leftist insurgencies."[61]

The Scope of Narco-Terrorism in the Hemisphere

The Reagan Administration and its supporters have, in general, tried to pin a Marxist label on the narcotics industry and to link Marxist movements and regimes to narcotics trafficking. The narco-guerrilla stereotype is one aspect of this policy. Another dimension is reflected in charges that communist governments—specifically the governments of Cuba and Nicaragua—deliberately facilitate drug smuggling through their territories. Evidence does suggest that individual Cuban and Nicaraguan officials were involved in the transshipment of drugs. Moreover, Cuba and Nicaragua probably adopt a policy of benign neglect (perhaps malign neglect would be a better term) toward the traffic—that is, they do not devote scarce resources to combatting what they see as a U.S. problem. However, it is not clear whether there has been a state-sanctioned policy of encouraging or protecting the transshipment of drugs to the United States. Even less compelling is the assertion, made in a May 1985 Senate hearing by then-Senator Paula Hawkins, that the goal of Cuban and Nicaraguan leaders is to "destroy American youth, cripple American society, by flooding our country with drugs."[62] Finally, and most important, the Reagan Administration exhibited a double standard in dealing with countries in the Hemisphere; for years, the Administration ignored evidence that noncommunist governments were providing safe havens and support for shipping drugs to the United States and elsewhere.

Colombian traffickers began cultivating ties with Caribbean and Central American countries with a vengeance in 1984, following the assassination of the Colombian Justice Minister, Lara Bonilla. The resulting government crackdown forced many leading traffickers into exile in Panama. There, as Bruce Bagley notes, they "strengthened already existing relations with General Noriega."[63] They set up a large cocaine processing laboratory in Panama's Darien province and transformed that country into the world's foremost center for laundering drug money.

From their vantage point in Panama, the Colombians began planning the establishment of new transshipment routes and money-laundering countries. They cultivated ties with both the Sandinistas and with the Contras in Nicaragua. They made deals with Mexican traffickers and officials to transship cocaine through Mexico. Using Juan Matta Ballesteros, a Honduran agent of the Medellín mafia who had escaped from a Bogotá jail in 1986, they subverted members of the Honduran military. They augmented their networks of corrupt officials in the Bahamas. They "developed new ties in Cuba, Haiti, Belize, and several smaller island countries."[64] It is nearly impossible to find governments in the Caribbean and Central America that have not been tainted to some degree by drug money. Yet, Reagan Administration officials have hammered on "the complicity of communist governments in the drug trade" in isolation from this pattern of Hemisphere-wide corruption.[65]

First, consider Nicaragua. A U.S. government affidavit filed in U.S. District Court in Miami in July 1984 charged that two major Colombian traffickers, Pablo Escobar and Jorge Ochoa, and a Nicaraguan official were conspiring to smuggle cocaine. The official, Frederico Vaughn, was an assistant to Nicaraguan Interior Minister Tomás Borge. According to the indictment, these men conspired to smuggle roughly 1.5 tons of cocaine from Colombia to the United States via Nicaragua. Vaughn allegedly was paid $1.5 million for providing the traffickers with secure facilities. The indictment was supported by photographs, which showed Vaughn and Escobar loading a Miami-bound aircraft with unidentified boxes, thought to contain cocaine. The photographs also showed Sandinista troops helping to load the plane, suggesting that, in addition to Vaughn, other Nicaraguan officials may have participated in the drug smuggling scheme.[66] The Nicaraguan government, not surprisingly, denied the charges. In a statement issued in July, it said, "At no time has there been any connection on the part of high government officials or anyone else with drug traffickers."[67] Furthermore, there are contrary allegations that the Medellín syndicates funneled $10 million to the Nicaraguan Contras between 1982 and 1985. The purpose of the donation, according to unpublished testimony before the Senate Foreign Relations Committee, was to buy "a little friendship" from the CIA.[68]

In the case of Cuba, reports of a triangular relationship involving Colombian drug smugglers, M-19, and Cuban officials surfaced in the 1983 Congressional testimony of Deputy Assistant Secretary of State for Inter-American Affairs James Michel, who said, "In exchange for Colombian drug runners smuggling arms to Cuban-backed insurgents, Cuba offered safe passage for ships carrying narcotics to the United States through Cuban waters." Evidence of the Cuban connection stemmed from a 1982 federal indictment against 14 persons, including four high-ranking Cuban officials and a Colombian smuggler named Jaime Guillot-Lara, for importing drugs into the United States by way of Cuba. The Cubans, who allegedly were paid off by Guillot for their part in the deal, included a former Cuban ambassador to Colombia, a Cuban communist party official, a vice admiral in the Cuban navy, and the president of Cuba's Institute of Friendship with the People.[69]

The extent of this alleged drugs-for-weapons connection—or whether it ever existed or still exists—is not known. State Department officials insist, however, that Cuba continues to facilitate narcotics trafficking, allowing smugglers to use Cuban ports, territorial waters, and airspace. U.S. law enforcement officials said in Congressional testimony that Colombians pay hard currency to Cuban authorities for the right to offload "mother ships" in Cuban waters, that is, to transfer their illicit cargo (apparently predominantly marijuana rather than cocaine) to smaller, faster boats for delivery to Florida. A former U.S. Army general contends that traffickers have "an assigned corridor which they can transit without challenge from Cuban air defenders."[70]

The Cubans, of course, disagree: "We have been trying to help in control of the drug traffic," said a Cuban press attaché in Washington in 1984. "Every plane, every ship or yacht which we catch in our waters or in our airspace we have detained." Charges of Cuban complicity in drug running were, in his words, "unfounded." Moreover, he said, at any given time, 15 to 30 U.S. traffickers were in Cuban jails. "We have been freeing

some of them at the request of [U.S.] Congressmen as a goodwill gesture,''
the attaché added. In an interview in November 1985, Fidel Castro said
that Cuba has had an "unimpeachable" record of fighting drugs since the
revolution and also—referring to the Guillot-Lara indictments—said that
he knew of "not one such case" in which Cuban officials were involved
with the drug business. Castro also noted that small civilian aircraft
frequently violate Cuban airspace and pay no attention to signals from
Cuban interceptors.[71]

Recent events, however, forced the Reagan Administration to retreat
from its policy of singling out Cuba and Nicaragua. It has become painfully
clear that many Caribbean countries—for example, Panama, Costa Rica,
Jamaica, Mexico, the Bahamas, Honduras, and the Turk and Caicos
Islands—serve as money-laundering centers or staging areas for drugs.
The role played by Cuba and Nicaragua in drug smuggling is minuscule
compared to the role played by countries that are friends and allies of the
United States. Official collusion with traffickers is widespread in these
countries, reaching a level as high if not higher than that in the two
communist countries.

For example, the army commander of Panama, General Manuel Noriega,
was indicted by federal grand juries in Tampa and Miami in February 1988.
The indictments accused Noriega of turning Panama into a virtual free
trade zone for drug shipments, payoffs, and the manufacture of cocaine.
Ironically, in earlier years, Noriega received several letters of commenda-
tion from top U.S. officials, praising him for his aid in the war against
drugs. A letter written in May 1986 to Noriega by DEA Chief John Lawn
expressed "deep appreciation for the vigorous antidrug policy you have
adopted."[72]

According to the indictment, Noriega accepted $4.6 million in payoffs,
enabling the Medellín cartel to ship more than 4 tons of cocaine through
Panama into the United States. He permitted Colombian traffickers to
set up a cocaine processing plant in a province near the Colombian-
Panamanian border. He laundered hundreds of millions of dollars of drug
profits through Panama's banks. (According to U.S. intelligence officials,
Noriega reportedly owns a substantial interest in a bank in Colón, Panama's Free Zone, which launders money for the M-19 as well as for
narcotics dealers.) He allowed Medellín cocaine barons to establish a
temporary headquarters in the country after the assassination of Colombia's Justice Minister in April 1984, when the Betancur government's
crackdown on drugs following the murder forced many traffickers into
hiding or exile.[73] Noriega had been both an intelligence and a military
asset. According to various accounts, he provided the CIA with information on Cuban activities and was in fact on the CIA's payroll, he allowed

the agency to operate an electronic surveillance station in Panama, and he let the United States train Nicaraguan Contra soldiers in the country. (Noriega bragged that as long as he helped the Contras, he could manipulate the Americans like "monkeys at the end of a chain.") Finally, Noriega was valuable to the U.S. military, which maintained bases in the former Canal Zone. Specifically, according to former U.S. Ambassador to Panama Ambler Moss, he allowed the U.S. Southern Command (SouthCom) to station more troops than were permitted under the Panama Canal treaties. Obviously, General Noriega had, and no doubt still has, his defenders within the U.S. government.[74]

In addition, the indictment mentioned a Cuban connection, saying that Castro had mediated a conflict between Noriega and the Medellín syndicates over the Panamanian government's raid on a cocaine laboratory (probably the above-mentioned laboratory) owned by the syndicates. This part of the indictment was based entirely on testimony by a former Panamanian counsel in New York, José Blandon. (Several U.S. law enforcement and intelligence officials have indicated that they do not regard Blandon as a credible witness.) According to Blandon, the raid resulted in the impounding of the laboratory as well as the confiscation of helicopters and aircraft. In addition, 23 Colombians associated with the operation were jailed. To add insult to injury, the Medellín syndicates already had paid $5 million to Panamanian officials—including $1 million to Noriega himself—to protect the laboratory. According to Blandon's account, Castro clearly did not mediate at all, but rather transmitted a demand from the Medellín traffickers to Noriega: Make good the losses that we suffered in the raid. Noriega complied, freeing the 23 prisoners, returning the laboratory equipment and the aircraft, and giving back the $5 million that the traffickers had paid in bribes. The Cuban Interests section in Washington dismissed Blandon's story as science fiction, and, indeed, it does seem somewhat farfetched. Conceivably, though, the Medellín mafia—knowing of Castro's friendship with Noriega—decided to send a message through the leader. Castro may have acted as a conduit, because he did not want to see his friend assassinated by the cartel.[75]

The Noriega affair exposed some serious contradictions between the war against drugs and U.S. security policy in Central America. Indeed, as suggested in the preceding pages, fighting communism and combatting drugs are often incompatible objectives. No resolution of the affair is now in sight. U.S. economic sanctions—which included cutting off aid to Panama, freezing Panamanian bank accounts, and stopping the flow of laundered money from Panama to the United States—have failed to unseat Noriega (although they have severely damaged Panama's economy). In May 1988, U.S. officials apparently offered Noriega a deal—the United

States would drop the drug indictments if the Panamanian leader would step down. Negotiations are apparently continuing, but there is as yet no sign that Noriega will leave. The Medellín mafia also reportedly seeks Noriega's departure, because he is an "obstacle to the functioning" of Panama's money laundering system.[76] The mafia is said to have put out a $1-million contract on the dictator. Shortly after his indictment, according to a rumor circulating in Panama, Noriega received a large package from Medellín containing a coffin—an unmistakable sign of the mafia's displeasure.

Noriega, however, is just one of several noncommunist leaders in the region who are allegedly implicated in drug trafficking. In the Bahamas, several cabinet ministers and public officials, including Prime Minister Lyndon Pindling, were investigated in 1984 for allegedly taking bribes from drug smugglers. The official Commission of Inquiry's report led to a cabinet shuffle: Three ministers resigned, and two were dismissed. According to information that surfaced during the trial of Carlos Lehder in 1988, Lehder paid Pindling $88,000 a month for the right to use Norman's Key as a drug-smuggling base.[77] In March 1985, the then Chief Minister of the Turks and Caicos Islands, Norman Saunders, was arrested in Miami on drug trafficking charges. He subsequently was convicted and sentenced to 8 years in prison.[78] In early 1988, a Miami jury indicted one of Haiti's top military strongmen, Colonel Jean Paul Alende, for conspiring to import 100 kilos of cocaine into Miami. According to one report, Colonel Paul rented out a dirt airstrip at his ranch 90 miles north of Port-Au-Prince to Colombian cocaine traffickers; for about $250,000, the Colonel provided military protection for the shipments and fuel for the planes.[79]

Finally, some allegations suggest that the Nicaraguan Contras used profits from drug running to pay for their war. A book published in 1987 by a former CBS news correspondent, Leslie Cockburn, describes the elements of alleged Contra drug connections in some detail. According to Cockburn, professional drug pilots "with ties to the CIA" flew weapons from the United States to Contra supply bases in Honduras and Costa Rica and carried cocaine and marijuana back to Florida on their return flight. (In one such flight, a DC-6 loaded with over 25,000 pounds of marijuana reportedly flew into Homestead Air Force Base in South Florida.) Reagan Administration officials, Cockburn suggests, helped maintain the arms-for-drugs link. In her view, this was part of a pattern of extra-budget support for the Contras; the diversion of funds from the arms sales to Iran (Irangate) was part of the same pattern. Cockburn's thesis of U.S. complicity in the drug trade is, to say the least, controversial; however, her account of the Contra connection itself cites a sufficient number of anecdotes to be credible at least in part.[80]

None of this denies that Cuba and Nicaragua play a role in the movement of drugs from South America to the United States. Cuban air traffic controllers, members of the Cuban navy and coast guard, Nicaraguan army officers, and officials of the Nicaraguan Ministry of Interior probably have at various times been involved in drug smuggling. Yet, this involvement, such as it is, is part of a much larger international pattern of narcotics-related corruption. For the Reagan Administration, the Cuban and Nicaraguan connections served roughly the same political purpose as the narco-guerrilla connection in Colombia and Peru, discrediting communism and the narcotics trade simultaneously. Unfortunately, the Administration's ideological and security concerns in the Hemisphere led it to ignore a more fundamental reality: the increasing penetration by drug traffickers of noncommunist governments, regimes, and movements.

This drugs-insurgency nexus constitutes a troubling phenomenon. Segments of the cocaine industry contribute financially to forces that are destabilizing Latin American societies. However, there are important qualifying factors. Cocaine traffickers in Colombia and Peru are increasingly resisting guerrillas' shakedown attempts—indeed, the relation between the two groups seems to be more hostile than cooperative, especially in Colombia. The cocaine mafia retaliates against guerrillas in Colombia by massacring visible members of the revolutionary left. Colombia's cocaine elite, with perhaps the exception of Carlos Lehder, bears many of the characteristics of an arriviste class, seeking social status and a modicum of political power, but not fundamental changes in the rules of the game. Finally, narcotics control itself can be a two-edged sword. In theory, it can eliminate one of the wellsprings of support for subversive movements. At the same time, the economic and social dislocation resulting from drug control measures, especially those directed against peasant farmers, can play into the hands of extremist groups.

On balance, the cocaine industry is more a conservative than a revolutionary political force. In South America, Central America, and the Caribbean, the cocaine industry's money and power support established political regimes. (Funding for the Nicaraguan Contras may be an interesting exception.) To pretend otherwise, as some Reagan Administration officials have done, is either to carry on an exercise in self-deception or to make a deliberate misrepresentation of reality.

Notes

1. "In a Clearing," *Time*, April 16, 1984, p. 35.
2. "Jacobo Arenas Discusses Lehder," *Semana*, March 10, 1987, pp. 22–25.
3. Guy Gugliotta, "Colombia's Drug Runners, Guerrillas: Friends or Foes?" *Miami Herald*, May 21, 1984.

4. "M-19's Navarro Wolff Interviewed on Truce, Drugs," Panama City Panavision, August 14, 1985.
5. Alan Riding, "Colombia Says Drug War Won't Bar Rebel Pact," *The New York Times,* May 22, 1984.
6. Fernando Cepeda Ulloa, "La lucha por la autonomía, la gran encrucijada de la política exterior de Betancur," unpublished paper, 1986, p. 27.
7. "La conexión," *Caretas,* September 7, 1987, p. 36.
   "Crack Secret Police Outfit to Combat the Shining Path's New Offensive," *The Andean Report,* March 1987, p. 39.
   "Jacobo Arenas Discusses Lehder," pp. 22–25.
8. Raúl González, "Coca and Subversion in the Huallaga," *Quehacer,* Lima, September–October 1987, pp. 55–72.
9. "18 sindicados por masacres de Uraba," *El Espectador,* September 6, 1988.
10. Ibid.
    "El prontuario," *Semana,* September 19, 1988, pp. 26–34.
11. "Masacre," *Semana,* April 12, 1988, pp. 28–34.
12. "La mafia asesinó a Pardo Leal," *El Tiempo,* November 13, 1987.
    For a good discussion of the mafia's links to the right, see Merrill Collett, "Colombia's Drug Lords Waging War on Leftists" ("Colombia's Drug Lords"), *The Washington Post,* November 14, 1987.
13. Ayatollah, "Guerrillas y narcos: cuentas pendientes," *El Tiempo,* November 15, 1987.
14. Paul Eddy et al., *The Cocaine Wars* (New York: W. W. Norton, 1988), p. 287.
15. Ibid., p. 288.
16. "The Medellín Cartel: World's Deadliest Criminals" ("The Medellín Cartel"), Special Report, *Miami Herald,* February 1987, p. 8.
    Fabio Castillo, *Los Jinetes de la Cocaína (Los Jinetes)* (Bogotá: Documentos Periodisticos, 1987), pp. 111–114.
17. Merrill Collett, "The Myth of the Narcoguerrillas," *The Nation,* August 13, 1988, p. 132.
18. "El gobierno reconoce existencia de 128 grupos paramilitarios," *El Espectador,* October 1, 1987.
19. "Guerra cruzada afronta el cartel de Medellín," *El Tiempo,* September 28, 1988.
20. Interviews with CORAH officials in Tingo María, October 12, 1987.
    Interviews with U.S. pilots, Upper Huallaga Valley trip, October 13, 1987.
    Interview with U.S. narcotics official in Lima, October 15–16, 1987.
    Interview with General Juan Zarate of DIPOD in Lima, October 16, 1987.
    "Turf War Over Coca-Growing Territory Leaves 34 Dead, 11 Wounded in Peru," *Miami Herald,* October 14, 1987.
21. "Invasión de narcotraficantes colombianos," *El Tiempo,* February 22, 1988.
22. Alfredo Molano, *Selva Adentro* (Bogotá: El Ancora, 1987), p. 134.
23. For an account of this operation, see *Los Jinetes,* p. 235.
    Fabio Castillo, "Operación encubierta para proteger laboratorio de coca," *El Espectador,* August 1, 1985, pp. 1A, 13A.
24. "Los barrios pobres y la erradicación de la probreza," *Medellín Cívico,* October 1986, p. 3.
    "La paz es la justicia social," *Medellín Cívico,* November 1986, p. 3.
    "Mientras el pueblo padece hambre, varias industrias se enriquecen," *Medellín Cívico,* April 1987, p. 4.

"Letter to Fabio Castillo," *Medellín Cívico*, p. 13.
"Existen más de dos milliones de desempleados," *Medellín Cívico*, May 1987, p. 6.

25. "Belisario no entregará a ningún colombiano," *Quindío Libre*, October 1, 1983, p. 8B.
Mario Arango Jaramillo and Jorge Child Vélez, *Los Condenados de la Coca: El Manejo Político de la Droga (Los Condenados)* (Medellín: J. M. Arango, 1985), reports on a January 1985 interview with Lehder.
"Text of Drug Traffickers' Terms for Ending Activities," *El Tiempo*, July 7, 1984.
26. Jorge Eliecer Orozco, *Lehder . . . El Hombre* (Bogotá: Epoca, 1987), p. 235.
27. Bruce Bagley, "The Colombian Connection: The Impact of the Drug Traffic on Colombia" ("The Colombian Connection"), in Deborah Pacini and Christine Franquemont (eds), *Coca and Cocaine* (Peterborough, New Hampshire: Transcript Printing Company, 1986), p. 96.
28. *Los Jinetes*, p. 234.
Interviews with U.S. narcotics experts in Bogotá, March 1986.
29. "La cocaína está empacada en latas de verduras," *El País*, Cali, September 28, 1988.
"¿Estamos perdiendo la guerra?" *El Tiempo*, March 6, 1988.
30. "Mannesmann Comes Under Attack; Firm Accused of Buying Protection from Rebels," *Latin American Weekly Report*, July 26, 1985, p. 10.
"Mannesmann Row Claims Victim; Company Head Gets His Marching Orders," *Latin American Weekly Report*, August 2, 1985, p. 5.
Sam Dillon, "Oil Firms, Guerrillas, in Uneasy Coexistence in Colombia," *Miami Herald*, September 18, 1985, pp. 1A, 3A.
"Compañías petroleras financian la guerrilla," *El Tiempo*, July 16, 1985.
31. José Suarez, "Desconocemos cualquier hecho entre petroleras y guerrillas," *El Tiempo*, July 18, 1985.
"Terminó Viacrucis de Mannesmann," *La República*, Bogotá, August 24, 1985.
32. "Veto a transnacionales que financian terrorismo," *La República*, August 15, 1985.
33. R. W. Lee, "The Latin American Drug Connection," *Foreign Policy*, No. 61 (Winter 1985–1986), p. 156.
34. "The Colombian Connection," p. 96.
35. See, e.g., "9 mil millones ganaron las FARC por venta de cocaína," *El Tiempo*, February 11, 1984, p. 6B, report of an interview with Ambassador Lewis Tombs.
For an eyewitness description of a FARC cocaine base laboratory, see Russell Stendahl, *Rescue the Captors* (Barnsville, Minnesota: Ransom Press, 1984), pp. 107–108.
36. "FARC to Cooperate in Coca Eradication in Guaviria," *Clarion*, Buenos Aires, January 11, 1987.
37. "Crops to Replace Coca Cultivation in Caqueta Region," *El Espectador*, February 18, 1986.
Jaime Jaramillo et al., *Coca Colonización y Guerrilla* (Bogotá: Universidad Nacional de Colombia, 1986), pp. 135–157.
38. "Huge Coke Bust Was Like an Invasion," *Miami Herald*, March 23, 1984, pp. 1A, 4A.
"The Medellín Cartel," p. 8.

39. "Statement of Special Agent Michael Fredericks," President's Commission on Organized Crime, *Organized Crime and Cocaine Trafficking* (Washington, D.C.: U.S. Government Printing Office, 1984), pp. 614, 616.
40. "Pruebas de vínculos FARC-narcotraficantes," *El Espectador,* April 11, 1984.
41. *Organized Crime and Cocaine Trafficking,* p. 617.
42. See, e.g., "Colombia's Drug Lords," pp. 14A, 22A.
43. *Los Jinetes,* p. 234.
44. Ibid., p. 235.
45. Elaine Shannon, *Desperados, Latin Drug Lords, U.S. Lawmen, and the War America Can't Win (Desperadoes)* (New York: Viking, 1988), pp. 173–176.
46. "Justice Minister on Narcotrafficker Financing of Guerrillas," *El Espectador,* November 9, 1985, pp. 1-A, 12-A.
47. Timothy Ross, "Colombia Goes After Drug Barons," *Christian Science Monitor,* January 12, 1987, p. 9.
48. Quoted in *Desperados,* p. 176.
49. "Sandinista Role in Justice Palace Takeover Detailed," *El Tiempo,* December 20, 1985, p. 8A.
    See also *Desperados,* pp. 174-176.
50. "Siege Report Quashed by Attorney General," *Latin American Newsletter,* July 3, 1986, p. 3.
    See also *Desperados,* p. 176.
51. "M-19 Leader Justifies Actions," Paris AFP, November 8, 1985.
    Peter Nares, "A View from the Inside of Colombia's M-19 Guerrillas," *Wall Street Journal,* July 29, 1988.
52. Joseph Treaster, "Guard Did Not Stop Colombian Rebel," *The New York Times,* November 12, 1985.
    "M-19 Defends Court Siege," *Miami Herald,* November 12, 1985.
53. "Comienza a destaparse 'olla mágica,' " *El Espectador,* March 3, 1988.
54. *Los Condenados,* p. 140.
55. William Montalbano, "Battling Cocaine, Guerrillas in an Amazon Valley War of Drugs, Rebels Rages in Peru," *Los Angeles Times,* August 2, 1987.
56. Merrill Collett, "Maoist Guerrilla Band Complicates Anti-Drug War in Peru," *The Washington Post,* June 4, 1988.
57. See, e.g., "UMOPAR Chief Calls Tocache 'Sea of Coca,'" *El Comercio,* June 17, 1985.
    "Se acentúa relación entre narcos y guerrillas," *El Comercio,* May 10, 1984.
    "Por dinero Sendero colabora con 'narcos,' " *El Comercio,* December 12, 1983.
58. "Prepared Statement of Clyde B. Taylor," in *International Insurgency and Drug Trafficking: Present Trends in Terrorist Activity (International Insurgency and Drug Trafficking)* (Washington, D.C.: U.S. Government Printing Office, 1986), Joint Hearings before the Committee on Foreign Relations and the Committee on the Judiciary, U.S. Senate, p. 133.
59. Joel Brinkley, "In the Drug War Battle Won and Lost," *The New York Times,* September 13, 1984.
    "Sendero Fans Out to Jungle Areas; Coca Eradication Schemes Help Them Win Support," *Latin American Weekly Report,* August 17, 1984.
60. "The New Coca Boom Boosts the Balance of Payments as U.S. Anti-Narcotics Efforts Flop," *The Andean Report,* April 1985, p. 42.
61. Ted Galen Carpenter, "The U.S. Campaign Against International Narcotics

188   The White Labyrinth

Trafficking: A Cure Worse than the Disease?'' Cato Institute for Policy Analysis, December 9, 1985, p. 15.

62. "Prepared Statement of Paula Hawkins," *International Insurgency and Drug Trafficking*, p. 104.
63. Bruce Bagley, "Colombia and the War on Drugs," *Foreign Affairs*, Fall 1988, p. 83.
64. Ibid.
65. Speech by George Schultz to the Miami Chamber of Commerce, September 11, 1984, quoted in *Desperados*, p. 159.
66. "Prepared Statement of Clyde B. Taylor," p. 9.
   General Paul F. Gorman, "Illegal Drugs and U.S. Security," in President's Commission on Organized Crime, *America's Habit: Drug Abuse, Drug Trafficking and Organized Crime* (Washington, D.C.: U.S. Government Printing Office, March 1986), Appendix G, pp. 18-26.
67. "No ha habido vinculación con los narcotraficantes," *El Tiempo*, July 24, 1984.
68. "Reports CIA Received Cocaine Cartel Cash," United Press International, Washington News, June 30, 1987.
   Leslie Cockburn, *Out of Control: The Story of the Reagan Administration's Secret War in Nicaragua, the Illegal Guns Pipeline, and the Contra Drug Connection (Out of Control)* (New York: Atlantic Monthly Press, 1987), pp. 154–155.
69. "Statement of Francis M. Mullan" and "Statement of James Michel," in *The Cuban Government's Involvement in Facilitating International Drug Traffic* (Washington, D.C.: U.S. Government Printing Office, 1983), Joint Hearings before the Committee of the Judiciary and the Committee on Foreign Relations, U.S. Senate, pp. 81–86.
70. "Smugglers of Drugs from Colombia to U.S. Are Protected by Cuba," *Wall Street Journal*, April 30, 1984, p. 1.
   "Illegal Drugs and U.S. Security," p. 20.
71. "Smugglers of Drugs," p. 14.
   INCSR, 1986, pp. 102–103.
72. "Drugs, Money, and Death," *Newsweek*, February 15, 1988, p. 34.
73. "Miami Jury Indicts Noriega," *Miami Herald*, February 5, 1988.
   "Noriega Indicted by U.S. for Links to Illegal Drugs," *The New York Times*, February 6, 1988.
   Seymour Hersh, "Panama Strongman Said to Trade in Drugs, Arms, and Illicit Money," *The New York Times*, June 12, 1986.
74. "Drugs, Money, and Death," p. 38.
75. Committee on Foreign Relations, U.S. Senate, *Drugs, Law Enforcement, and Foreign Policy: Panama* (Washington, D.C.: U.S. Government Printing Office, 1988), Hearings before the Subcommittee on Terrorism, Narcotics, and International Communications, February 8–11, 1988, pp. 101–107.
76. Committee on Foreign Relations, U.S. Senate, *Drugs, Law Enforcement, and Foreign Policy: The Cartel, Haiti, and Central America* (Washington, D.C.: U.S. Government Printing Office, 1988), Hearings before the Subcommittee on Terrorism, Narcotics, and International Communications, April 4–7, 1988, pp. 28–29.
77. "Bahamas Leader Tied to Drug Probe," *The New York Times*, January 14, 1988.

78. "The Latin American Drug Connection," p. 149.
79. Charles McCoy, "Cocaine Trade Snares Haitian Strongman," *Wall Street Journal,* March 15, 1988.
80. *Out of Control,* pp. 169–188.

5

The Enforcement Picture

*Who knows where our country would be without
drugs? Who knows how much common crime we
would have if it were not for the breathing space
accorded by the drug traffic?*
—Gabriel García Marquez, 1984

U.S. and Latin American curbs on the supply of cocaine have failed
abjectly. Between 200 tons and 300 tons of cocaine may flow into U.S.
markets yearly. As one observer notes, "The supply of cocaine has never
been greater in the streets, the price has never been lower, and the drug
has never been purer."[1] The United States supports a number of supply-
side programs in the Andean countries. Funding for these programs
amounts to perhaps $50–$60 million a year, compared to the South
American cocaine industry's earnings of $5–$6 billion a year. A massive
infusion of antidrug aid, however, might not be the answer. As the
preceding discussion shows, breaking the power of narcotics lobbies in the
Andean countries will be extremely difficult. Furthermore, some serious
structural barriers impede drug law enforcement in these countries, including weak central governments, the lack of strong public support for
narcotics control, divisions within governments over antidrug policy, and
tension between civilian and military authorities. As the following discussion demonstrates, Andean nations are poorly equipped politically and
administratively to control cocaine trafficking within their borders.

The Control Problem

Governments often exercise little or no effective control over territories
where drug production flourishes. Such areas are remote from metropolitan centers, relatively inaccessible (characterized by mountainous or jungle terrain), and patrolled by guerrillas or other hostile groups. Vast

sections of northern Bolivia, eastern and southeastern Peru, and southern Colombia are in effect a no-man's-land where government forces vie for political control with drug traffickers and anti-government guerrillas.

Nor is this lack of control limited to Latin American governments. The rapidly growing narcotics trade is symptomatic of the failures of political modernization in much of the developing world. In Burma, for example, central government authority is virtually non-existent in that country's northern Shan state, a major world center of opium and heroin production. Control in the region, rather, is exercised by an assortment of tribal separatists, revolutionary organizations, and insurgent groups. In Pakistan, narcotics production is concentrated in quasi-independent tribal areas along the border with Afghanistan. In the most important production center, the Northwest Frontier province, armed tribesmen oppose the government's antinarcotics programs and call for "freedom in developing the area's national resources"[2]—a reference to opium and heroin.

In South America, the cocaine industry represents a force for colonization, bringing a human presence, road penetration networks, airstrips, satellite industries, and some licit agriculture (mainly subsistence farming) to regions that previously were virtually uninhabited. However, cocaine trafficking tends to weaken governments' already tenuous hold on their territories. As shown in Chapter 4, guerrilla movements finance their activities by taxing the cocaine trade, especially in its upstream phases. Movements such as Colombia's FARC and Peru's Sendero Luminoso apparently created a mass following among the coca-growing peasantry. In Peru's Upper Huallaga Valley, another distintegration process seems to be at work. The region ships coca paste, by far its most important export, to Colombia and receives in return money, weapons, and a degree of economic leadership. Colombian aircraft maintain this connection, flying in and out of Peruvian airspace with virtual impunity. Colombian middlemen increasingly buy paste directly from peasants in the Valley rather than through Peruvian dealers. In terms of the value and volume of transactions, the Upper Huallaga is becoming less a part of Peru and more a part of Colombia.[3]

The obverse of the territorial integration problem is official corruption. Bribery, it can be argued, has long been the cement of political and social interaction in much of Latin America. However, drug traffickers, especially cocaine traffickers, capitalize on this tradition to transform the existing power structure, to create networks of compliant officials at national-department and local levels. These networks vitiate the effectiveness of criminal justice systems. In Bolivia during 1986, for example, Chapare traffickers reportedly were paying police $20,000 to $25,000 for a 72-hour window of impunity for loading coca paste into airplanes or for moving major shipments by land or by river.[4] In Peru, the pattern of corruption can be very complex. In mid-1988, according to an informed U.S. source, traffickers paid roughly $12,000 in bribes for a load of cocaine base flown out of the Uchiza district in the Upper Huallaga Valley: $5,000 went to the military command in the district, $5,000 to local offices of the civil guard (the national police), and $2,000 to various community organizations thought to be fronts for Sendero Luminoso.

In Colombia, Medellín's famous Olaya Perrera International Airport, located in the center of the city, was for several months in 1986 the scene of a major cocaine smuggling operation that apparently was carried out with the full knowledge of a 12-man police commando unit on permanent guard at the airport.[5] As noted in Chapter 3, the Colombian mafia's network of informants enables its chief executives to escape police dragnets and to live a fairly comfortable existence in major cities such as Medellín and Cali. On the rare occasion when traffickers are arrested, they usually can bribe their way out of jail. At this time—1988—no major traffickers are in jail anywhere in Colombia. Law enforcement in Latin American countries often functions simply as a way to share in the proceeds of the drug trade. The police take bribes not to make arrests and seizures. When the police do make successful busts, the confiscated drugs are often resold on the illicit market.

In Bolivia, the problem of corruption may be especially serious. The advent of democratic government in 1982 somewhat weakened the direct political influence of the cocaine mafia. Yet, according to both U.S. and Bolivian government estimates, the cocaine trade has expanded enormously since García Meza's day. Cocaine traffickers, who account for as much as one-half of Bolivia's yearly inflow of foreign exchange, retain widespread influence in government institutions, the military, and the various peasant federations that produce coca. Traffickers probably control local politics in much of the Beni region. The level of corruption in Bolivia is simply extraordinary, even by Latin American standards. A 1988 U.S. General Accounting Office report noted:

> According to several U.S. and Bolivian officials, corruption exists within all levels of the Bolivian government and very few government officials are to be trusted—corruption is widespread and generally accepted within the Bolivian police, military, and judicial systems.[6]

Bolivia's cocaine superstate may have passed from the scene, but the narcotics control environment is fundamentally no better than it was in the early 1980s.

Corruption has devastating effects on drug law enforcement in South

America. Unfortunately, the disease has no cure. In the Andean countries, the cocaine industry represents one of the few important sources of wealth. At the same time, poverty in these countries is rampant, economic oportunities are circumscribed, and salaries of public servants often barely exceed the subsistence level. Under such conditions, cocaine dealers find it easy to co-opt parts of the state apparatus. A Colombian official who conducted a 1986 investigation of the Medellín Metropolitan Police observed, "Only corruption can explain how a second lieutenant earning 35,000 pesos a month [about $175] can make a million-peso deposit in his account and live in an 18-million-peso apartment."[7] For the legions of underpaid policemen, judges, and government officials in Colombia and elsewhere in the Andean world, the price of honesty may seem excessively high.

Public Opinion

Success in drug control in any society requires, among other things, a high level of political consensus. The top leadership level in Colombia, Bolivia, and Peru evidences this will. Leaders talk harshly about the drug trade. Former Colombian President Betancur says that "drugs are the worst problem that Colombia has had in its history" and rails against "the multinationals of crime that have aspired domestically to ever-higher positions of political power." President Barco calls drug traffickers "a total challenge to our institutions, our traditions and our values." Peru's Alan García says that Peru cannot "be identified as an exporter of poison" and that drug trafficking "corrupts institutions and degrades man." Victor Paz Estenssoro calls drug trafficking a "flagrant crime against mankind" and says that it causes Bolivia "moral damage in the eyes of the rest of the world."[8]

These leadership concerns, however, are not reflected at the grass roots level. There is not yet an awakened public consensus against drugs in the Andean countries. For example, opinion surveys commissioned in late 1987 by the U.S. Information Agency (USIA) show that drug trafficking ranks near the bottom of public concerns in Colombia, Bolivia, and Peru. The drug trade is outranked by problems such as unemployment; poverty; terrorism (in Colombia and Peru); and the lack of housing, education, and health care (in Colombia and Bolivia).[9] In a national survey conducted in late 1988 of more than 1,500 adults in 50 Colombian cities, respondents mentioned guerrillas as an important national problem five times as frequently as they mentioned narcotic trafficking; unemployment was mentioned six times as frequently. USIA surveys and other polling data from the Andean countries suggest a moderate level of concern about drug addiction—in contrast to drug trafficking. Yet, in general, Andean publics do not view either aspect of the drug problem as a survival issue.

Furthermore, the cocaine industry is not usually a prime target of politicians seeking election to public office. For example, drugs were hardly mentioned by candidates in the 1986 or the 1982 presidential campaigns in Colombia. The Liberal Party platform for the 1986 elections included only one weak plank on drugs—support for an "international strategy for combatting the traffic of drugs." A 222-page book by Virgilio Barco, *Toward a New Colombia,* that appeared just before the presidential election in May managed to make only one passing reference to drug trafficking.[10] The candidates evidently did not perceive the subject as being important to voters, or they felt that they would lose more votes than they would gain by staking out a position on drugs in their campaigns. In the United States, in contrast, drugs ranked second as a presidential campaign issue in 1988, according to a Gallup poll of 2,113 adults conducted in the spring of that year.[11] One reason for the difference in attitudes is the difference in patterns of drug consumption. An extensive study conducted in 1987 by the University of Antioquia reported that only 2 percent of the population could be classified as regular users of cocaine products or marijuana, compared to about 10 percent of the U.S. population.[12] In Colombia, office-seekers also have to worry about reprisals from cocaine traffickers—The Extraditables' kidnapping of Andres Pastrana, who did take a strong anti-mafia stance in his campaign for mayor of Bogotá, is a case in point.

In addition, the prevailing attitude toward drug control is characterized by ambivalence, pessimism, and hostility. There is a widely held perception in Latin American countries that the drug traffic is good for the economy even if it is harmful in other respects. Top leaders and officials appear to share this perception. For example, Bolivia's President Victor Paz Estenssoro remarked in 1986, "Cocaine has gained an importance in our economy in direct response to the shrinking of the formal economy." Alan García once called cocaine "the only successful multinational" that had emerged in the Andean countries. Leading bankers in Peru talk about the importance of cocaine earnings in stabilizing Peru's currency. Colombia's Controller General Rodolfo González attributes what he calls the "reactivization" of the Colombian economy during 1987 to the inflow of narco-dollars.[13]

These and other leaders are well aware of the debilitating effects of drug trafficking on government institutions, on public morals, and on their countries' international relations. Yet, they may be as afraid of narcotics control as they are of the narcotics industry itself. The crises of debt, economic stagnation, and rampant unemployment that haunt most countries in the region reinforce this perception. In Bolivia, for example, officials warn privately that compliance with U.S. dictates on narcotics could precipitate a military coup in that country.[14] Indeed, if the cocaine industry disappeared tomorrow, the results could be catastrophic, at least in Peru and Bolivia: the evaporation of hard-currency reserves, massive unemployment, an increase in crime and subversion in rural areas, a flood of new migrants to the cities, and so on. Such a situation could only play into the hands of extremist groups on both the left and the right. For example, how long would democracy last in Bolivia if 200,000 dispossessed coca farmers decided to march on La Paz?

Latin Americans also resent U.S. interference in their affairs. Narcotics lobbies consistently equate drug control with a loss of national sovereignty; and leftist intellectuals see it as reinforcing U.S. domination of Latin America's political, military, and public institutions. Moreover, earlier drug control measures have been broadly unpopular. In Colombia, the extradition of drug traffickers under a 1979 treaty with the United States has long been a cause célèbre for nationalists of all political leanings. Although President Barco and most of his cabinet supported the treaty, it was opposed by a powerful coalition of legislators, jurists, labor leaders, government officials, and (behind the scenes) cocaine traffickers. Such opposition proved overwhelming. In June 1987, Colombia's Supreme Court, by a vote of 13 to 12, invalidated legislation that would have made it possible to implement the treaty. Now the government cannot extradite Colombian citizens even if it wants to do so. The Colombian Congress could theoretically pass new implementing legislation, but it displays little support for such a move. Apparently, public support is not significant either. A December 1987 survey conducted by a Colombian polling organization showed that two-thirds of the Colombian population opposes extraditions to the United States.[15] A USIA poll taken at the same time reported that 58 percent of urban Colombians disapproved of the February 1987 extradition of Carlos Lehder.[16]

In Bolivia, Operation Blast Furnace—the use of troops and helicopters against cocaine laboratories in the summer of 1986—provoked a nationalist outcry across the entire political spectrum. Leftist, centrist, and rightist leaders alike condemned the operation as an affront to the nation and as a violation of its constitution. Mindful of the political lessons of Blast Furnace, the Bolivian government rejected in April 1988 as "unacceptable for national sovereignty" a U.S. proposal to create a multinational police force that would operate in Bolivian territory.[17]

Finally, Latin Americans question both the legitimacy and the effectiveness of Washington's supply-side approaches to drug control. In Colombia, Belisario Betancur referred to "the high income countries which, with their unlimited demand, stimulate in a permanent manner the cultivation and sale" of drugs. Peru's Alan García, in a 1987 television interview, said, "I have always thought of drug trafficking as the final stage of capitalist consumerism." He went on, "The problem does not lie in the fact that a poor town in my country . . . produces coca leaves in the Peruvian jungle. The basic problem lies in the world's big consumer markets, consisting of the richest societies."[18] USIA surveys in Colombia, Bolivia, and Peru show that huge majorities in these countries see the United States as the country most to blame for the drug problem.[19]

Latin American leaders and publics recognize that narcotics industries take a serious political, social, and moral toll on their societies. The issue, however, is where to draw the battle lines against the drug menace. Most Latin Americans are skeptical that the war against drugs can be won by implementing controversial policies such as spraying herbicides on South American coca fields, sending U.S. troops or multinational forces to raid Bolivia's cocaine laboratories, or extraditing the chief executives of Colombia's cocaine industry. As a former Colombian Justice Minister, Enrique Low Murtra, remarked, "It won't do any good if we capture the big capos, because, as long as there is a strong consumer market abroad, other people will appear with the same objectives and the same power. The names change, but the problem remains."[20] Similarly, many Peruvian and Bolivian leaders argue that until the industrialized countries curb their voracious appetite for cocaine, peasants will continue planting coca, and coca will continue producing higher returns than most other crops.

Furthermore, Latin Americans are demoralized by what they see as an unequal struggle. Government officials in Bolivia, Peru, and Colombia make a point of comparing the billions of dollars earned each year by cocaine traffickers with the few million dollars in drug-fighting aid that their countries receive each year from the United States. In Colombia, a national survey conducted in late 1988 showed that Colombians believe by a margin of 4 to 3 that their government is losing the war against drugs.

In sum, U.S. antidrug policies in the Andean countries do not enjoy wide popular or official support. Latin American publics see drug control programs as a low national priority. Governments likewise are inclined to feel that the war against drugs interferes with more pressing priorities, for example, coping with inflation and unemployment, servicing foreign debt, and fighting guerrillas. Moreover, Latin Americans from top government officials on down are afraid that cracking down on drugs will hurt the economy. Many people in the Andean countries would probably agree with the Nobel-prize-winning Colombian novelist Gabriel García Marquez, who, in a 1984 interview, asked rhetorically, "Who knows where our country would be without drugs? Who knows what level of common crime we would have if it were not for the breathing space accorded by the drug traffic?"[21] Latin American nationalism also colors attitudes on the drug issue, and policies that are perceived as the product of U.S. pressure are apt to be widely unpopular. Finally, there is a tendency to view drugs as a North American problem: The solution, many Latin Americans believe, lies not in waging war against drug farmers or cocaine barons, but in getting North Americans to reduce their intake of illicit drugs.

Behind these attitudes lies a pervasive fear that antidrug programs may be destabilizing—that they may entail serious threats to public order and pose new political challenges to clearly frail democratic regimes. As the discussion in the previous chapters suggests, such a fear is not entirely groundless. Of course, economic and social dislocations in South America will occur however the cocaine industry meets its demise, whether production is eliminated at the source, or whether the six million Americans who now use cocaine switch to other drugs or engage in healthier forms of recreation. Yet, for Andean governments, the issue of responsibility is crucial. They are reluctant to make a frontal attack on their cocaine constituencies, just as many U.S. politicians are reluctant to implement demand-side strategies to catch and punish the 5 million to 6 million regular cocaine users in the United States. Such are the politics of drug control. The question therefore is, on what side of the cocaine equation— demand or supply—can the costs of stopping the traffic be more easily absorbed?

The Role of Governments

Andean governments find themselves in an uncomfortable position in the war against drugs. On the one hand, the cocaine trade injects needed dollars into Andean economies and employs hundreds of thousands of people. Drug enforcement measures generally have little popular appeal; indeed, they arouse substantial opposition, although it should be emphasized that the opposition does not all come from people who make a living from the narcotics industry. Governments themselves are apt to feel (with some justification) that the war against drugs conflicts with other priorities; for example, coping with inflation and unemployment, promoting economic growth, and combatting crime and subversion.

At the same time, Latin American governments are under some domestic and international pressure to control drug trafficking. The public consensus on drugs is perhaps not very highly developed, but there is concern—especially over increased consumption of coca products among young people. Moreover, Latin American governments face the threat of reprisals by the United States for not taking strong action. U.S.

Congressional attitudes hardened in recent years, and legislation (especially since 1983) has endorsed progressively stiffer and more wide-ranging sanctions against governments that are uncooperative on drug control.

These contradictory tendencies condition the ways that governments approach narcotics control. There have been several distinct approaches. First, governments set up elaborate bureaucratic structures for fighting the drug traffic. Second, they sought to maximize the inflow of international aid for this purpose and to minimize their own outlays. Third, in Peru and Bolivia especially, they tried to refocus drug control strategy, stressing interdiction over eradication. Governments find it politically easier to raid cocaine laboratories than to destroy peasants' coca fields. Finally, continuing controversy over narcotics policy within the bureaucracy and within the society at large has immobilized governments in important ways. They cannot implement enforcement measures that could materially advance the cause of drug control. Significant measures apparently on hold include the use of herbicides to eradicate coca and the extradition of leading cocaine traffickers to the United States.

The Policy Context

Formal structure.   Colombia, Bolivia, and Peru all have bureaucratic infrastructures for narcotics control. In Colombia, a multi-ministry policymaking body—the National Council of Dangerous Drugs (CNE)—is chaired by the Ministry of Justice. The Minister of Justice and the Commander of the National Police more or less coordinate Colombia's antidrug effort, although they frequently disagree on policy. Most operational responsibility for eradication and interdiction is vested in an 1,800-man Directorate of Anti-Narcotics of the National Police (DAN), which includes a technical operation branch, an air wing, and an investigation and intelligence branch. The Ministries of Health and Agriculture and subordinate institutes play a key role in enforcement, because they are charged with evaluating the effects of herbicides, both on illicit crops and on the surrounding environments. The Ministry of Health also holds the main responsibility for prevention, rehabilitation, and media awareness programs. An agency under the Ministry of Health that reports directly to the presidency—the National Institute for Family Welfare (ICBF)—is the lead agency for prevention, rehabilitation, and media awareness programs. Two Ministry of Agriculture agencies—the Institute for Agrarian Reform (INCORA) and the National Institute of Natural Renewable Resources (INDERENA)—are primarily responsible for whatever minimal efforts are being made in Colombia to help coca farmers switch to other occupations.

In Peru, a somewhat similar policymaking structure exists, the Multisec-toral Committee for Control of Drugs (COMUCOD). This committee is chaired by the Ministry of Interior and, under the Belaunde administration at least, the Peruvian president was also a member. Responsibility for anti-cocaine operations is split between two police agencies under the Ministry of Interior, the Peruvian Investigation Police (PIP) and the Civil Guard (GC), which both have specialized drug-fighting units. GC, however, is the lead agency in Peru's drug control effort—or, at least, the United States has designated it as such. Between 1984 and 1986, GC's investigative and rural mobile police units received $3.8 million in U.S. aid, but PIP received only $200,000. (This figure does not include over $2 million in funding for UMOPAR, which is now subordinate not to DIPOD but to a different GC division, the Head Office for Special Affairs.) One reason for the disparity is that PIP has been riddled with corruption. Many senior officers have been charged with accepting payoffs from cocaine traffickers. As noted earlier, one major Peruvian trafficker, Reynaldo Rodríguez, actually worked as an adviser to the PIP high command and maintained an office in PIP headquarters while he was running his cocaine ring.

Eradication of coca is a police function in Peru, as it is in Colombia and (formally) in Bolivia. The CORAH program in the Upper Huallaga is under the Ministry of Interior. (Until late 1987, it was part of the Ministry of Agriculture.) The GC's rural mobile police (UMOPAR) are an essential adjunct to the program, because they provide protection for eradication teams. Other actors in Peru's antidrug effort are described briefly below. The National Coca Enterprise (ENACO) is supposed to exercise the government's legal monopoly over the purchase and sale of coca leaves. In practice, ENACO can capture less than five percent of the leaves—most of the rest go to traffickers. The Ministries of Health and Education share responsibility for fighting domestic drug addiction. The Ministry of the Presidency supervises the Special Upper Huallaga Project (PEAH)—a $41.8-million agricultural development program in the Valley, largely paid for by the U.S. Agency for International Development (AID).

The organization of Bolivia's drug-fighting effort now is in a state of flux. By October 1987, a multiagency body, the National Drug Council, had been created that was roughly similar to Peru's COMUCOD and Colombia's NCDD. This Council included the Ministers of Interior, De-fense, Foreign Affairs, Planning, Health, Agriculture, and Information. Under this body were two subsecretariats, one for social defense and the other for alternative development. The former had responsibility for anti-cocaine missions; the latter was responsible for crop reduction, regulation of the legal coca market, and crop substitution and rural modernization programs. Confusingly, the Sub-Secretariat for Social Defense was at the same time subordinate to the Ministry of Interior; likewise, the Sub-Secretariat for Alternative Development and Substitution of Coca was under the jurisdiction of the Ministry of Agriculture. To muddle matters even further, the Sub-Secretariat for Social Defense comprised representatives of both the military and the national police. The military representatives took orders from their respective services—that is, not from the Council or the Ministry of Justice—and military-police relations within the Sub-Secretariat were extremely strained. The system, said one U.S. narcotics expert in La Paz, "has no chance of working."[22]

Since that time, there has been discussion in Bolivia about establishing a cabinet-level department to take charge of drug problems—the first such department to be created in the Hemisphere. Presumably the new organization, which would incorporate the Sub-Secretariat for Social Defense, would streamline the implementation of antidrug policy. Problems are likely to persist, however, if active military men hold leadership positions within the new entity.

Paying for drug control.   Latin American governments see the war on drugs as a drain on scarce resources and as underfunded by the international community. They cite the awesome economic and military power of international cocaine mafias and the relatively low levels of international support as reasons for their failure to control the drug traffic. In addition, governments in varying measure perceive narcotics control as imposing economic and social side effects—principally in the form of lost income and jobs. The rich drug-consuming countries, in their view, should compensate for their losses with major new infusions of money and development assistance.

In Peru and Bolivia, governments have kept their expenditures on narcotics control to a minimum. Essentially, Peru and Bolivia allow the United States to conduct antidrug operations on their national territory at U.S. expense. U.S. antinarcotics aid to the two countries—about $20 million in FY 1988—is spent on almost everything but weapons: food, fuel, aircraft, vehicles, equipment, housing, tents, bathrooms, showers, salary supplements, and training. The coca eradication program in the Upper Huallaga Valley is funded almost entirely by the United States, according to officials familiar with the program. The U.S. role is probably even more prominent in Bolivia; as one U.S. narcotics official in La Paz put it, "The Bolivians lack any resources whatsoever to contribute other than personnel."[23]

The pattern is somewhat different in Colombia. The Colombian economy is stronger than those of the other Andean nations, and Colombia is combatting the twin evils of cocaine and marijuana. Colombia's DAN maintains a fleet of 18 to 19 helicopters, and its 1,800-man police force, whose salaries are fully paid by the government, is much larger than the antidrug force in either Peru or Bolivia. Colombia's antinarcotics budget is said to fall between $20 million and $25 million a year. Colombia supposedly contributes one-half of that amount, and the United States provides the rest. Colombia's financial outlays for drug control are almost certainly greater, both absolutely and relatively (as a percentage of total antidrug expenditures), than those of Peru and Bolivia. Furthermore, the drug war in Colombia has been waged with greater intensity. Between 1985 and 1988, Colombian traffickers reputedly killed more than 400 police and military men, scores of judges, more than a dozen journalists, and several top government officials.[24] Such a death toll is unmatched in the other Andean countries—indeed, it is probably unprecedented in the annals of world crime.

Government leaders and officials in Andean countries recognize that the war against drugs in their societies has failed, but they blame a lack of resources rather than an absence of will. The struggle, they emphasize, is grossly unequal. Government officials in Andean countries constantly stress in interviews and in briefings that traffickers have faster airplanes, more automatic weapons, and more sophisticated communication gear than police agencies. In a 1986 interview with the magazine *Caretas,* Peru's Minister of Interior Abel Salinas compared the $4–$5 million "including foreign aid" that Peru spends on drugs each year with the estimated $2 billion earned yearly by cocaine traffickers in the Upper Huallaga Valley. In an August 1988 interview, Bolivia's Foreign Minister, Guillermo Bedregal, said that the amount of aid that the United States has contributed to fight drug trafficking in Bolivia "is minimal and absolutely ridiculous."[25] The message is clear: International drug trafficking organizations are extremely powerful, producer countries do not possess the means to fight them, and nothing short of a massive infusion of international aid can alter the situation.

Finally, Andean governments take the position that drug trafficking programs inflict socioeconomic losses on the society and that it is the responsibility of the international community to compensate for these losses. The compensation theme is a permanent feature of the U.S.-Latin American dialogue over narcotics. For example, in the summer of 1983, the Belaunde government in Peru asked the United States for $200–$300 million to develop the Upper Huallaga Valley and to create income alternatives for coca growers. In 1987, the García government asked for $750 million for the Valley, and the García administration indicated that it will not push eradication very quickly unless the United States comes up with a better aid package for coca farmers. The Bolivian government's "Triennial Plan for the Struggle Against Drug Trafficking" envisages an

agricultural reconstruction program comprising direct and indirect payments of $300 million to the nation's coca growers. Of that sum, the
international community is responsible for contributing $260 million. (Bo-
livian officials now indicate that the package of economic measures for
growers will cost at least $350 million.) In Colombia, which now receives
almost no U.S. economic aid, top narcotics officials stress that coca
farmers need both help in planting substitute crops and air transport
networks to bring the products from the remote Llanos and Amazon
regions to markets in the cities. The pressure of insurgent movements in
Colombia's coca-growing areas, say these officials, makes such programs
an urgent necessity.[26]

Furthermore, the compensation game is not limited to coca cultivation;
Andean countries want the United States to provide foreign exchange to
substitute for cocaine earnings. For example, at the end of July 1986, the
Bolivian Ambassador to the United States, Fernando Illanes, told a U.S.
Senate subcommittee that his country would need a $100-million emer-
gency bridge loan to defray the loss of hard currency in Bolivia because of
reduced cocaine exports.[27] Cocaine exports at the time were down because
of Operation Blast Furnace, the joint U.S.-Bolivian attacks on the country's cocaine processing infrastructure. Bolivia did not get the loan.

Given the cocaine industry's powerful economic and political foothold
in these countries, such desires are understandable—but also unrealistic.
In these days of Gramm-Rudman and $200-billion budget deficits, the U.S.
Congress is unlikely to show much interest in funding safety net programs
for coca farmers or compensating Latin American countries for lost
cocaine income. Furthermore, many U.S. lawmakers do not understand
why the United States should reward countries for not doing what they
should not be doing anyway. Consequently, South America will probably
lose the compensation game. However, in the absence of safety-net programs for coca farmers and others whose economic survival is tied to the
cocaine industry, countries in the region will continue to have little stake
in the success of drug control programs.

Policy Debates

The eradication tangle. The United States exerts the strongest pressures on Latin American governments over coca eradication. U.S. legislation makes aid to Peru and Bolivia contingent on those countries' progress
toward eradicating illicit coca. The U.S. government has long viewed
eradication as a relatively cheap solution to the U.S. drug problem. U.S.
officials believe it is easier to locate and destroy crops in the field than to
locate and destroy laboratories (which are fairly easily concealed) or to
interdict processed drugs on the streets of U.S. cities.[28]

Yet, Latin American governments see the physical destruction of illicit crops, which pits the state directly against tens of thousands of farmers, as posing major political problems. In Bolivia, the sheer size of the coca lobby, which encompasses the country's main peasant and labor organizations as well as the coca farmers themselves, constitutes a major deterrent to eradication. Furthermore, as recounted in Chapter 2, the coca lobby has demonstrated its political muscle in ways that the Bolivian authorities find hard to ignore—by shutting down the nation's highway system, for example.

In Peru and Colombia, concerns about eradication are linked to the government's struggles against left-wing guerrilla movements and leftist subversion. Many Peruvian military and political leaders see eradication as generating anti-government feeling in rural areas and playing into the hands of radical leftist groups such as Sendero Luminoso. In the Upper Huallaga Valley, such programs reportedly provoked coca farmers and other disaffected Valley residents into joining or supporting local Sendero forces. In Colombia, despite public government rhetoric about the narco-guerrilla alliance, officials privately express similar concerns. A high Justice Ministry official interviewed in April 1986 said that the spraying of Colombia's main coca fields, located in the Llanos and the Amazon Basin, would create serious economic and social problems in these regions. Possible consequences, said the official, would be an increase in violent crime and an expansion of local guerrilla activity.[29]

These political forces have kept eradication efforts almost at a standstill. In 1987, about 1,800 hectares of coca were destroyed in the Andean countries out of a total Andean cultivation that the United States estimates at between 162,000 hectares and 211,000 hectares. (South American estimates, as noted in Chapter 1, are much higher.) Meanwhile, the amount of coca under cultivation in South America keeps growing. A 1988 State Department report estimated that between 1986 and 1987, net cultivation (that is, total cultivation after subtracting eradicated hectares) rose 4 percent in Peru and eight percent in Bolivia. A General Accounting Office report in that year estimated that for each of the 1,040 hectares of Bolivian coca eradicated in 1987, nearly 3 new hectares were planted. The same report shows net cultivation in Colombia increasing 61 percent between 1985 and 1987—from 15,500 hectares to 25,000 hectares. In 1988, according to the State Department, the unfavorable trends continued; net coca cultivation increased by 1 percent in Peru, 8 percent in Colombia, and 24 percent in Bolivia.[30]

In Bolivia, neither the Siles nor the Paz government dared to destroy coca plantations and risk confrontations with large numbers of campesinos. A 1983 agreement between the United States and Bolivia to eradicate

4,000 hectares of coca was never implemented. As a result, Bolivia lost some $17.4 million in U.S. economic and military aid in FY 1986 and FY 1987—hardly a significant sum given the likely economic and political costs of complying with U.S. demands. In 1987, Bolivia did manage to eradicate 1,000 hectares, a fairly remarkable feat, but this was accomplished through a complex process of negotiation with the Chapare Peasants' Federation. In other words, the government did not destroy the plots, the peasants themselves did. The government's strategy, as discussed in Chapter 2, is to maintain pressure on the cocaine processing infrastructure and, by so doing, to make it hard for farmers to find buyers for their leaves. The strategy works up to a point: Leaf prices have fallen dramatically from the 1984–1985 high. Yet, for farmers in the Chapare, the Yungas, and the Santa Cruz regions, coca still offers better returns than any alternative crop.

In Peru, the CORAH eradication program has been confined entirely to the Upper Huallaga Valley, one of several growing regions in Peru (most of the rest of Peru's coca grows in the south, in the provinces of Cuzco and Ayacucho). CORAH's labors resemble those of Sisyphus. It eradicated 11,600 hectares between 1983 and 1987, but U.S. and Peruvian officials believe that net coca cultivation in the Valley more than doubled during that period. Peruvian agricultural experts interviewed in Tingo María say that for every hectare of coca destroyed by CORAH, three to four new hectares have been planted, mostly in remote locations beyond the effective reach of eradication teams.

CORAH teams eradicate coca manually, plant by plant, a highly inefficient method. Logistically speaking, it may be impossible for CORAH to continue operating this way. In Leoncio Prado, most coca fields near the main jungle highway have been eradicated, and CORAH is forced to go ever farther afield to destroy plants. CORAH laborers spend up to 5 hours a day walking to and from the distant coca fields still remaining in the zone assigned to the project.[31] The project zone includes Tocache, where there is not only ample coca but flatter and more accessible terrain; however, penetrating Tocache has proved to be a supremely difficult task (see the discussion in Chapter 2). In the summer of 1987, the Peruvian government established a large camp for CORAH eradication workers at a site called Santa Lucia, several miles from Tocache City, but dangerous security conditions in the Valley kept the workers virtually confined to the camp. As noted in Chapter 2, in all of 1987, Peru only eradicated 355 hectares of coca, compared to 2,575 hectares in 1986 and 4,830 hectares in 1985. The Peruvian government, like the Bolivian government, is concentrating on attacking the cocaine industry downstream, in the hope of disrupting markets for coca leaves. However, as in Bolivia, the strategy makes little impact on the farmers' choices.

At this point, the last hope for winning the war against cocaine in South America is the large-scale application of herbicides against coca plants. However, governments fear a social convulsion and damage to the jungle environment and thus seem unwilling to take this step. The Bolivian government more or less has ruled out the spraying option. In June 1988, the country's Foreign Minister, Guillermo Bedregal, said, "Bolivia will not be the guinea pig for experimentation with herbicides that may have adverse effects on other vegetation and do damage to the inhabitants." In the same month, the Interior Minister, Juan Carlos Duran, said, "We have rejected the use of herbicides . . . The manual eradication of coca is backed by the peasants and avoids ecological harm."[32] These particular comments were prompted by a highly publicized controversy over the use of herbicides in Peru (which will be discussed below). However, as noted in Chapter 2, the Bolivian government for several years has taken the position that it will never use chemical means of eradicating coca.

In Peru, the García administration was at one time receptive to the idea of using herbicides against coca. Beginning in October 1987, the government authorized some backpack (manual) test spraying of plants in the Upper Huallaga Valley. One herbicide, tebuthiuron, which was manufactured by Eli Lilly under the trade name Spike, proved in the tests to be especially effective against coca. There were plans to move ahead in mid-1988 with crucial tests of Spike and one other herbicide, hexazinone (Velpar), manufactured by DuPont.[33]

However, Peru's spraying program suffered a possibly fatal setback in May 1988, when Eli Lilly announced that it would no longer supply tebuthiuron for the program. "A number of practical and policy considerations prevent our participation," said a Lilly spokesman. Lilly was almost certainly afraid of lawsuits stemming from improper use of the chemical. A company representative quoted by the Lima daily *El Comercio* said that Spike "could cause irreversible harm to flora and fauna and even affect human beings if it is not applied with extreme caution." The Peruvian press reprinted sections of a brochure that Lilly distributed with Spike: The folder warned that the compound could destroy the roots of trees, shrubs, and other vegetables and cause vomiting and pulmonary and heart damage in humans.[34]

Lilly's decision to withdraw from the program precipitated an angry debate in the United States over the ecological effects of Spike and other herbicides. U.S. Assistant Secretary for Narcotics Matters, Ann Wrobleski, called the decision "surprising" and said that Spike was "less toxic than aspirin, nicotine, and nitrate fertilizers." On the other hand, U.S.

environmental advocates such as Jay Feldman, the head of the National
Coalition against Abuse in the Use of Pesticides, disagreed. In a television
debate with Wrobleski, he said that using Spike would be equivalent to
"unleashing an atomic bomb in the zone." Said Feldman, "We are talking
about an agrarian society which depends on the earth for subsistence and,
if we destroy the agricultural base, we can't promote economic development with harvests of legal products."[35] Feldman's remarks were echoed
by other U.S. environmentalists. Dr. Peter Kurtz of the California Food
and Agriculture Department warned, "The major danger of tebuthiuron is
that it eradicates vegetation completely, that is, creates deserts where it is
used in sufficient quantity, and that it is very persistent" in soils. Dr.
Richard Wiles of the National Academy of Sciences warned of "ecological
devastation" from the application of Spike.[36]

These and other negative comments by U.S. environmentalists were
faithfully reported in the Peruvian press. The U.S. debate, needless to say,
intensified the concerns of Peruvian environmentalists and agricultural
experts over the possible hazards of using Spike and other chemical
herbicides against coca. A major concern, voiced by coca experts such as
Edgardo Machado, was that the heavy rainfall in the Upper Huallaga
Valley would wash the chemical off the leaves before it even killed the
plant. Furthermore, they argued, the rain would carry the chemical into
streams and rivers, with disastrous effects on licit crops and other plant
life. (Machado, incidentally, strongly advocates biological control of coca,
for example, the use of insects such as the "Malunya" butterfly, the larvae
of which feed on coca leaves.)[37] Peruvian proponents of spraying argued
(correctly) that the cocaine industry itself causes ecological damage, that
coca farming results in deforestation and erosion, and that the chemicals
used in processing coca leaves (such as kerosene and sulphuric acid)
pollute the river system in the Huallaga Valley. However, the debate over
Spike has left the impression in Peru that even worse damage to the
ecosystem could result from the application of toxic herbicides to the
country's vast coca plantations.[38]

The antispraying lobby seems at this point to have the upper hand.
Peru's most outspoken advocate of spraying, Interior Minister Jose Bar-
sallo, was removed from his post in June 1988. In July, the Peruvian
government decided not to initiate the aerial testing of herbicides, although
the State Department apparently stockpiled enough Spike to continue the
tests. By the end of 1988, Peru still had not proceeded with aerial spraying.
In December, the government created a committee of experts to study the
problem, but the committee's findings probably will not be issued for
months. The García government ultimately may conduct some aerial

spraying tests; however, the chances that it will ever use herbicides extensively against coca do not appear to be very strong.

In Colombia, as in Peru, the geographical remoteness of coca-growing areas and the presence of anti-government guerrillas in many of these areas virtually preclude the manual eradication of coca. Colombia is not opposed in principle to spraying; since 1984, the Colombian government has (with mixed success) been using herbicides against marijuana. However, a combination of factors—public reaction to the marijuana spraying program, protest by coca farmers and communist groups, and high-level opposition within the government itself—have effectively derailed efforts to use herbicides against coca.

Shortly after the April 1984 death of Lara Bonilla—in many respects a watershed in Colombian antidrug efforts—the government started spraying marijuana fields in northeastern Colombia and began preparations to use herbicides on coca. Colombia's National Council on Dangerous Drugs (CNE) in December 1983 made a tentative decision to "study the possibility of using paraquat and other herbicides, principally in the destruction of marijuana cultivation."[39] This decision raised two main issues: whether spraying should use paraquat or some other herbicide and, more fundamentally, whether the government should spray at all.

Fairly broad agreement within the key evaluating ministries—Health and Agriculture—suggested that paraquat was toxic to human health. By mid-1984, the CNE decided to drop paraquat in favor of a supposedly safer herbicide, glysophate.

However, opposition to using glysophate arose as well. The Institute of Health (INS), part of the Ministry of Health, issued a preliminary report on the herbicide in May 1984, saying that "its aerial use for destruction of marijuana and coca cultivation is not recommended."[40] A Ministry of Agriculture organization, the National Institute of Natural Renewable Resources (INDERENA)—a sort of Colombian EPA—lobbied strongly against the use of glysophate, citing possible harmful effects on plants, animals, and humans.[41] (INDERENA, in the words of a spokesman, is "philosophically opposed" to spraying in general.) Another organization in the same Ministry, the Agricultural Livestock Institute (ICA), supported spraying with glysophate, arguing that any environmental damage that could result from using the compound was minor compared to the destruction of the forests and woodlands to clear lands for planting marijuana.[42]

Against this rather confused background, the CNE announced at the end of June 1984 that it would begin spraying an undetermined number of hectares of marijuana in the Sierra Nevada region of Santa Marta, an area that is inhabited by several Indian communities and also is a national park. The decision provoked widespread opposition, much of it from people who had nothing to do with the marijuana trade—from scientists, ecologists, local farmers' organizations, coffee and banana growers, youth groups, and well-known journalists (such as German Castro Caycedo of *Radio Television Interamericana* and *El Tiempo's* Enrique Santos Calderón). The extreme left also took a dim view of the government's policy: The April 19th guerrilla movement (M-19) threatened to fire on any government helicopters that came to spray marijuana fields.[43]

In July 1984, after spraying had commenced, a lawyer named Antonio Nieto filed a suit with the attorney general's regional office in Baranquilla against Enrique Parejo, the Minister of Justice and the Chairman of the CNE. The principal charge against Parejo was that the spraying of marijuana had been carried out without authorization from Colombia's Council of Ministers. Such authorization would have required a verdict from the INS on the herbicide's effect on the ecosystem. INS' preliminary recommendation, as noted above, was negative, and a later September report also recommended against aerial spraying. The primary INS concern was "drift"—the movement of particles of spray onto crops and vegetables in surrounding areas—a concern apparently shared by the manufacturer of glysophate. Monsanto spokesmen warned that even "small quantities of the herbicide can cause severe damage or destruction" of desirable vegetation and that the risk of environmental damage was greater when the chemical was sprayed in winds of more than 8 km per hour—which is a relatively permanent condition of the Sierra Nevada range.[44]

Nieto's lawsuit precipitated a full-scale investigation by the nation's Attorney General, Carlos Jiménez Gómez, and in December 1984, Jiménez took the unprecedented step of denouncing Parejo before the Committee of Indictments of the House of Representatives. Jiménez said that Parejo— as the head responsible for the spraying program—had violated five separate provisions of Colombia's penal code. The thrust of Jiménez's accusations was that Parejo abused his authority in acting without the sanction of the Council of Ministers and that he permitted the contamination of the country's natural resources. None of this controversy, however, made any impact on the government's policy. The Committee on Indictments shelved the charges against Parejo. The spraying continued and by the end of 1985 had destroyed or forced the abandonment of approximately 8,000 hectares, representing 60–80 percent of the country's marijuana crop, according to State Department estimates.[45]

However, spraying remains a divisive issue in Colombia. INDERENA and other opponents charge that glysophate destroyed food crops and poisoned fish and livestock. A Bogotá TV correspondent claims that the chemical caused anemia among local Indian populations. Anti-marijuana spraying reportedly did $10 million worth of damage to licit crops in the

Sierra Nevada de Santa Marta region. Among the reported losses are 5,000 cacao plants, 6,300 yucca plants, 4.5 hectares of coffee, and 2 hectares of sugar cane. The affected farmers plan to sue the national government.[46]

INDERENA is also concerned about the socioeconomic effect of spraying and has proposed various forms of compensation for marijuana farmers who lose their crops. On the other hand, proponents such as ICA downplay the health and environmental consequences of spraying, saying that marijuana cultivators have done greater damage to the environment by tearing up forests to plant their illicit crops. Nor is ICA interested in alternative income schemes for marijuana farmers. In early 1986, the attorney general again stepped into the debate by ordering or pressuring the CNE to set up an expert commission to review Colombia's entire herbicide program for marijuana and for coca. By mid-1988, the commission had completed its work, although two of its members, ICA and INDERENA, were reportedly at loggerheads on the environmental effects of marijuana spraying.

The debate over marijuana spraying has obviously carried over into the government's deliberations on coca spraying. Colombia began spraying coca experimentally in late 1984, and, according to the State Department, eradicated 2,000 hectares by the end of 1985—perhaps 10–15 percent of Colombia's crop at the time—through a combination of aerial and backpack spraying.[47] The program as a whole was shrouded in secrecy. The location of test sites was not revealed, although they seemed to be in the southern Llanos region. At least one site was near the Llanos town of San José del Guaviare. Rumors circulated about spraying in the Serrania de Macarena, a national park in Meta department. Approximately ten different herbicides were tried, separately and in combination, but the environmental effects of the tests were never publicized.

The program was troubled from the start. "It was all highly improvised," said one U.S. official. "We had minimal resources and no scientific support."[48] One U.S. chemical manufacturer, Dow Chemical, demanded indemnification against lawsuits if the State Department decided to use the company's herbicide Garlon-4 in Colombia. Indemnification was not forthcoming, and Dow consequently refused to sell more than token quantities of the herbicide to the State Department. Within the Colombian government, INDERENA and the Minister of Health expressed serious reservations about the spraying program. INDERENA representatives were especially enraged over the apparent spraying of coca in the Serrania de Macarena, because the organization conceives of itself as a protector of Colombia's national parks. Furthermore, there were strong reactions from local campesino groups. A U.S. narcotics expert writing in early 1986 from the town of San José del Guaviare suggested that the coca-growing population had begun to mobilize against spraying. His internal memorandum stated:

> The civilian population in San José is more hostile than ever. Many campesinos
> are threatening legal action and scream about losing their livelihood and against
> police abuses at every opportunity . . . [Large] scale demonstrations and other
> problems could be on the horizon. Intelligence sources also claim an increase in
> guerrilla activity in the San José area.

Sometime in early 1986, Colombia's National Council on Dangerous Drugs suspended the test-spraying program. In 1988, the program was still on hold. The government told the U.S. State Department and the Colombian National Police that they will have to grow the plants themselves if they want to spray coca in Colombia. A U.S. State Department official interviewed at the end of May, however, thought that there was still hope for the program, especially if Peru made the decision to proceed with aerial spraying tests.

The extradition mess.   Extradition is by far the most important of the drug law enforcement issues in Colombia. The 1979 U.S.-Colombian treaty on extradition was an obviously important tool of drug enforcement. The purpose of the instrument, as one DEA official in Bogotá puts it, is to show that there is "no safe haven in Colombia" for Colombian traffickers who violate U.S. drug laws. After the death of Lara Bonilla in April 1984, the Colombian government cooperated up to a point in implementing the treaty. By June 1987, when the treaty ceased to be operative, the U.S. had submitted 140 extradition requests for drug trafficking and related offenses: 24 of these requests had been approved, and 16 persons (14 Colombians and 2 foreigners) had actually been extradited.[49]

The rationale for the treaty stemmed from Colombia's porous system of criminal justice. The system convicts only a small percentage of those tried for narcotics offenses, and those who are convicted are small fry. No leading traffickers are now serving time in prison. The drug mafia's use of bribes and threats successfully neutralizes many judges. Judges are often poorly trained or incompetent, the judicial system is overloaded, and drug crimes may be reduced to misdemeanors to expedite cases and get people out of jail. What conspiracy laws there are in Colombia are seldom applied in practice. It is extremely difficult to prosecute anyone not actually caught in possession of drugs.

Fernando Cepeda, former Dean of the University of the Andes and currently Colombia's Ambassador to Great Britain, strongly favors extradition as a counterweight to Colombia's judicial system, which he describes as "a disaster." The *El Tiempo* columnist D'Artagnan calls extradition "the only way to convince the North American people that we are in a struggle to the death with the mafia and are not tolerating its actions and incursions." Other notables such as the director of *El Espectador,* Guillermo Cano, favored application of the treaty because of the pervasive corruption of the judiciary in Colombia, which allowed drug criminals there to operate with impunity.[50]

Yet, many Colombians see extradition as an example of "colonial" justice and a renunciation of sovereignty. Opposition has been widespread and sometimes violent. The narcotics lobby has mounted an intense propaganda campaign against extradition and may well have resorted to stronger measures. As described in a previous chapter, Colombian Supreme Court justices received anonymous threats that they would be killed unless they declared the treaty unconstitutional. Government officials received death threats for implementing the treaty. As noted in Chapter 3, a Colombian Supreme Court judge who approved extradition of drug trafficking suspects to the United States was assassinated in Bogotá in July 1986. The extreme left—the Unión Patriótica (which represents the FARC) and M-19 guerrillas—also has taken a strong stance against extradition. M-19 guerrillas destroyed records of extradition cases when they staged an attack on the Palace of Justice in November 1985, although they might have done so at the behest of drug traffickers.

It is important to note, however, that antiextradition sentiment was not just confined to the ultranationalist fringe. Many people took a stand against the treaty: distinguished jurists, the leaders of Colombia's two major labor unions, prominent writers and journalists, congressmen, and even government officials. In January 1985, a report of *Noticiero TV-Hoy* in Bogotá showed three extradited Colombians being delivered to Miami Federal Court in handcuffs, chains, and leg irons. The image of the three traffickers "chained like beasts," in the words of *Semana* magazine, provoked wide public outrage as well as official protest from Colombia's Foreign Ministry. A former Colombian foreign minister remarked shortly after the incident, "President Betancur, in allowing the extradition of Colombians to the United States, has effectively sacrificed his nationalism."[51]

The focal point for opposition within the Betancur administration was the Attorney General, Carlos Jiménez Gómez—also an opponent of spraying and an advocate of negotiations with drug traffickers. Jiménez wrote a letter to President Betancur in November 1984 saying that "Colombia must neither practice nor allow the surrender of its nationals to foreign justice." Also, Jiménez petitioned the Colombian Supreme Court on eight separate occasions—each involving an extradition case—to declare the treaty unconstitutional. In four of the cases, Jiménez argued that the treaty violated Colombian sovereignty and in four others challenged the instrument on various technical grounds.[52]

Jiménez's stance set him apart from the rest of the cabinet; however, as time went on, the Betancur administration's attitude toward the treaty became increasingly equivocal. In early 1986, the Colombian government—via Enrique Parejo—began threatening to break the treaty unless the U.S. agreed to changes. Colombia had two key complaints: One was that the list of extraditable offenses included activities—such as money laundering—that were not clearly crimes in Colombia. (One of the original groups of extradited Colombians exhibited in the NBC report had, in fact, been charged with laundering $55 million through Florida banks.) A second complaint concerned the compulsory nature of the treaty. Article 8 of the treaty appears to require that extradition of nationals be granted in the following cases: (1) "where the offense involves acts taking place in the territory of both States with the intent that the offense be consummated in the Requesting State" (the case, for example, of a trafficker planning a shipment of cocaine from Colombia to the United States), and (2) "where the person for whom extradition has been sought has been convicted in the Requesting State of the offense for which extradition is sought."[53] It is this particular clause, more than any other, that has offended nationalist sentiment in Colombia: The Colombian government wanted to change the language of Article 8 to make extradition discretionary rather than binding.

The administration of Virgilio Barco seemed prepared to uphold the 1979 treaty (Barco himself had negotiated the treaty for Colombia when he was Colombia's Ambassador to the United States). However, in December 1980, Colombia's Supreme Court dealt the treaty a strong setback: It overturned Law 27, which the Colombian Congress had passed in 1980 to give legal force to the treaty. The court took the action on the technical ground that the law had not been signed by the President—at the time Julio Cesar Turbay Ayala—but rather by a "Minister delegate" (German Zea Hernández). Barco's response, which was both intelligent and courageous, was to give the implementing legislation a new number—it became Law 68—and to sign it. The antiextradition forces challenged this move, however; the Colombian Congress, they said, would have to pass a new law. The chances of this happening were virtually nil; congressional sentiment, like public sentiment, ran overwhelmingly against the treaty.

In June 1987, the Colombian Supreme Court voted on the legality of Law 68. The result was a 12-12 tie and an outside jurist, Alfonso Suarez de Castro, was brought in to resolve the deadlock. Suarez voted to overturn the law; he stressed in doing so that his vote did not address the legality of the treaty itself, but that the decision was made on narrow technical grounds. The President of the Court, Juan Hernández Saenz, explained the ruling, "Law 68 was not in reality a new law, but the same law on which a new number and a presidential signature were placed." The court advised Barco to submit new implementing legislation to the Colombian Congress for approval. The treaty was, for practical purposes, defunct. As a headline in the July 1987 issue of *Medellín Cívico* read, "Triumph of the people; extradition has collapsed."[54] No doubt death threats from drug traffickers influenced the court's decision, but public opinion was also a factor; the majority of Colombians do not favor extradition.

Following the demise of the 1979 treaty, the Colombian government was left with two possible legal options for extraditing drug traffickers: One was a U.S.-Colombian extradition treaty that had been signed in 1888, and the other was a multinational accord on extradition that the United States and Colombia had signed in Montevideo in 1933. Attorney General Carlos Mauro Hoyos favored the 1888 treaty, which had the advantage of not requiring Colombian Supreme Court approval for each extradition. However, others of the cabinet, including Justice Minister Enrique Low Murtra, argued that the 1888 treaty had been superseded by the instrument signed in 1979; they favored the Montevideo accord, although this would have required the Colombian Supreme Court to share responsibility for extraditions.[55] In early January 1988, the Colombian government issued warrants "with the intention to extradite" for Escobar, the Ochoa brothers, and Gonzalo Rodríguez Gacha. However, in March, the nation's supreme administrative tribunal, the State Council—responding to a legal challenge from the traffickers themselves—declared the extradition warrants invalid. The extradition process had effectively ceased to function in Colombia.[56]

The Role of the Military

Andean military establishments do not have a major antinarcotics mission. Rather, they provide occasional logistical support, such as helicopters and pilots, for operations planned, executed, and controlled by antidrug units of the national police. Historically, the military has not sought a major role in the war against drugs; in fact, it has tended to perceive the drug war as running counter to both its mission and its institutional interests.

In Peru and Bolivia, the military has contributed almost no resources and manpower to fight the drug traffic. Indeed, the military sometimes has hindered the effort—for example, by establishing a cordon sanitaire around major trafficking zones and by denying the police in Bolivia access to advanced weapons. The Colombian military, which falls under the same ministry as the national police, has been somewhat more involved.

However, according to Army General Paul Gorman, most military officers "disbelieve that the narco-traffickers threaten Colombia's national security"[57] and probably resent being distracted from their main missions. Colombia's Defense Minister Rafael Samuel Molina observed, "The Army would have better results in the antiguerrilla struggle if it were not tied down in antinarcotics activities."[58] To be sure, the military has struck some blows against the mafia. For example, the IV Brigade in Antioquia raided a Medellín residence of Pablo Escobar in March 1988—failing, however, to capture the trafficker. (The alleged links of the Brigade's intelligence chief to the Medellín mafia might have occasioned an information leak.) In early May, the Brigade raided some large CHCL laboratories in southern Antioquia that apparently were controlled by Escobar's organization.[59] Such episodes, however, are the exception rather than the rule; the Army's resources and manpower by and large are dedicated to chasing guerrillas, not to attacking the mafia's installations.

Furthermore, there have, in fact, been episodes of collaboration between military factions and cocaine traffickers throughout the Andean world. The linkages may derive from corruption, from strategic considerations, or even from shared political and ideological values. Also, the inherent nationalism of the armed forces has been a barrier to increased international cooperation against narcotics: The attitude of the Peruvian military toward the initial Condor operations with Colombia (discussed below) is a case in point. Finally, there is rivalry and historical animosity between the military and the national police in the Andean countries. Military establishments seek effective control over the legitimate use of force in their societies; for this reason, they have resisted efforts by the national police to develop an independent drug-fighting capability.

Interactions

U.S. and Latin American rhetoric about the "narco-guerrilla alliance" tends to overshadow another important relationship of the 1980s: the one involving drug traffickers and elements of the military. The military, like many other institutions in Andean countries, has been corrupted by the drug trade; yet, corruption is not the entire story. Individual military commanders, for example, may see coca growers or cocaine traffickers as potential allies in the struggle against subversion. There may be a commonality of values—for example, nationalism, hostility toward subversion and toward the left generally, and (for completely different reasons) a dislike of the narcotics police.

In Colombia, to quote the U.S. scholar Bruce Bagley, there has been a "linkage between drug money, death squads, anti-left activity, and the military."[60] Cocaine dealers and military men appear to be associated via common membership in right-wing vigilante groups. The most prominent of these groups is known as Death to Kidnappers (Muerte a Los Secuestradores, or MAS). The history of MAS deserves some attention here. According to one report, MAS was founded in a general assembly of over 200 drug barons in December 1981. Pablo Escobar and Carlos Lehder were said to be among the founders (although they both deny it). MAS offered rewards to public-spirited citizens who would cooperate in a clean-up campaign against kidnappers and subversives. A MAS communiqué also notes that the mafia had brought "progress and employment" to Colombia by paying for schools, hospitals, and other social services.[61]

The impetus for the creation of MAS, as noted in Chapter 4, was said to be the kidnapping of Marta Nieves Ochoa, the daughter of one of Colombia's best known trafficking families, in November 1981. The girl was eventually returned, safe and sound, without ransom being paid, but MAS survived and thrived. The organization expanded to include members of the rural elite—large landowners and cattle ranchers, right-wing businessmen, and military men who brought with them an expanded definition of undesirables. Over the past 5 years, it has been linked to the systematic assassination of labor union organizers, intellectuals, students, amnestied guerrillas, and left-wing political party leaders. MAS and its offshoots—one of which is called MASCO, or Death to Kidnappers and Communists—have probably been responsible for the death of several hundred "leftists" of various stripes.

In the 1984 meetings with Alfonso López Michelson in Panama, Pablo Escobar and Jorge Ochoa indicated that members of the armed forces had worked together with cocaine traffickers after the Ochoa kidnapping. Carlos Lehder may have been referring to this narco-military entente when he sought the support of the "nationalist sector of the army" in building an anti-imperialist alliance.[62] Betancur's Attorney General Carlos Jiménez Gómez was convinced of the relationship. In 1983, he indicted 59 active-duty army personnel, including 11 officers, for crimes associated with membership in MAS. This precipitated an angry civilian-military confrontation. Fernando Landazabal Reyes, then the Minister of Defense, when presented with the details of the investigation, denounced Jiménez indirectly for "attempting to blacken the reputation of the armed forces." The cases were turned over to the military courts.[63] It would appear that Betancur simply had too many important policies that depended on at least a minimally supportive military to risk a costly conflict on this issue. As Bruce Bagley notes, "Because of the delicate balance between the executive and the military, civilian courts were not deemed competent to judge these cases."[64] To date, there have been no convictions. Indeed, most of the cases have been thrown out of court for lack of evidence. Incidentally, the Colombian Army's high command reacted to the indictments by instructing all officers to donate 1 day's pay to the defense of the accused men and by decorating the highest-ranking accused, a lieutenant colonel who was a brigade commander in the department of Cundinamarca and one of the nation's top experts in counterinsurgency warfare.[65]

In addition to collaborating with cocaine traffickers via MAS or MAS-type organizations, the military has also protected the cocaine industry in various ways, mainly against FARC guerrillas. In one well-documented case that occurred at the end of 1983, a Colombian special forces company actually helped traffickers to relocate an entire cocaine laboratory. The First FARC Front operating in the area, somewhere in the department of Caqueta, had apparently attempted to extort $500,000 from the operators of the complex. The latter's response was to contact commanders of the Seventh Army Brigade in Villavicencio and ask for protection. The special forces were dispatched to the scene, where they formed a defense perimeter around the laboratory while it was being dismantled. Later, they accompanied the shipment of "drugs, means of production, and other elements" (transported apparently in private planes) to a site near the Brazilian border—one presumably out of reach of the guerrillas. The entire operation took 26 days, according to Colombian press reports.[66]

For these services, the 48 men of the company (6 officers and 42 NCOs) received payments ranging from 45,000 pesos to 200,000 pesos (roughly $500 to $2,250) from traffickers. The affair precipitated an internal investigation by the Colombian Army, and the results were curious. No one was jailed. Three officers were separated from the service, and three were suspended for a year. None of the NCOs—who were also paid off by the traffickers—received any penalty. The officers were disciplined, the army explained, not for helping the traffickers dismantle and move their laboratory but rather for taking bribes. Complicity in the drug traffic, apparently, was not a problem in itself.[67]

The Chief of Staff of the Seventh Brigade, who directly authorized the operation, was asked why the special forces did not impound the laboratory. His response was that "it is not the mission" of the army to control the cocaine problem but rather to combat guerrillas. A special forces captain, one of those dismissed from the army, blamed anonymous higher-ups and said, "I do not understand why the special forces of the army were placed in the role of protecting the mafia." Two Bogotá newspapers, El Espectador and Voz (a communist daily), suggested that the orders originated not from Villavicencio but from the army high command in Bogotá. Voz theorized that the special forces could not have been sent

without direct permission of the commandant of the armed forces himself—at the time General Miguel Vega Uribe.[68]

A similar call-in-the-army episode had occurred in January 1983 at one
of the six original Yari laboratory sites. The site was a ranch, called
Candilejas, owned by what the newspaper *El Tiempo* described as "an
industrialist and cattleman" named Camilo Rivera. The ranch seems to
have housed a large cocaine processing laboratory. On the night of January
14, guerrillas from the Third FARC Front raided Rivera's ranch, kidnapping 18 people and impounding 4 airplanes; the guerrillas demanded
$425,000 for the return of the hostages and the property. Several days
later, soldiers from the Colombian Army's Seventh Brigade rescued the
hostages and recovered two of the airplanes. The entire operation was
described in the Colombian media as a rescue of kidnapped cattlemen.
After the Yari complex was raided by police in March 1984, police
redesignated the site as El Diamante. It was only about 30 km from
Tranquilandia, the administrative center of the Yari complex.[69]

The rescuing units, according to Colonel Jaime Ramírez Gómez, whom
the author interviewed in April 1986, probably knew about the existence
of the cocaine laboratories; however, said Ramírez, the Colombian Army
high command was not informed, and the complex was, in effect, "redis-
covered" in early 1984. The rediscovery was the result of DEA investigations tracing the route of precursor chemicals—ether and acetone—origi-
nating in West Germany. (DEA's version is that the chemicals were
tracked from Chicago and Miami.) One informed U.S. source in Bogotá,
however, claimed that the Army had long been aware of the existence of
Yari. Military leaders, he said, withheld the information from the antidrug
police and even refused to let police overfly the area. Possibly the military
or other powerful people in Colombia had a financial stake in Yari,
although there is simply no way to corroborate such a conclusion. Yet, the
sheer size of the Yari complex suggests high-level complicity. To disguise
the operation would have been difficult; Yari reportedly produced over 3
tons of cocaine a month, and Tranquilandia itself had a 3,500-foot airstrip.[70]

In Peru, the struggle against insurgency—perhaps more clearly than in
the case of Colombia—provided the framework for collaboration between
the military and cocaine traffickers. The setting was the Upper Huallaga
Valley, and the sequence of events there may be recalled briefly. In 1983,
CORAH began eradicating coca, and the police stepped up their operations
against drug traffickers. These activities threatened to depress the economy in the Valley, which was (and still is) largely centered around the
cocaine trade. The result was widespread local resentment against the
government and against the United States. According to many accounts,
the Sendero Luminoso guerrillas took advantage of this situation to set up

a second front in the Upper Huallaga section in late 1983. Sendero began a recruitment drive against coca growers and other disaffected Valley residents, and as many as 2,000 people may have joined its ranks. By mid-1984, the guerrillas were making their presence known. They dynamited police stations, attacked banks and schools, and even laid siege for a while to the PEAH compound in Aucayacu.

The Belaunde government reacted to this situation by declaring a state of emergency in the Upper Huallaga zone. In late August 1984, the army and marines entered the zone and assumed full political and military control. The military government lasted for 1 year and 4 months; the state of emergency was not lifted until December 1985. The armed forces always took the view that they were sent to the Alto Huallaga to safeguard national security against guerrilla subversion, not to police the drug trade. Military patrols took no action when they passed through places where coca paste transactions were in progress. Moreover, they saw the activities of CORAH and UMOPAR as alienating the local population and, in general, as complicating the counterinsurgency effort.[71]

The military's response was to confine UMOPAR to barracks for 5 months (from August 1984 to January 1985). Thereafter, UMOPAR was allowed to work, but only with prior approval of each operation by the political-military command. The military also put a tight rein on CORAH. In practice, eradication teams and the UMOPAR team guarding them were restricted to areas of low coca density. In major producing centers (such as Tocache, Uchiza, and Monzón), plantations, laboratories, and clandestine airstrips proliferated. The army commander of the Upper Huallaga zone, Julio Carbajal, issued reassuring statements to coca farmers (see discussion in Chapter 4).[72] He also said in off-the-record briefings to reporters that coca cultivation meant work for poor people and that the cocaine trade provided desperately needed foreign reserves for a poor country such as Peru. Cocaine, he said, was really the gringo's problem.[73]

The military regime also formed what one Peruvian congressman termed an "alliance" with drug traffickers. The military made contact with known drug dealers in an effort to get information on the whereabouts of guerrillas—that is, it used the traffickers as intelligence assets. Meanwhile, it prevented the police from acting firmly against the drug traffic. The alliance spawned corruption; U.S. law enforcement officials claim that military commanders provided protection for Colombian traffickers flying in and out of the zone. UMOPAR units were ordered to chase subversives, that is, they were deflected from their antidrug mission. In September 1985, the head of the marine detachment in Uchiza issued a memorandum to UMOPAR contingents in that district. The memorandum, in effect, told police that they would only be allowed to confiscate "arms, munitions, subversive propaganda, and military clothing." Cocaine and other elements linked to drug trafficking, it seemed, would be exempt from confiscation.[74]

The armed forces were popular in the Valley, and the local residents did their best to delay their withdrawal. Petitions were signed in early 1985 asking the government to keep the military in control of the region. "Terrorist" attacks were staged by drug traffickers to highlight the need for continued militarization. Fake guerrillas and real guerrillas may have been acting in the Valley simultaneously. For whatever reason—corruption or a perceived security threat—the military stayed in the Valley until the end of the year. The withdrawal, when it occurred, was greeted with almost universal dismay. During a visit to Peru in February 1986, politicians representing the Valley were lobbying hard to have the state of emergency reintroduced.

In Bolivia, there was a pattern of military collaboration with drug traffickers that extended at least until the end of the military regime in October 1982. Bolivian politics in the 1970s and early 1980s, as the U.S. sociologist Kevin Healy points out, was dominated by an alliance of military men and two rural elite groups: cattle and rubber barons in the Beni and an agribusiness elite whose wealth and income derived largely from cotton, sugar cane, and assorted processing industries in Santa Cruz department. The economic elites launched themselves into cocaine production in the 1970s, partly with the help of state bank loans arranged by the military governments of the period. Individual military officers also became de facto members of the economic elite; they "carved out" various economic interests through public land grants, bank credits, and timber and mineral rights concessions from the state. They established their own private development corporations and even their own bank, the Banco de Progreso. Kevin Healy concludes that the military, like the economic elite, was well-positioned to become a key actor in the cocaine trade.

> Under the leadership of Meza and Gómez [General García Meza and Colonel Arce Gómez]—with well-organized political protection, private guards, financial resources, outposts, private landing strips, aircraft, trucks, and access to abundant cheap labor—this military group, similar to the two other strategically placed elite groups, possessed comparative advantages for seizing the lucrative opportunities of the illicit drug trade.[75]

The actual participation of the Bolivian military in the drug trade is well documented and has already been discussed in a previous chapter. It is true that the axis of military men, rural economic elites, and cocaine traffickers more or less lost political power in Bolivia with the advent of democratic government in 1982. Since then, the military has pretty much stayed out of the limelight in Bolivia and has given little clue as to its attitude toward the drug trade. However, the Bolivian Army, which (unlike the police) recruits mainly from the campesino population, is thought by most U.S. and Bolivian observers to be a strong foe of coca eradication. Also, Bolivian political leaders talk nervously (although in private) about a prodrug faction in the armed forces and openly express their fear that dictatorship may return to Bolivia, especially if exceptionally harsh measures are taken against the cocaine trade. In the Beni, Roberto Suarez openly expresses his contempt for the democratic system and longs for a more ordered society run by generals. The axis, in other words, may still be alive and well, even if it no longer controls the formal trappings of government.

Other Problems: Nationalism; Military-Police Rivalry

South American military establishments generally see themselves as guardians of the nation. Also, they seek to monopolize the legitimate use of force within their territories. Both attitudes have posed a problem for narcotics control efforts in South America. The Peruvian military, for example, has been openly hostile to transnational collaboration against the drug traffic—in part because Peru traditionally has had bad relations with its neighbors and in part because the military's rival, the national police, has played a leading role in such collaboration. In all three countries, the military has been suspicious of U.S. narcotics assistance programs to the extent that they add to the overall capabilities of the police. Efforts by the United States to increase significantly its aid to the antidrug police could run afoul of the military and conceivably even work to destabilize civilian governments in these countries.

The main case in point of military nationalism was the Peruvian armed forces' opposition to the Condor I and II operations that occurred in 1985 just after García took power. Condor—a joint Colombian-Peruvian project—targeted cocaine laboratories and airstrips in the Peruvian Amazon, near the Colombian border. The operation, which involved overflights of Peruvian territory by Colombian air force helicopters (carrying Colombian police) was seen by the Peruvian military as a gross violation of Peru's sovereignty and air space. A bitter dispute ensued between the air force—backed by other elements of the Peruvian armed forces—and the Ministry of the Interior. In October 1985, the Lima newspaper *El Nacional* interviewed Augustín Mantilla, Peru's Vice Minister of Interior, and asked him about "confrontations in the Condor I and II operations." The following section of the interview suggests the seriousness of the affair.

Mantilla: There were some disagreements.
El Nacional: With General Enrico Praeli [of the Peruvian Air Force]?
Mantilla: General Enrico Praeli expressed his concern, because the helicopters of
    the air force of Colombia flew over our air space.
El Nacional: And how did you answer him?
Mantilla: We referred him to the president of the republic.[76]

García backed Interior's position, but at considerable risk to himself
politically. According to a DEA official on the scene in Lima, the incident
almost brought down the new government. Condor can be viewed as an
initial test of strength between García and the military (the air force
position was supported, to a greater or lesser degree, by the other
services). Luckily for democracy in Peru, García won that round.

Military nationalism also has worked to the detriment of antidrug
cooperation between Peru and Ecuador. In the wake of the Condor
operations referred to above, Peru and Ecuador—more specifically, the
police of the two countries—established plans for joint aerial surveillance
of each other's territory along their common border. The plane or planes,
to be supplied by DEA, would fly Ecuadorian police over Peru's territory
and Peruvian police over Ecuador's. The scheme was publicly announced
by Peruvian and Ecuadorian officials in early 1986, but was never implemented because of opposition from the military of both countries.[77] It
should be noted, by way of background, that there is a major territorial
dispute between Ecuador and Peru, stemming from a war between the
countries in 1941-1942, in which Ecuador lost about one-third of its
territory. Ecuador has never accepted the legitimacy of the so-called Rio
Protocol, which ended the war. Hostilities still flare up from time to time
along the border. The Peruvian military plans actively for a two-front war
against Ecuador and Peru's other major enemy, Chile. Given such constraints, any significant Peruvian-Ecuadorian collaboration in the near
future would appear unlikely.

Finally, in Peru, Bolivia, and Colombia, the military sees the national
police as a competitor. As the preceding paragraphs suggest, this attitude
colors the military's entire perception of the antinarcotics effort. It may
dislike the police a lot more than it dislikes drugs. In general, U.S. policy
is to channel narcotics assistance to the police, but resistance from the
military puts qualitative and quantitative limits on such assistance. For
example, the head of Peru's Senate Investigative Committee on Narcotics
noted in 1986, "The Air Force does not consider that the police should
have its own system of helicopters and planes."[78] As of mid-1986, the Civil
Guard's antidrug division (DIPOD) had only one working helicopter and a
few light aircraft captured from drug traffickers. Since then, the United
States has managed to reinforce DIPOD's airborne capability; however, it

has done so by *leasing* aircraft—a C123 and three Bell helicopters—to the police. The United States holds title to the aircraft, and U.S. pilots (from the Evergreen Corporation, based in Portland, Oregon) fly them on missions in the Upper Huallaga.

In Bolivia, institutional rivalry between the police and the armed forces is reinforced by historical antagonism. The police and the army fought on opposite sides of the Bolivian revolution of 1952, which resulted in the victory of the National Revolutionary Movement (MNR) and in Victor Paz Estenssoro's first presidency. The army, which was on the losing side, was for a while eliminated as a force in Bolivian politics. However, the ruling MNR coalitions crumbled in the early 1960s, and in November 1964, a military-led coup removed Paz and his movement from power. Military regimes dominated Bolivian politics for nearly two decades thereafter, until democracy was restored in October 1982.

The military's instinct has always been to keep the police in check, and it has acted accordingly. In a well-publicized incident in early 1984, the Bolivian army impounded a large shipment of French submachine guns that the Ministry of Interior had ordered for UMOPAR.[79] According to an informed U.S. source, the army also confiscated several hundred U.S. M-16 rifles that were imported for use in antidrug operations. The Bolivian Air Force monopolizes the use of helicopters and fixed-wing aircraft, and the navy similarly dominates the use of its river patrol craft. The navy has established what amounts to a fiefdom in Puerto Villaroel, a port city on the Rio Marmoré and one of the three ports of entry into the Chapare region. The navy does not permit antidrug operations in or around the port; it allegedly profits handsomely from traffickers' bribes to allow shipments of coca paste out of the region.[80] The Bolivian Air Force controls the six new HUEY helicopters that the United States gave Bolivia after Operation Blast Furnace for use in drug interdiction. Unfortunately, some Bolivian Air Force pilots are reputedly corrupt. A report by the Senate Caucus on International Narcotics Control notes:

> There have been several missed opportunities to seize cocaine laboratories because of the pilots' refusal to fly. UMOPAR and DEA personnel strongly suspect that the excuses pilots give for not flying (e.g., bad weather and lack of fuel) are covers for the fact that the pilots had been paid off to prevent missions from taking place.[81]

The air force will not let UMOPAR pilot the helicopters, and the police are not qualified to fly them in any case.

In Colombia, military-police relations are on the surface smoother than in Bolivia or Peru. A major reason is that both institutions are under the same umbrella ministry—the Ministry of National Defense. In the other countries, the police are subordinate to the Ministry of Interior, which is completely separate from the military. The Colombian military has not objected to the police's having helicopters and airplanes, as have the military establishments in Peru or Bolivia (the United States has transferred nearly 20 helicopters to CONAN since the early 1980s). Yet, the military has drawn the line on the issue of firepower. In the Foreign Assistance Act of 1986, Congress authorized $1 million to "arm, for defensive purposes, aircraft used in narcotics control eradication or interdiction efforts."[82] There was a U.S. plan in early 1986 to use some of this money to arm Colombian police helicopters with light machine guns; however, under pressure from the armed forces, the project was disapproved by the Defense Ministry. So the police still must rely on military gunships to escort them on antinarcotics missions in insecure areas.

Assessment

The events of the 1980s suggest that the U.S.-sponsored narcotics control effort in South America is to some extent a hostage of the military. The police must depend on the military for mobility and firepower. There are problems of coordination: Military support, according to police commanders in Colombia and Peru, is often too little and too late. In addition, the military's own source of priorities may simply preempt narcotics control efforts. During the state of emergency in the Upper Huallaga, the military formed what amounted to an alliance with drug traffickers. In Colombia, despite the "narco-guerrilla alliance," military commanders may find it expedient to cooperate tactically with cocaine dealers against the FARC and other revolutionary groups. International collaboration against drugs is clearly a sensitive issue for military establishments, in part because it is a "police" function and in part because it runs counter to the military's own nationalist agenda. Finally, the cocaine mafia and right-wing elements of the military may find common cause in vigilantism and anticommunism.

Drugs have clearly emerged as a problem in civil-military relations in Andean countries. The military sees antidrug programs as a tool of civilian politics—and with some justification. Civilian leaders in Andean countries may be tempted to build up the power of the police as a counterweight to the armed forces and may see drug fighting as a convenient excuse for doing so. A police force that was adequately equipped to cope with the drug traffic—and this is nowhere the case in South America—would be a very powerful force indeed. As of this writing (July 1988), the military-logistical capabilities of national police forces are slowly improving, especially in Peru. (Some UMOPAR units have been outfitted with North Korean AK-47s; also, as mentioned above, antidrug units have the use of three Bell helicopters and one C-123.) However, the police are still woefully ill-equipped to perform their mission.

Creating an effective antinarcotics strike force without antagonizing the military is not impossible, but the chances are not particularly good. The problem perhaps can be addressed by buying off the military with new equipment or by orchestrating aid programs in such a way as not to upset existing force ratios. For such a solution to work, however, the military would have to be willing to sacrifice its monopoly over the significant tools of war-fighting. Another option would be to build an antinarcotics unit within the armed forces. The disadvantage of this idea is that drugs are not the military's main mission. Arms and equipment supplied to such a unit might be deployed elsewhere—along the Peruvian-Chilean border, for example, or against the FARC in Colombia. The dilemma, in other words, will not be an easy one to resolve.

Notes

1. Phillip Boffey, "Drug Users, Not Suppliers, Held Key Problem," *The New York Times,* April 12, 1988.
2. Hussein Haqqani, "Truce with the Tribes," *Far Eastern Economic Review,* March 20, 1986, p. 50.
3. For a discussion of the strategic implications of drug trafficking for Peru, see Alejandro Destua, *El Narcotráfico y el Interés Nacional* (Lima: CEPEI, 1987), pp. 32–46.
4. Bureau of International Narcotics Matters, U.S. Department of State, *International Narcotics Control Strategy Report (INCSR)* (Washington, D.C., 1987), p. 70.
5. "El Dossier de Medellín," *Semana,* January 27, 1987, p. 25.
6. U.S. General Accounting Office, *Drug Control: U.S. Supported Efforts in Colombia and Bolivia (U.S. Supported Efforts)* (Washington, D.C., November 1988), p. 54.
7. "El Dossier de Medellín," p. 24.
8. "Paz Delivers State of Union Address to Congress," La Paz Domestic Service, August 6, 1986.
   Alan García, "To the Immense Majority," in Alan García, *Three Speakers for History* (Lima, 1985), p. 34.
   Alan García, "Debt or Democracy," in *Three Speakers for History,* p. 68.
   "Barco Speaks on Law and Order," Bogotá Inravision, Cadena 1, January 14, 1988.
   "Betancur Speaks at Opening Session of Congress," Madrid EFE, July 21, 1984.
   "Betancur Addresses Nation," Bogotá Cadena Radial Super, May 1, 1984.
9. "Urban Colombians Favor International Cooperation Against Drugs, but Re-

ject Extradition and Fear Herbicides" ("Urban Colombians"), USIA Research Memorandum, Washington, D.C., February 22, 1988, p. 3.

"Urban Peruvians Applaud Their Government's Anti-Narcotics Efforts and Support International Cooperation Against Drugs" ("Urban Peruvians"), USIA Research Memorandum, Washington D.C., May 5, 1988, p. 16.

"Urban Bolivians Applaud Their Government's Anti-Narcotics Effort and Want Other Countries' Help to Control Production" ("Urban Bolivians"), USIA Research Memorandum, Washington, D.C., May 4, 1988, p. 17.

10. Virgilio Barco, *Hacia Una Colombia Nueva* (Bogotá: Lerner, 1986), p. 12.
    Programa del Partido Liberal Colombiano, Bogotá, December 4, 1985.

11. "NEA Poll Finds Education, Drugs, Concern Public Most," *Washington Times,* July 6, 1988.

12. "6 de cada mil colombianos son consumidores de basuco," *El Occidente,* Cali, February 11, 1988.

13. "Reactivación económica por dinero caliente," *El Tiempo,* October 3, 1987.
    "Directivo de BCR habla sobre narcodólares," *El Comercio,* October 8, 1987, p. B13.
    "Debt or Democracy," p. 68.
    Bradley Graham, "Bolivia Runs Risk in Drug Drive," *The Washington Post,* July 16, 1986.

14. R. W. Lee, "The Drug Trade and Developing Countries," Overseas Development Council, *Policy Focus,* June 1987, p. 7.

15. Bradley Graham, "Colombians Stunned by Audacity, Firepower of Major Traffickers," *The Washington Post,* February 2, 1988.
    Interview with staff of Invamer, March 1988.

16. "Urban Colombians," p.15.

17. "Bolivia no aceptará fuerza multinacional contra drogas," *El Comercio,* April 13, 1988.

18. "President García Grants Interview to TV Latina," Panama City Panavision, July 5, 1987, p. R1.
    "Frente común internacional contra la droga pide B. B.," *El Espectador,* August 21, 1984.

19. "Urban Colombians," p. 17.
    "Urban Bolivians," p. 10.
    "Urban Peruvians," p. 16.

20. Alan Riding, "A Drug Problem for All the Americas," *The New York Times,* July 31, 1988.

21. "El tráfico de drogas es mecanismo de autodefensa, dice García Márquez," *El Espectador,* July 3, 1984.

22. Interviews with U.S. narcotics experts in La Paz during March 1986, May 1986, and October 1–2, 1987.
    Interview with the Sub-Secretary of Social Defense, La Paz, October 6, 1987.

23. Interviews with U.S. narcotics officials in Lima and La Paz during March 1986, May 1986, and October 1987.

24. Michael Isikoff and Eugene Robinson, "Colombian Drug Kings Becoming Entrenched," *The Washington Post,* January 8, 1989.

25. "Exorcizando a la policía," *Caretas,* May 5, 1986, p. 30.
    "Antidrug Aid Ridiculous," Madrid EFE, August 5, 1988.

26. Interviews with the Ministry of Interior and the Colombian National Police, April 1986.

27. Joel Brinkley, "Bolivia Asks U.S. for Big Loan to Make Up Lost Cocaine Income," *The New York Times,* July 31, 1986.
28. Rafael Perl, "International Narcotics Control," Congressional Research Service Issue Brief, July 11, 1988, p. 5.
29. Interviews at the Ministry of Justice in Bogotá, April 1986.
30. *INCSR,* 1988, pp. 63, 75, 89.
    "U.S. Supported Efforts," pp. 23, 56.
31. "Mixed Signals from the Huallaga Cocaine Belt" ("Mixed Signals"), *The Andean Report,* December 1985, p. 235.
32. "Bolivia Will Not Allow Use of Herbicides to Kill Coca Plant," Reuters Library Report, June 17, 1988.
    "Bolivia también dice no," *El Comercio,* June 15, 1988.
    James Smith, "Aerial Attack on Coca? Peru Stalls U.S. Plan" ("Aerial Attack on Coca"), *Los Angeles Times,* June 30, 1988.
33. Alan Riding, "In War on Coca, U.S. Weapon Is Bogged Down in a Dispute" ("In War on Coca"), *The New York Times,* June 28, 1988.
34. "Aerial Attack on Coca," p. 12.
    "Herbicida Spike podra causar daños ecológicos irreversibles," *El Comercio,* June 22, 1988.
35. "Herbicida contra cocales es una bomba atómica," *El Comercio,* June 15, 1988.
    "In War on Coca," see note 33.
    "Niegan a EE. UU. venta de producto contra cocales," *El Comercio,* May 25, 1988.
36. "Nos escriben y contestamos," *Caretas,* June 20, 1988, p. 6.
37. Hernán Velarde, "La Malunya," *Estampa,* Lima, April 10, 1988, pp. 2–3.
38. For a discussion of the proherbicide position, see "Narcotraficantes están contaminando los ríos," *El Comercio,* June 22, 1988.
39. Rodrigo Lara Bonilla, "Comunicado del Consejo Nacional de Estupefacientes," Bogotá, Ministry of Justice, 1983, p. 1.
40. Instituto Nacional de Salud, "Informe: Comité de Expertos en Herbicidas," Bogotá, May 7, 1984, p. 18.
41. Ulilo Acevedo, "El glisofato destruirá a la Sierra Nevada y al Tayrona," *El Heraldo,* Barranquilla, June 30, 1984.
42. Orlando Brínez Ramírez, "Informa ICA comisión observación aplicaciones glisofato en la Sierra Nevada de Santa Marta," Bogotá, April 2, 1986, p. 10.
43. Enrique Santos Calderón, "Drogas y triunfos morales," *El Tiempo,* October 24, 1985.
    "M-19 Opposes Fumigation Plan," Bogotá Radio Cadena Super, July 12, 1984.
44. "Unauthorized Spraying of Marijuana Investigated," *Cromos,* Bogotá, January 29, 1985, pp. 22–25.
    ICA, "Round-Up: Herbicida de Monsanto," translation of company's instructions, p. 5.
45. "Despacho del procurador general," document describing Nieto lawsuit, December 21, 1981, pp. 1–11, 40–42.
46. "Coffee, Coca Crops Damage Attributed to Glysophate," *El Tiempo,* September 15, 1986.
47. *INCSR,* 1986, p. 90.
48. "In War on Coca," see note 33.
49. Interviews with U.S. narcotics experts in Bogotá, October 22, 1987.

50. D' Artagnan, "Cocalombia: así nos ven," *El Tiempo*, September 7, 1983.
    Guillermo Cano, "Liberta de Apuntes," *El Espectador*, January 20, 1985.
51. Mario Arango Jaramillo and Jorge Child Vélez, *Los Condenados de la Coca (Los Condenados)* (Medellín: J. M. Arango, 1985), pp. 232–240.
    "Narcotráfico y nacionalismo," *Visión*, February 25, 1985, p. 37.
52. "Narcotráfico y nacionalismo," p. 37.
    "Por octava vez procurador pide tumbar extradición," *El Tiempo*, October 10, 1985.
53. Fabio Rincón, *La Extradición* (Bogotá: Pensar, 1984), pp. 54–55.
54. "Triunfo del pueblo: cayó la extradición," *Medellín Cívico*, July 1987, pp. 1, 8.
55. Alan Riding, "Intimidated Colombian Courts Yield to Drug Barons," *The New York Times*, January 11, 1988.
56. "Suspenden capturas del cartel de Medellín," *El Tiempo*, March 24, 1988, p. 1.
57. Committee on Foreign Relations, U.S. Senate, *Drugs, Law Enforcement, and Foreign Policy: Panama* (Washington, D.C.: U.S. Government Printing Office, 1988), Hearings before the Subcommittee on Terrorism, Narcotics, and International Communications, Part 2, p. 2.
58. "¿Estamos perdiendo la guerra?" *El Tiempo*, March 6, 1988.
59. *Mid-Year Update, INCSR*, pp. 8–9.
60. Bruce Bagley, "The Colombian Connection," in Deborah Pacini and Christine Franquemont (eds), *Coca and Cocaine: Effects on People and Policy in Latin America* (Petersborough, New Hampshire: Transcript Printing Company, June 1986), p. 95.
61. "The Medellín Cartel: World's Deadliest Criminals" ("The Medellín Cartel"), Special Report, *Miami Herald*, February 1987, p. 9.
62. *Los Condenados*, p. 140.
    "El país tiene que hacerse cargo de la magnitud del problema de la droga," *El Tiempo*, July 19, 1984.
63. "Colombia: MAS Report Raises New Political Storm," *Latin American Weekly Report*, February 18, 1983, p. 5.
64. "The Colombian Connection," p. 95.
65. Terri Shaw, "Death Squad Members Face Trial in Colombia," *The Washington Post*, July 11, 1983.
66. Fabio Castillo, "Operación encubierta para proteger laboratorio de la coca," *El Espectador*, August 1, 1985.
67. Ibid.
68. Ibid.
    "Militarismo y narcotráfico: matrimonio sin divorcio," *La Voz*, Bogotá, August 15, 1985.
69. This account has been pieced together from various sources:
    "Rescatan rehenes y aviones: muertos tres guerrillas," *El Tiempo*, January 26, 1983.
    "Rescatados otros 37 secuestrados," *El Tiempo*, January 27, 1983.
    "Statement of Special Agent Michael Fredericks," in President's Commission on Organized Crime, *Organized Crime and Cocaine Trafficking* (Washington, D.C.: U.S. Government Printing Office, 1984), p. 610.
70. "The Medellín Cartel," p. 3.
71. "Mixed Signals," pp. 246–248.
72. "The New Coca Boom Boosts the Balance of Payments as United States Anti-Narcotics Efforts Flop," *The Andean Report*, April 1985, p. 42.

73. William Montalbano, "Coca Valley: Peru Jungle Surrealism," *Los Angeles Times,* December 2, 1985.
74. Carlos Noriega Espejo, "La guerra de la coca," *Caretas,* January 27, 1986, pp. 10A, 20B.
75. Kevin Healy, "The Boom Within the Crisis," in *Coca and Cocaine,* p. 106.
76. "Interior Official on Anti-Narcotics Plans, Scope of Problem," *El Nacional,* Lima, October 20, 1985.
77. "Perú y Ecuador inician lucha conjunta contra narcotráfico," *Hoy,* Quito, February 6, 1986.
    "Habrá acción conjunta de Colombia Perú y Ecuador contra narcotráfico," *El Siglo,* Bogotá, January 9, 1986.
78. "Se tienen que investigar los coca dólares," *El Nacional,* February 2, 1986.
79. "Caged Leopards of the Drug War," *The New York Times,* September 12, 1984.
80. On this point, see "Se hace investigación dentro la armada en Puerto Villaroel," *Hoy,* October 12, 1988.
81. Senate Caucus on International Narcotics Control, *On Site Examination of Narcotics Control Efforts in Bolivia: A Staff Report* (Washington, D.C.: U.S. Government Printing Office, 1987), p. 187.
82. U.S. House of Representatives and U.S. Senate, *Legislation on Foreign Relations Through 1987* (Washington, D.C.: U.S. Government Printing Office, 1988), Volume 1, p. 331.

6

Conclusion: The U.S. Policy Dilemma

A 1988 Department of State report noted that Latin American governments do not yet recognize that coca and cocaine trafficking "pose serious threats to their own survival."[1] Indeed, many Andean leaders have reason to believe that the cure is worse than the disease, because crackdowns on the drug industry pose severe economic and political hazards. To a degree, these concerns coincide with U.S. concerns: The United States wants to encourage stable, economically viable governments in the region, to promote democracy, and to suppress leftist insurgent movements. The war against drugs is not necessarily compatible with these other priorities, at least in the short run. In fact, the argument can be made that the United States and its Latin American allies share a common interest in minimizing the intensity of the drug war. After all, narcotics control, although an important concern, is not the only issue on the Hemisphere's agenda.

This perspective proved hard to maintain in an election year. The Reagan Administration was pilloried by its opponents for not making drug control its top foreign policy priority. Legislators and local officials demanded reprisals against governments that tolerate the narcotics industry; U.S. Senator John Kerry (Democrat, Massachusetts) and New York City Mayor Edward Koch wanted to send troops to Colombia to root out the Medellín syndicates. The Nicaraguan Contras were accused of taking money from Colombian cocaine syndicates ($10 million between 1982 and 1985), and U.S. intelligence agencies were accused of helping the Contras smuggle drugs into the United States.[2]

These critics responded to real public pressures. An April 1988 New York Times/CBS News poll reported that U.S. citizens perceive drug trafficking as a more important international problem than arms control, terrorism, Palestinian unrest in Israel, or the situation in Central America. Another poll showed that Americans feel that thwarting the drug dealings

231

of anticommunist leaders in Central America is more important (by a vote of three to one) than fighting communism in the region. A third poll noted a public preference for U.S. government policies that reduce the supply of illicit drugs entering the United States over policies that focus on persuading U.S. users to stop taking drugs.[3]

Certainly the status quo does not work in the long-term interests of the Latin American countries. At issue is not so much the fate of democracy as the deterioration and the demodernization of political and economic institutions. As U.S. Ambassador to Colombia Charles Gillespie recently remarked, "The traffickers have already penetrated the fabric of Colombian life . . . this penetration will lead not to the downfall of Colombia and its institutions but rather to a serious and lasting corruption."[4] The traffickers also cause other political problems: The hold of governments on their territories is weakened, the reputation of drug-exporting countries is damaged, and citizens and products are the victims of international discrimination.

Yet, there may be no useful way to upgrade the war against cocaine and other narcotics industries overseas. Virtually every prescription under discussion carries major disadvantages.

Enhancement of Drug-Fighting Capabilities in Producer Countries

Under this approach, Andean governments would be provided with firepower, transport, communications, and intelligence support to establish their authority in drug-trafficking zones and to destroy the infrastructure of the cocaine industry. However, as the discussion in Chapter 5 suggests, this approach risks exacerbating civilian-military tensions in the Andean countries. Furthermore, the prevailing pattern of corruption in the region makes many U.S. observers skeptical of the utility of such buildups. RAND economist Peter Reuter suggested that infusions of U.S. aid may do little more than change the distribution of profits between drug cartels and governments.[5]

In the view of many U.S. officials, the main hope for controlling the cocaine coming from source countries lies in the aerial spraying of coca. Some herbicides have proved effective against coca in tests (Eli Lilly's Spike is one such compound). Bolivian leaders, however, now rule out the use of chemical tools for eradication. Colombia's National Council on Dangerous Drugs suspended the government's test spraying program in early 1986 and seems unlikely to permit spraying any time soon. Peru's Alan García calls for an "exhaustive, profound, and lengthy study" of anti-coca herbicides to demonstrate that there are no harmful consequences for the ecology or for humans. García also wants to know how the substitution of coca cultivation would be financed if Peru did agree to use herbicides.[6] The spraying approach probably will not be politically acceptable in South America. Governments fear ecological damage from the use of toxic chemicals, and current U.S. debates on the environmental consequences of spraying, which are widely reported in the South American press, have done much to inflame these concerns. However, governments are even more concerned with the social effects—the prospects of massive rural unemployment and (in Colombia and Peru) the aggravation of a festering insurgency problem.

"Americanization" of the War on Drugs

This strategy calls for the United States to receive permission to take over drug enforcement functions that producer countries cannot perform. Examples of this approach include Operation Blast Furnace, the U.S. Army-supported operation against cocaine laboratories in Bolivia in the summer of 1986, and the trial of Colombian drug traffickers in U.S. courts. Americanization works to a point—Blast Furnace virtually shut down Bolivia's cocaine industry for 3 months—but such operations carry extreme political risks for host governments. All segments of Bolivia's political establishment condemned the operation, and a leader with less stature than Victor Paz Estenssoro could not have survived the political fallout. The Colombian and Peruvian governments have pointedly declined U.S. offers of military assistance. Even U.S. officials closely associated with Blast Furnace realize that U.S. military intervention was a mistake. Says David Westrate, DEA's Assistant Administrator for Operations, in Congressional testimony in June 1988, "What we learned at the end ultimately is that we cannot do that again . . . .I do not see the U.S. military being deployed in an enforcement context, particularly in Latin American countries, in the future."[7] Ultimately, Americanization could land the United States in a Vietnam-type morass, with U.S. troops and law enforcement agents pitted against Third World peasants in a struggle that is unwinnable, both strategically and politically.

Extradition also appears to be a dead issue. In June 1987, the Colombian government nullified legislation enabling the government to extradite drug traffickers to the United States. Efforts by the government to extradite under a different legal formula (the 1933 Montevideo convention) were struck down by the Council of State. In Bolivia, the government rebuffed a U.S. request to deliver Roberto Suarez, the "King of the Beni," who has been indicted in Florida and Bolivia on cocaine smuggling charges. Extradition is widely unpopular in Colombia and anathema in much of

Latin America: It has been a cause celebre for Latin American nationalists of all political stripes.

Income Replacement

"If we are to make a difference in cocaine control," declares a recent State Department report, "a massive infusion of economic assistance will be required."[8] Such assistance compensates countries for the economic and social costs of shutting down cocaine production. Possible income-replacement measures include supplying hard-currency loans to compensate for the reduced flow of narco-dollars and lowering import barriers for legitimate products (such as textiles and sugar).

In general, strengthening the legal economies of the Andean countries should be an aim of U.S. policy. Economic progress in the region can limit the relative economic power—and consequently the relative political power—of the cocaine industry. However, reducing countries' economic or socioeconomic dependence on cocaine will be a complex, arduous, and expensive task. Take, for example, the hundreds of thousands of small farmers who cultivate coca. A coca farmer in the Bolivian Chapare can net up to $2,600 per hectare per year, more than four times the income he can earn from cultivating the next most profitable traditional crops (oranges and avocadoes). Consequently, crop substitution offers few attractions.[9] The U.S. government is now indirectly paying $2,000 for each hectare of coca eradicated in Bolivia, but the Bolivian government estimates that the social costs of eradication—the costs of redirecting farmers into the licit agricultural economy—would total at least $7,000 per hectare.[10] For Bolivia, where coca grows on between 50,000 hectares and 70,000 hectares, the cost of total eradication would run a mind-boggling $350 million to $490 million. Even if such funding were available, misspending is a risk. Persistent rumors suggest that some coca farmers in the Upper Huallaga Valley and the Chapare used the cash payments for eradication to underwrite the costs of planting new coca fields. Said Freddy Vargas, an MNR deputy in the Bolivian Congress, "We know that in the Chapare the peasants cut back on the coca leaf crop to get $2,000 and then use that money to expand their planting in more remote locations."[11]

Sanctions

Perennially popular with Congress, sanctions include withholding aid, denying trade benefits, cutting off international lending, and restricting the flow of travelers. A few U.S. law enforcement officials advocate (perhaps not entirely seriously) branding Colombia, Bolivia, and Peru as international outlaw states and imposing a near-total embargo on those countries. Unfortunately, the record shows few cases where sanctions achieved the desired objective. Cutting off aid to the Andean countries would probably be counterproductive, arousing intense anti-Yankee feeling, poisoning the diplomatic atmosphere, and reducing the resources available for antidrug campaigns. Furthermore, the countries may simply be incapable of taking the enforcement action demanded by the United States. The Bolivian government, for example, does not dare eradicate coca plantations without the consent of the powerful growers' federations. To do so would risk provoking a civil war in Bolivia.

Moreover, sanctions are too blunt an instrument for specific problems. Thus, when Jorge Ochoa was released from a Colombian jail on December 30, 1987 (the second such release in 16 months), the United States singled out Colombian passengers and products for special customs checks at U.S. ports of entry. According to Bruce Bagley, Colombian exporters of perishable products—for example, shrimp, avocadoes, and bananas—lost an estimated $25 million when their products rotted because of customs delays.[12] Yet, the Colombian government had no jurisdiction over the criminal court judge who ordered Ochoa's release. (The Colombian government, however, did take extraordinary measures to ensure that Ochoa could not escape from jail.) The U.S. sanctions therefore were misplaced: They will not put Ochoa back in jail, nor will they make Colombia's criminal justice system any less porous. Worse, such sanctions undoubtedly intensified the unpopularity of the war against drugs. As Carlos Mauro Hoyas, Colombia's recently murdered attorney general, remarked, "Reprisals against innocent tourists create anger and resentment as well as a sort of solidarity with the drug bosses, not as traffickers but as fellow Colombians."[13]

Negotiations of Cutbacks in Drug Production

Negotiating would require a dialogue with the Escobars, the Ochoas, the Rodríguez Gachas, and the other chief executives of the cocaine industry. The idea of such a dialogue as a prelude to stopping the drug trade—or, alternatively, to legalizing it—attracts enormous public support in Colombia. Supporters include a number of distinguished figures: a former head of Colombia's State Council (the country's top administrative court), a former acting attorney general, two Catholic bishops (of Popayan and Pereira), and several congressmen and academics.[14] The traffickers themselves made a formal offer to the government in 1984, agreeing to withdraw from the cocaine industry, dismantle their laboratories and airstrips, and repatriate their capital. In return, they wanted guarantees against extradition, which would have been tantamount to a safe haven in Colombia. The Colombian government officially says that it will not negotiate with traffickers. In the fall of 1986, according to a July 1988 *Washington Post* report, three Colombian traffickers—Pablo Escobar, Jorge Ochoa, and, curiously, Carlos Lehder—made an informal proposal through a Miami lawyer to the U.S. government: In return for amnesty from prosecution—presumably, the United States would drop requests for extradition—they would abandon the drug trade and provide "sensitive intelligence about leftist guerrillas in Colombia." (Lehder, as noted earlier, did not support the 1984 Panama proposals.) U.S. officials were not sympathetic to the proposal. In an interview, Ann Wrobleski, referring to the traffickers' offer, remarked, "We do not do business with international outlaws—these people are the scum of the Earth."[15]

Certainly, selective amnesty arrangements for criminals can and have been tried as tools of law enforcement. (The United States manages its own witness protection program, for example.) Cocaine chiefs could reveal much about the structure and operations of the international cocaine industry—its supply channels, distribution networks, personnel policies, financing, and names of corrupt U.S. officials who abet the trade. Cocaine capos also could provide information about guerrilla operations, because the two often use the same territory, the same clandestine methods, the same smuggling channels, and even the same overseas banks.

Yet, it is hard to see how the Colombian traffickers' proposal would work in practice. One problem is timing: When the traffickers made their original offer to the Colombian government in 1984, they were under great pressure. Colombia had a functioning extradition treaty with the United States, and traffickers were being tried in military courts, which have a higher conviction rate than civilian courts. Thanks to Colombian Supreme Court decisions, neither of these conditions is operative today, and the Barco government does not possess a great deal of bargaining leverage vis-à-vis the country's cocaine syndicates.

Furthermore, monitoring an amnesty arrangement—the repatriation of capital and the shutting down of a multibillion-dollar industry—presents fundamental problems. How many Colombian law enforcement officials would be necessary to oversee such a program, and who would monitor the monitors? Too, the traffickers might be unable to deliver on their promises. Is the cocaine industry so tightly structured that a few kingpins can command a larger number of lieutenants to order an even larger number of contractors and subcontractors to stop producing a product that earns so much? Possibly, but an amnesty might constitute little more than a retirement program for the chief executives of the cocaine industry.

They would have to make a practical demonstration of their market power, say, by shutting down 80 percent of Colombian cocaine production for 6 months. Amnesty at best represents a futuristic option; the idea has some theoretical merit, but would be extremely difficult to implement. Preparing public opinion for the idea of a détente with drug barons would itself be a challenging task.

These difficulties suggest that curbing the supply of cocaine from producer countries thus may not be effective, regardless of the level of funding that the United States government devotes to overseas programs. U.S. antidrug programs have yielded some useful results in some countries. They have helped to keep the cocaine industry (or much of it) underground, to raise the prices of coca products to Andean consumers, and to limit the inroads that cocaine traffickers can make in the political system. Yet, even if such programs were much more successful than they are now, they would probably have little effect on the consumption of cocaine in the United States. Cocaine traffickers find it all too easy to shift their sources of supply from region to region, from country to country (and, if necessary, from continent to continent). For example, although Operation Blast Furnace made a major dent in Bolivian cocaine production for about 10 weeks, U.S. drug supplies and prices were virtually untouched.[16]

Are there better ways to spend the U.S. drug enforcement dollar? The options seem to be increased interdiction, stepped-up enforcement against drug dealers and pushers, and demand-reduction efforts such as stiffer penalties for users, "Just Say No" programs, and massive and involuntary drug testing. For example, interdiction of drugs at U.S. borders poses some formidable challenges. The U.S. coast line is 90,000 miles long. Approximately 600 commercial and noncommercial vessels, 700 private aircraft, 1,200 commercial flights, 20,000 containers, 25,000 motor vehicles, and 800,000 people enter the United States *each day*. The U.S. Customs Service can detect at most 15 percent of the drug-smuggling flights that enter the United States; less than 5 percent are actually caught.[17] Of the boats stopped on the high seas by the Coast Guard, "with prior information that the boats are suspected of carrying drugs," only one out of eight actually has drugs on board.[18] Enormous Congressional pressure favors getting the U.S. military involved in policing U.S. borders, but the military views such a responsibility as a corruption of its main mission. A Marine lieutenant general in charge of drug policy and enforcement for the Office of the Secretary of Defense asks rhetorically, "What would you give up if you decided to enlist the army, navy, and air force in interdicting the flow of drugs into the United States? Are you going to give up NATO? Are you going to give up our contracts with our friendly allies?

Are you going all of a sudden to say I can't be bothered defending us against missiles?"[19]

In theory, there are four ways to make cocaine less available to users in the United States. One option is going to the source, destroying coca plantations, cocaine laboratories, and trafficking networks in foreign countries. A second option is preventing or restricting cocaine imports. A third approach is destroying drug dealing and money laundering networks within the United States. A fourth option is deterring potential users and convincing those now consuming the drug to stop. The first two options are not likely to affect cocaine imports, short of drastic remedies—for example, destroying all plant life in the Upper Huallaga Valley and the Chapare, saturation-bombing Colombian cocaine laboratories continually, suspending most commerce with South America, imposing martial law at U.S. ports of entry, or shooting down suspected drug-smuggling aircraft on sight. However, the solution to America's cocaine problem—if there is indeed a solution—seemingly lies on the domestic front.

Increasing repression of the cocaine trade domestically does not seem to be a very promising approach. The U.S. court system and prison system are already overloaded with drug cases. Drug law violators account for almost 40 percent of inmates in federal prisons and for about 10 percent of those in state prisons and local jails. In New York City, almost one-half of the felony indictments were for drug offenses, and in Washington, D.C., the figure was more than 50 percent.[20] The vast repressive apparatus of drug enforcement, however, is not a particularly effective deterrent. As Baltimore mayor Kurt Schmoke says, traffickers "care very little about the sanctions of the criminal justice system. Going to jail is just part of the cost of doing business. It's a nuisance, not a deterrent."[21] Measures that attack the financial underpinnings of the drug trade, that focus on the proceeds rather than on the dealer or the product, could constitute a more effective enforcement weapon. Yet, the methods and channels for laundering narco-dollars are numerous and varied. To track the flow of this money could impose intolerable reporting and recordkeeping requirements on banks and on other U.S. institutions that handle large amounts of cash and could represent an intolerable regulatory burden on the IRS, the DEA, and other U.S. enforcement agencies.

Reduction of Demand

The best strategy is to reduce demand, "to punish those who use cocaine, do what we can to break their habit, and try to persuade everyone else not to use it in the first place."[22] Of course, there are political and legal limits to controlling drug consumption, just as there are political and legal limits to controlling production in the Andean countries. One obvious punishment option is imposing mandatory prison sentences on cocaine users. Such a tactic would doubtless produce some deterrent effect, as it did before the trend toward decriminalizing drug use that characterized the late 1960s and 1970s. But the social costs in wrecked careers and lives and the massive expansion in prison capacity required to accommodate the new prisoners make such an approach repugnant to a democracy. Massive compulsory drug testing represents, in the opinion of many Americans, a severe threat to individual freedom. Such testing is being challenged in the courts as a violation of the Fourth Amendment, which affords U.S. citizens protections against unreasonable searches and seizures.

Cleaning up the drug mess undoubtedly will require some restriction of personal liberty as a counterweight to the threat that drug users pose to innocent citizens or to the security of the nation. For example, testing may be warranted for airline pilots, railroad engineers, surgeons, and military commanders. And there is a case to be made for civil penalties to discourage middle-class and upper-middle-class users, who constitute a large percentage of the cocaine-consuming population. Taking away drivers licenses, denying access to federal loans, suspending security clearances, withholding government contracts, and levying large fines such as those that the current drug law authorizes (up to $10,000 for possession of drugs) could make some inroads into the yuppie drug culture. Yet, the main emphasis of demand reduction should be on persuasion rather than coercion. Education and "Just Say No" programs and media campaigns featuring prominent celebrities can at least alert people to the dangers of drug use, although they might not do much to help the hundreds of thousands of people who are already dependent on cocaine. For those people, detoxification via a network of government-run or private treatment facilities is probably the only answer.

Legalization: Benefits and Risks

A completely different approach is removing prohibitions altogether and establishing a structure for the legal sale of drugs, with exceptions such as restricting sales to minors. Advocates of legalization emphasize the social costs of harsh criminal penalties for drug use, costs that can be measured "not just in tax dollars but also in individual lives, personal liberty, political stability, social welfare, and moral well-being."[23] Advocates also stress that drug use is most frequently a crime of self-harm whose solution lies in education, not criminalization. Moreover, advocates contend that the harms ascribed to the sale and use of drugs stem primarily from the *illegality* of the drug; for example, murders associated with the illegal drug trade, overdoses attributable to contaminated or unexpectedly high-dosage drugs, and violent *narcotraficantes* in Latin America. Legalization of drugs, especially cocaine—which is dangerously addictive, particularly when smoked as crack—commands little public support. Few politicians take the career risk of going on record as favoring such a step. Yet, it represents a serious alternative to the current drug war and draws support from a number of scholars, journalists, jurists, and law enforcement officials. Legalization, in combination with a serious drug-use education campaign, deserves serious consideration, if only in the abstract—particularly when no effective solutions have as yet been tried.

Legalizing cocaine and other illicit drugs would clearly produce some positive effects, such as simply saving billions of dollars that are now spent on drug law enforcement. Ethan Nadelmann, a scholar at Princeton University, estimates that U.S. federal, state, and local agencies spent $8 billion in 1987 on "all aspects of drug enforcement, from drug eradication in foreign countries to imprisonment of drug users and dealers in the United States." Moreover, the state could tax the sales of cocaine, heroin, and marijuana. As Nadelmann notes, the net benefit of reduced law enforcement expenditures and of revenues raised by taxing drug consumers and producers could add billions of dollars a year to the U.S. Treasury.[24] Some of this money could conceivably be used to combat drug abuse, for example, to fund long-term programs of drug education, prevention, and rehabilitation. Or the money could be reallocated to other law enforcement targets, such as violent crimes against people and property (which might decline under a legalization program, as noted below).

A second effect of legalization is a drastic lowering of the price of now-illicit drugs. A legal gram of pharmaceutically pure cocaine now costs about $15, but a gram of cocaine that is 50–65 percent pure costs between $80 and $100 on the illicit market.[25] The huge markup is, of course, a function of the costs and risks associated with illicit marketing. Legalization would remove the huge clandestine profits from the drug trade and obviously also would lower operating costs—bribes, elaborate security systems, and private armies. But legalization would drive down drug prices even more noticeably. Falling prices and profits, as legalization advocates argue, would generate several benefits for society. First, if drugs such as heroin or cocaine were significantly cheaper, the number of crimes committed by drug users to support their habits—crimes such as armed robbery, prostitution, and burglary—would probably decline. Criminal organizations would have less financial incentive to operate in the drug trade. The power of criminal networks to corrupt police and judges and (in South America) to manipulate entire governments would wane. Finally, there would be a reduction in the violence that plagues many North

American and South American cities because of internecine warfare among drug dealers. The shootouts between Medellín and Cali cartels, the machine-gun battles between rival gangs in Dadeland and Queens, and other such turf disputes occasionally kill innocent citizens and in general contribute to urban decay.[26]

A third effect of legalization would be a significant reduction of tension, at least initially, in U.S. relations with most drug-exporting countries, especially those nations in Latin America. The era of drug diplomacy would end. The United States would no longer need to certify drug-source countries as eligible to receive foreign aid. The United States would no longer impose sanctions on countries that fail to reduce their coca crop, to stop money laundering, or to control official corruption. The "de-cocainization" of U.S. relations with Latin America would make it easier for the United States to pursue its traditional diplomatic interests in the region. However, narcotics would not disappear as an issue in U.S.-Hemispheric relations. On the contrary, new problems would arise. The decline of prices for cocaine, marijuana, and heroin in U.S. markets could impose major economic and social hardships on producer nations—for example, reduced inflows of foreign exchange, lower prices for drugs all along the production-logistics chain, and some increase in unemployment. Latin American countries would doubtless demand compensation: It is U.S. demand, Latin Americans say with some validity, that created the problem in the first place, distorting economic development and creating huge populations dependent on the production and export of illicit drugs. Legalization undoubtedly would increase the U.S. foreign aid bill and would involve the United States directly in rehabilitating the economies of drug-exporting countries. A more fanciful idea is that the Andean countries would try to maintain prices by cartelizing the cocaine trade—by forming an organization of cocaine-exporting nations, an OCEC. Of course, legalization and the potential for legal profits might mobilize U.S. companies into producing organic or synthetic cocaine and thus competing with OCEC.

Despite these apparent benefits, opponents worry about one major overriding risk: that the number of drug users will expand, perhaps substantially, and will impose a cost on innocent as well as knowing victims and on the moral and productive fiber of the country. Proponents of legalization admit this risk, but argue that it does not justify the current machinery of repression and the consequent social and individual costs. They argue that the risk can be addressed through education and selective drug testing applied under probable-cause criteria. Nonetheless, it seems likely that more people would at least try cocaine if it could be purchased freely or under minimum controls—in liquor stores or drug stores—rather than procured covertly, sometimes in dark alleys and seedy hotel rooms, with the threat of arrest hanging constantly over the buyer and dealer. In the United States today, an estimated 20 million people have tried cocaine. Of these people, between five million and six million use cocaine once a month. Some 200,000 to one million people are compulsive users—addicts who consume the drug every day.[27] Legal sales would almost certainly increase the number of addicts and recreational users, even if only temporarily. Furthermore, legalization would be a very difficult step to reverse—the larger the market, the more formidable the problem of control. As one U.S. commentator recently remarked, "Proposals for legalizing some or all drugs amount to an admission of defeat and invite social catastrophe."[28] Of course, such a prediction could have been made about the repeal of Prohibition—and some would argue that the prediction has been fulfilled—but a continuing system of Prohibition might well be producing economic and social distortions of its own.

Then there is the issue of timing. A successful demand-reduction effort can achieve much the same benefits as legalization, and there are now signs that the appeal of the drug culture in the 1960s and 1970s is beginning to fade. Perhaps the so-called war on drugs may be gaining ground. According to a University of Michigan survey, there was a significant drop in demand for cocaine among adolescents and young adults between 1986 and 1988. Cocaine use had been relatively stable in these groups between 1979 and 1986. For example, the number of high school seniors reporting cocaine use in the year before the survey fell by 38 percent between 1986 and 1987 (from 13 percent of respondents to 8 percent). The same drop occurred among U.S. young adults (high school graduates) between the ages of 19 and 29—respondents reporting use in the last year fell from 20 percent of the sample to 14 percent. Among college students, the decline was from 17 percent to 10 percent of respondents. In all cases, the changes were statistically significant.[29] The Michigan study also shows a long-term decline in marijuana use among high school seniors and young adults since the late 1970s.

The reasons for such turnarounds are not entirely clear, but one possible determinant is a dramatic increase in the number of young people who believe that cocaine is a dangerous drug. For example, the percentage of high school seniors who associate "great risk" with trying cocaine once or twice increased from 34 percent in 1986 to 51 percent in 1988. The number of respondents perceiving occasional use as risky rose from 54 percent to 67 percent. The tragic deaths of sports stars such as Len Bias and Don Rogers—and the well-publicized problems of repentant celebrities—undoubtedly influenced this shift in perception. However, the change also reflects the intensifying attention that political leaders and the news media have given to the cocaine menace.[30]

Do such shifts represent the beginning of a long-term trend? Will use resurge soon or in the future? Obviously, it is too early to tell—and national policies that criminalize 1 out of every 5 or 10 young people must be thoroughly evaluated. Nonetheless, the question must be asked: If Americans, for whatever reasons, are losing their taste for illicit drugs, why legalize them? Individuals with an appetite for drugs will never entirely disappear from U.S. society or other industrialized societies. However, there are grounds for believing that the number of such people can be contained and that the secret of that containment lies in changing the habits and preferences of the U.S. consumer. Destruction of the insidiously appealing drug culture cannot be accomplished overnight—it will take years, perhaps a generation or more, particularly if our experience with alcohol and nicotine is any index.

Should the United States, then, just abandon the idea of controlling cocaine at the source? For political and moral reasons, the United States cannot simply withdraw from the drug war in South America. Antidrug measures, however, will make little headway without improvements in the political and economic infrastructure of producer nations. Prerequisites include stronger law enforcement and judicial systems, better government control over drug-producing zones, and a pattern of self-sustaining economic growth. This suggests that the United States must be prepared to take a comprehensive and long-term view of its narcotics control objectives in South America. For now, North American political leaders and statesmen should attempt to lower the profile of the cocaine issue in U.S. relations with the Andean countries and should encourage normal processes of economic and political development in these countries.

Notes

1. Bureau of International Narcotics Matters, U.S. Department of State, *International Narcotics Control Strategy Report (INCSR)*, 1988, p. 8.
2. Leslie Cockburn, *Out of Control* (New York: Atlantic Monthly Press, 1987), chs. 9, 10.
3. Elaine Sciolino and Stephen Engelberg, "Drive Against Narcotics Foiled by Security Fears," *The New York Times*, April 10, 1988.
4. Quoted in William Long, "Powerful Medellín Cartel Safe in its Colombian Base," *Los Angeles Times*, February 21, 1988.
5. Congressional Research Service, *Combatting International Drug Cartels: Issues for U.S. Policy* (Washington, D.C.: U.S. Senate, 1987), Report for the Caucus on International Narcotics Control, p. 13.
6. "Perú vera con EE. UU. solución al problema de los cocales," *El Comercio*, August 4, 1988.

7. Committee on Armed Services, U.S. House of Representatives, *Narcotics Interdiction and the Use of the Military: Issues for Congress* (Washington, D.C.: U.S. Government Printing Office, 1988), Report of the Defense Policy Panel and Investigation Subcommittee, p. 7.
8. *INCSR*, 1988, p. 8.
9. Gerald Owens, "Costs of Production: Coca," unsolicited report to AID, December 31, 1986, p. 6.
10. Peter McFadden, "New Eradication Program Winning Over Coca Farmers," Associated Press, Business News, December 31, 1987, p. 8.
11. Roberto Fernandez O., "The Reduction of Chapare Coca Plantations: A Farce or Fact," *Los Tiempos*, March 8, 1988.
12. Conversation with Bruce Bagley in Biloxi, Mississippi, June 17, 1988.
13. Alan Riding, "Colombia Says U.S. Reprisals Weaken Support for Drug Fight," *The New York Times*, January 13, 1988.
14. See, e.g., "Hay que hablar con los narcos dicen 2 obispos," *El Tiempo*, February 13, 1988.
    "Lo único que hacemos es el oso," interview with Gutierrez Marquez, *El Tiempo*, February 22, 1988.
    Richard Craig, "Illicit Drug Traffic Implications for South American Source Countries," *Journal of Interamerican Studies and World Affairs*, Volume 29, No. 2 (Summer 1987), p. 4.
15. Michael Isikoff, "Medellín Cartel Leaders Offered U.S. a Deal," *The Washington Post*, July 20, 1988.
16. Inter-American Dialogue, *The Americas in 1988: A Time for Choices*, Washington, D.C., April 28, 1988, pp. 22–23.
17. Barbara Bradley, "From School Yards to High Seas; U.S. Wages War on Drugs," *Christian Science Monitor*, March 7, 1988.
    Committee on Government Operations, U.S. House of Representatives, *National Narcotics Law Enforcement Strategy* (Washington, D.C.: U.S. Government Printing Office, 1988), Hearings, March 3, 1988, p. 10.
18. Peter Reuter, "Intercepting the Drugs; Big Cost, Swift Results," *The Washington Post*, May 18, 1988.
    Peter Reuter et al., *Sealing the Borders: The Effects of Increased Military Participation in Drug Interdiction* (Santa Monica: The RAND Corporation, 1988), p. 44.
19. Stephen Olmstead, "The Role of the Military in the Nation's War on Drugs," paper delivered at a conference on "The Latin American Narcotics Trade and United States National Security," June 16–17, 1988, Biloxi, Mississippi, pp. 8–9.
20. Ethan Nadelmann, "U.S. Drug Policy: A Bad Export," ("U.S. Drug Policy") *Foreign Policy*, No. 70 (Spring 1988), pp. 98–99.
    Ethan Nadelmann, "Shooting Up," *The New Republic*, June 13, 1988, p. 17.
21. Kurt Schmoke, "Decriminalizing Drugs," *The Washington Post*, May 15, 1988.
22. James Lieber, "Coping with Cocaine," *The Atlantic*, January 1986, p. 39.
23. "U.S. Drug Policy," p. 83.
24. "U.S. Drug Policy," p. 105.
25. "Coping with Cocaine," p. 44. This argument is based on the work of Steven Wisotsky, a law professor at the University of Wisconsin.
26. "Shooting Up," pp. 11–17.
27. National Institute of Drug Abuse, "Cocaine Use in America," *Prevention Network*, April 1986, p. 1.

National Narcotics Intelligence Consumers Committee (NNICC), *The NNICC Report 1985-1986* (Washington, D.C., June 1987), p. 26.
28. Jeffrey Eisenach, "Why America Is Losing the Drug War," *Backgrounder* (Washington, D.C.: The Heritage Foundation, June 9, 1988), pp. 9, 11.
29. University of Michigan, "Details of Annual Drug Survey," *News and Information Services*, January 13, 1988, pp. 1, 2.
University of Michigan, "Teen Drug Use Continues Decline," *News and Information Services,* February 24, 1989, pp. 1–5.
30. Ibid.

Selected Bibliography

Books

Albani, Joseph L. *The American Mafia: Genesis of a Legend*. New York: Appleton-Century-Crofts, 1971.

Amado, Canelas Orellana and Juan Carlos Canelas Zannier. *Bolivia: Coca Cocaína*. La Paz: Los Amigos Del Libro, 1983.

Ashley, Richard. *Cocaine: Its History, Uses and Effects*. New York: Warner Books, 1975.

Aspiazu, Rene Bascope. *La Veta Blanca: Coca y Cocaína en Bolivia*. No location listed: Ediciones Aquí, 1982.

Bakalar, James B. and Lester Grinspoon. *Drug Control in a Free Society*. Cambridge: Cambridge University Press, 1984.

Barco, Virgilio. *Hacia una Colombia Nueva*. Bogotá: Editorial La Oveja Negra, 1986.

Briceno, Carlos Alberto. *Las Drogas en El Perú*. Lima: Sesator, 1983.

Cabieses, Fernando. *Etnología, Fisiología y Farmacología de la Coca y la Cocaína*. Lima: Sociedad de Beneficiencia Pública de Lima, 1985.

Carter, William E. (cómpilador). *Ensayos Científicos Sobre la Coca*. La Paz: Librería Editorial Juventud, 1983.

Castillo, Fabio. *Los Jinetes de la Cocaína*. Bogotá: Editorial Documentos Periodísticos, 1987.

Caycedo, Germań Castro. *El Karina*. Bogotá: Plaza & Janes, 1985.

Cockburn, Leslie. *Out of Control*. New York: Atlantic Monthly Press, 1987.

Deustua, Alejandro. *El Narcotráfico y El Interés Nacional*. Lima: Centro Peruano de Estudios Internacionales, 1987.

Eddy, Paul, with Hugo Sabogal and Sara Walden. *The Cocaine Wars*. New York: W. W. Norton & Company, 1988.

Grinspoon, Lester and James R. Bakalar. *Cocaine: A Drug and Its Social Evolution*. New York: Basic Books Inc., 1978.

Guizado, Alvaro Camacho. *Droga Corrupción y Poder: Marihuana y Cocaína en la Sociedad Colombiana*. Cali: Universidad del Valle, Centro de Investigaciones y Documentación Socioeconómica (CIDSE), 1981.

Instituto de Estudios Políticos Para América Latina (IEPALA). *Narcotráfico y Política Militarismo y Mafia en Bolivia*. Madrid: Graficas Margaritas, 1982.

Jaramillo, Jaime, Leonidas Mora, and Fernando Cubides. *Colonización, Coca y Guerrilla*. Bogotá: Universidad Nacional de Colombia, 1986.

Jaramillo, Mario Arango. *Impacto del Narcotráfico en Antioquia*. Medellín: J. M. Arango, 1988.

Jaramillo, Mario Arango and Jorge Child Vélez. *Los Condenados de la Coca: El Manejo Político de la Droga*. Medellín: J. M. Arango, 1985.

Jaramillo, Mario Arango and Jorge Child. *Narcotráfico Imperio de la Cocaína*. Medellín: Editorial Percepción, 1984.

Jeri, F. R. (ed). *Cocaine 1980: Proceedings of the Interamerican Seminar on Coca and Cocaine*. Lima: Pacific Press, 1980.

Kelly, Robert J. (ed). *Organized Crime: A Global Perspective*. Totowa, N.J. Roman & Littlefield, 1986.

Lara, Patricia. *Siembra Vientos y Recogerás Tempestades*. Bogotá: Editorial Punto de Partida, 1982.

Medina, Samuel Doria. *La Economía Informal en Bolivia*. La Paz: EDOBOL, 1986.

Mills, James. *The Underground Empire: Where Crime and Governments Embrace*. Garden City, New York: Doubleday & Company, 1986.

Mitchell, Christopher. *The Legacy of Populism in Bolivia: From the MNR to Military Rule*. New York: Praeger Publishers, 1977.

Molano, Alfredo. *Selva Adentro*. Bogotá: El Ancora Editores, 1987.

Musto, David F. *The American Disease: Origins of Narcotics Control*. New Haven, Connecticut: Yale University Press, 1973.

Orozco, Jorge Eliecer. *Lehder . . . El Hombre*. Bogotá: Plaza & Janes, 1987.

Pacini, Deborah and Christine Franquemont (eds). *Coca and Cocaine: Effects on People and Policy in Latin America*. Peterborough, New Hampshire: Transcript Printing Company, June 1986.

Pardo, Rodrigo and Juan G. Tokatlian. *Política Exterior Colombiana*. Bogotá: Tercer Mundo Editores, 1988.

Phillips, Joel L. and Ronald D. Wynne. *Cocaine: The Mystique and the Reality*. New York: Avon Books, 1980.

Reid, Michael. *Peru: Paths to Poverty*. London: Latin American Bureau, 1985.

Reuter, Peter, *Disorganized Crime, The Economics of the Visible Hand*. Cambridge, Massachusetts: MIT Press, 1983.

Reuter, Peter, Gordon Crawford, and Jonathan Cave. *Sealing the Borders: The Effects of Increased Military Participation in Drug Interdiction*. Santa Monica: The RAND Corporation, 1988.

Rincon, Fabio. *Ochoa: La Extradición La Captura*. Bogotá: VEA, no date listed.

———. *La Extradición*. No location listed: Imarchar Editores, 1984.

Shannon, Elaine. *Desperados: Latin Drug Lords, U.S. Lawmen, and the War America Can't Win*. New York: Viking, 1988.

Stendal, Russell. *Rescue the Captors*. Burnsville, Minnesota: Ransom Press International, 1984.

Tanzi, Vito (ed). *The Underground Economy in the United States and Abroad*. Lexington, Massachusetts: Lexington Books, 1982.

No author listed. *Narcotráfico y Política II: Bolivia 1982–1985*. Cochabamba: No publisher listed, 1985.

Articles

Bagley, Bruce M. "Colombia and the War on Drugs." *Foreign Affairs*. Fall 1988.
———. "The Colombian Connection: The Impact of Drug Traffic on Colombia." In: Deborah Pacini and Christine Franquemont (eds), *Coca and Cocaine: Effects on People and Policy in Latin America*. Peterborough, New Hampshire: Transcript Printing Company, June 1986.
Block, Alan A. "A Modern Marriage of Convenience: A Collaboration Between Organized Crime and U.S. Intelligence." In: Robert J. Kelly (ed). *Organized Crime: A Global Perspective*. Totowa, New Jersey: Rowman and Littlefield, 1986.
Collett, Merrill. "The Myth of the 'Narco-Guerrillas.'" *The Nation*. August 13–20, 1988.
Craig, Richard B. "Illicit Drug Traffic: Implications for South American Source Countries." *Journal of Interamerican Studies and World Affairs*. Volume 29, No. 2, Summer 1987.
———. "Illicit Drug Traffic and U.S.-Latin American Relations." *The Washington Quarterly*. Volume 8, No. 4, Fall 1985.
———. "Domestic Implications of Illicit Colombian Drug Production and Trafficking." *Journal of Interamerican Studies and World Affairs*. Volume 25, No. 3, 1983.
———. "Colombian Narcotics and United States-Colombian Relations." *Journal of Interamerican Studies and World Affairs*. Volume 23, No. 3, 1981.
Gomez, Hernando. "La economía ilegal en Colombia: tamaño, evolución, características, e impacto económico," *Coyuntura Económica*, September 1988.
Gugliotta, Guy and Jeff Leen. "Medellín Cartel: The World's Deadliest Criminals." *Miami Herald* (Special Report). February 1987.
Healy, Kevin. "Bolivia and Cocaine: A Developing Country's Dilemmas." *British Journal of Addiction*. Volume 83, 1988.
———. "The Boom Within the Crisis: Some Recent Effects of Foreign Cocaine Markets on Bolivian Rural Society and Economy." In: *Coca and Cocaine: Effects on People and Policy in Latin America*. Cultural Survival Report 23, June 1986.
Junguito, Roberto and Carlos Caballero. "Illegal Trade Transactions and the Underground Economy of Colombia." In: *The Underground Economy in the United States and Abroad*. 1982.
Lee, Rensselaer W. III. "Why the U.S. Cannot Stop South American Cocaine." *ORBIS*. Fall 1988.
———. "The Drug Trade and Developing Countries." Overseas Development Council. *Policy Focus*. No. 4, May 1987.
———. "The Latin American Drug Connection." *Foreign Policy*. No. 61, Winter 1985–86.
Lieber, James. "Coping with Cocaine." *The Atlantic*. January 1986.
Lupsha, Peter A. "Organized Crime in the United States." In: Robert J. Kelly (ed). *Organized Crime: A Global Perspective*. Totowa, New Jersey: Rowman and Littlefield, 1986.
———. "Drug Trafficking: Mexico and Colombia in Comparative Perspective." *Journal of International Affairs*. Volume 30, No. 1, Spring–Summer 1981.
Massing, Michael. "The War on Cocaine." *The New York Review*. December 22, 1988.

Nadelmann, Ethan A. "U.S. Drug Policy: A Bad Export." *Foreign Policy*. No. 70, Spring 1988.

Perl, Raphael and Roy Surrett. Congressional Research Service. "Drug Control: International Policy and Options." Issue Brief #IB88093, August 31, 1988.

Plowman, Timothy. "Botanical Perspectives on Coca." In: F. R. Jeri (ed), *Cocaine 1980: Proceedings of the Interamerican Seminar on Coca and Cocaine*. Lima: Pacific Press, 1980.

Reuter, Peter. "Eternal Hope: America's Quest for Narcotics Control." *The Public Interest*. No. 79, Spring 1985.

Valcourt, Richard R. "Controlling U.S. Hired Hands." *International Journal of Intelligence and Counterintelligence*. Vol. 2, No. 2, 1988.

White, Peter T. "Coca—An Ancient Herb Turns Deadly." *National Geographic*. January 1989.

Hearings, U.S. Senate

Committee on Appropriations, U.S. Senate. *International Narcotics Control*. Hearings: January 10, 1985. Washington, D.C.: U.S. Government Printing Office, 1985.

Committee on Foreign Relations, U.S. Senate. Subcommittee on Terrorism, Narcotics and International Communications. *Drugs, Law Enforcement and Foreign Policy: The Cartel, Haiti and Central America*. Hearings: April 4–7, 1988. Washington, D.C.: U.S. Government Printing Office, 1988.

———. *Drugs, Law Enforcement, and Foreign Policy*. Hearings: February 8–11, 1988. Washington, D.C.: U.S. Government Printing Office, 1988.

Committee on Foreign Relations, U.S. Senate. Subcommittee on Terrorism, Narcotics and International Communications and International Policy, Trade, Oceans, and Environment. *Drugs, Law Enforcement and Foreign Policy*. Hearings: May 27, July 15, and October 30, 1987. Washington, D.C.: U.S. Government Printing Office, 1988.

Committee on Foreign Relations and the Committee on the Judiciary, U.S. Senate. *International Terrorism, Insurgency, and Drug Trafficking: Present Trends in Terrorist Activity*. Joint Hearings: May 13–15, 1985. Washington, D.C.: U.S. Government Printing Office, 1986.

Committee on Governmental Affairs, U.S. Senate. Subcommittee on Investigations. *Drugs and Money Laundering in Panama*. Hearings: January 28, 1988. Washington, D.C.: U.S. Government Printing Office, 1988.

———. *International Narcotics Trafficking*. Hearings: November 10, 12, 13, 17, 18, 1981. Washington, D.C.: U.S. Government Printing Office, 1981.

Committee of the Judiciary, U.S. Senate. Subcommittee on Security and Terrorism; the Subcommittee on Western Hemisphere Affairs of the Foreign Relations Committee; and the Senate Drug Enforcement Caucus. *The Cuban Government's Involvement in Facilitating International Drug Traffic*. Joint Hearings: April 30, 1983. Washington, D.C.: U.S. Government Printing Office, 1983.

Committee on Labor and Human Resources, U.S. Senate. Subcommittee on Alcoholism and Drug Abuse. *Drugs and Terrorism, 1984*. Hearings: August 2, 1984. Washington, D.C.: U.S. Government Printing Office, 1984.

Hearings, U.S. House of Representatives

Committee on Appropriations, U.S. House of Representatives. Subcommittee on Foreign Operations and Related Agencies. *Foreign Assistance and Related Programs Appropriations for 1986.* Hearings: March 27, 1985. Washington, D.C.: U.S. Government Printing Office, 1985.

Committee on Foreign Affairs, U.S. House of Representatives. *Narcotics Review in the Caribbean.* Hearings: March 9, 1988. Washington, D.C.: U.S. Government Printing Office, 1988.

———. *Worldwide Narcotics Review of the 1988 International Narcotics Control Strategy Report.* Hearings: March 3, 1988. Washington, D.C.: U.S. Government Printing Office, 1988.

———. *Narcotics Review in South America.* Hearings: March 17 and 22, 1988. Washington, D.C.: U.S. Government Printing Office, 1988.

———. *Recent Developments in Colombia.* Hearings: January 27, 1988. Washington, D.C.: U.S. Government Printing Office, 1988.

———. *Recent Developments in Colombian Narcotics Control.* Hearings: May 24, 1984. Washington, D.C.: U.S. Government Printing Office, 1984.

———. *U.S. Response to Cuban Government Involvement in Narcotics Trafficking and Review of Worldwide Illicit Narcotics Situation.* Hearings: February 21 and 23, 1984. Washington, D.C.: U.S. Government Printing Office, 1984.

Committee on Government Operations, U.S. House of Representatives. A Subcommittee Meeting. *National Narcotics Law Enforcement Strategy.* Hearings: March 31, 1988. Washington, D.C.: U.S. Government Printing Office, 1988.

President's Commission on Organized Crime. *Organized Crime and Cocaine Trafficking.* Hearings IV: November 27–29, 1984. Washington, D.C.: U.S. Government Printing Office, 1984.

Select Committee on Narcotics Abuse and Control, U.S. House of Representatives. *National Drug Policy Board Strategy Plans.* Hearings: April 14, 1988. Washington, D.C.: U.S. Government Printing Office, 1988.

———. *U.S. Foreign Policy and International Narcotics Control.* Hearings: March 16, 1988. Washington, D.C.: U.S. Government Printing Office, 1988.

———. *U.S. Foreign Policy and International Narcotics Control-Part II.* Hearings: March 29, 1988. Washington, D.C.: U.S. Government Printing Office, 1988.

———. *Colombian Drug Trafficking and Control.* Hearings: May 6, 1987. Washington, D.C.: U.S. Government Printing Office, 1987.

———. *International Narcotics Policy.* Hearings: June 22, 1983. Washington, D.C.: U.S. Government Printing Office, 1984.

Reports

United States International Development Cooperation Agency, Agency for International Development. *Bolivia: Chapare Regional Development.* Project paper, no dates given.

Central Intelligence Agency. *The World Factbook 1988.* Washington, D.C.: U.S. Government Printing Office, May 1988.

Committee on Armed Services, U.S. House of Representatives, Defense Policy Panel and Investigations Subcommittee. *Narcotics Interdiction and the Use of the Military: Issues for Congress.* Report: June 7, 1988. Washington, D.C.: U.S. Government Printing Office.

Committee on Foreign Affairs and Committee on Foreign Relations, U.S. House of Representatives and U.S. Senate. *Legislation on Foreign Relations Through 1987.* Joint Report. Volumes I and II: March 1988. Washington, D.C.: U.S. Government Printing Office, 1988.

Committee on Foreign Affairs, U.S. House of Representatives. *International Terrorism: A Compilation of Major Laws, Treaties, Agreements, and Executive Documents.* Report: August 1987. Washington, D.C.: U.S. Government Printing Office, 1987.

————. *Compilation of Narcotics Laws, Treaties, and Executive Documents.* Report: June 1986. Washington, D.C.: U.S. Government Printing Office, 1986.

Caucus on International Narcotics Control, U.S. Senate. *Narcotics-Related Foreign Aid Sanctions: An Effective Foreign Policy?* Report: July 30, 1987. Washington, D.C.: U.S. Government Printing Office, 1987.

————. *On-Site Staff Examination of Narcotics Control Efforts in Bolivia.* Report: July 1987. Washington, D.C.: U.S. Government Printing Office, 1987.

————. *Combatting International Drug Cartels: Issues for U.S. Policy.* Report: May 8, 1987. Washington, D.C.: U.S. Government Printing Office, 1987.

Comité Multiseccional de Control de Drogas (COMUCOD). *Plan Nacional de Prevencia y Control de Drogas, Mediano Plazo, 1986-1990.* Lima, 1986.

Bureau of International Narcotics Matters, United States Department of State. *Midyear Update, International Narcotics Control Strategy Report.* September 1988.

————. *Midyear Update, International Narcotics Control Strategy Report.* September 1987.

————. *International Narcotics Control Strategy Report (INCSR).* Washington, D.C., March 1, 1989.

————. *INCSR.* Washington, D.C., March 1, 1988.

————. *INCSR.* Washington, D.C., March 1, 1987.

————. *INCSR.* Washington, D.C., March 1, 1986.

————. *INCSR.* Washington, D.C., February 1, 1986.

————. *INCSR.* Washington, D.C., February 1, 1985.

————. *INCSR.* Washington, D.C., February 1, 1984.

Dirección de Policía de Drogas de la Guardia Civil de Peru. *Projecto de Ayuda Específica del Gobierno de EE. UU. de NA para la Guardia Civil del Peru.* Lima 1984.

Drug Enforcement Administration, U.S. Department of Justice. *Worldwide Cocaine Trafficking Trends.* Special Report: May 1985.

Earth Satellite Corporation. *Bolivian Coca: Technical Evaluations of Recent Aerial Survey Projects in the Chapare Region.* Washington, D.C., April 15, 1981.

General Accounting Office. *Drug Control: U.S. Supported Efforts in Colombia and Bolivia.* Washington, D.C.: U.S. Government Printing Office, November 1988.

Government of Bolivia. "Triennial Program of the Battle Against Narcotics Trafficking." La Paz, November 1986.

Government of Bolivia and Government of the United States of America. *Project Agreement: Control of Legal Coca.* La Paz, August 11, 1983.

International Monetary Fund (IMF). *International Financial Statistics.* Washington, D.C.: IMF, August 1988.

Instituto Nacional de Planificacion. *Plan Nacional de Eliminación del Narcotráfico.* (Proyecto). Lima, 1986.

Inter-American Development Bank (IADB). *Economic and Social Progress in Latin America, 1988 Report.* Washington, D.C.: IADB, 1988.

IRI Research Institute. *Huallaga Valley Agribusiness and Marketing Study.* A consultancy report to the United States Agency for International Development. Stamford, Connecticut, May 1985.

Ministerio de Planeamiento y Coordinación. *Acuerdo entre el Gobierno Constitucional COB, CSUTCB y Federaciones Campesinas Productoras de Coca Sobre el Plan Integral de Desarrollo y Substitución de los Cultivos de Coca y la Lucha Contra el Narcotráfico.* La Paz, June 6, 1987.

National Narcotics Intelligence Consumers Committee. *The NNICC Report 1987: The Supply of Illicit Drugs to the United States.* Washington, D.C., April 1988.

————. *The NNICC Report 1985-1986: The Supply of Illicit Drugs to the United States from Foreign and Domestic Sources in 1985 and 1986.* Washington, D.C., June 1987.

————. *Narcotics Intelligence Estimate 1984.* Washington, D.C., 1984.

————. *The Supply of Drugs to the U.S. Illicit Market from Foreign and Domestic Sources in 1980.* Washington, D.C., 1980.

President's Commission on Organized Crime. *America's Habit: Drug Abuse, Drug Trafficking and Organized Crime.* Report to the President and Attorney General. Washington, D.C.: U.S. Government Printing Office, March 1986.

Select Committee on Narcotics Abuse and Control, U.S. House of Representatives. *U.S. Congressional Delegation to the Andean Parliament, Paipa and Bogotá, Colombia.* Study Mission Report. Washington, D.C.: U.S. Government Printing Office, 1987.

————. *Latin American Study Missions Concerning International Narcotics Problems.* Report: August 3–19, 1985. Washington, D.C.: U.S. Government Printing Office, 1986.

————. *International Narcotics Control Study Missions to Latin America and Jamaica (August 6–21, 1983), Hawaii, Hong Kong, Thailand, Burma, Pakistan, Turkey, and Italy (January 4-22, 1984).* Report: August 2, 1984. Washington, D.C.: U.S. Government Printing Office, 1984.

————. *South American Study Mission.* Report: August 9–23, 1977. Washington, D.C.: U.S. Government Printing Office, 1977.

Glossary

AID: The U.S. Agency for International Development.

ANAPCOCA: Asociación Nacional de Productores de Coca, the National Coca Producers Association in Bolivia.

CALI CARTEL: Cali-based coalition of trafficking families.

CHAPARE: Bolivia's most important coca-growing area, encompassing the provinces of Chapare, Carrasco, and Tiraque in Cochabamba department.

COB: Central Obrera Boliviana, the Bolivian Workers Union.

CONAN: Comando Nacional Anti-Narcótico, the National Anti-Narcotics Police in Colombia.

COINCOCA: Comité de Industrialización de Coca, the Coca Industrialization Committee in Bolivia.

COMUCOD: Comité Multisectoral de Control de Drogas, Multisectoral Committee Control of Drugs, a Peruvian planning agency.

CONCOCA: Comité Coordinador Nacional de Productores de Coca, the National Coordinating Committee of Coca Producers in Bolivia.

CORAH: Control y Reducción de Cultivos de Coca en el Alto Huallaga. U.S.-financed Coca Reduction Agency in the Upper Huallaga, under Peru's Ministry of Interior.

CSUTCB: Confederación Sindical Unica de Trabajadores Campesinos de Bolivia, the Bolivian Peasants Union, affiliated with the COB.

DIPOD: Dirección de Policía de Drogas, the Anti-Drug Section of the Civil Guard (national police) in Peru.

DIRECO: Dirección de Reducción de Cultivos de Coca, the Coca Reduction Agency in Bolivia, under the Bolivian Ministry of Agriculture.

ELN: Ejército de Liberación Nacional, the National Liberation Army, a Colombian guerrilla group.

ENACO: Empresa Nacional de Coca, the National Coca Enterprise in Peru.

EPL: Ejército Popular de Liberación, the Popular Liberation Army, a Colombian guerrilla group.

FARC: Fuerzas Armadas Revolucionarias de Colombia, the Revolutionary Armed Forces of Colombia, Colombia's largest guerrilla group.

FEAT: Federación Especial de Trabajadores Campesinos del Trópico de Cochabamba, the main coca growers' federation in the Chapare.

FEDIPs: Frentes de Defensa de los Intereses del Pueblo, popular self-defense franís—loosely-organized coalitions of local interest groups in Peru.

ICA: Instituto Colombiano Agropecuario, the Colombian Agricultural Institute.

INDERENA: Instituto Nacional de Los Recursos Naturales Renovables, the Colombian National Institute of Natural Renewable Resources.

INM: The U.S. State Department's Bureau of International Narcotics Matters.

MAS: Muerte a Los Secuestradores, or Death to Kidnappers, a vigilante organization founded by Medellín traffickers in 1981.

M-19: The April 19th Movement, a Colombian revolutionary group.

MEDELLÍN SYNDICATES (OR MEDELLÍN CARTEL): Medellín-based coalition of trafficking families.

MRTA: Movimiento Revolucionario de Tupac Amaru, the Tupac Amaru guerrilla movement in Peru.

NNICC: National Narcotics Intelligence Consumers Committee, the federal coordinating body for drug estimates in the United States.

PEAH: Proyecto Especial del Alto Huallaga, the Special Upper Huallaga Project, a U.S.-financed development agency in the Upper Huallaga Valley.

QUINTÍN LAMÉ: A small, ethnically-based revolutionary group in Colombia.

SENDERO LUMINOSO: Shining Path, Peru's largest guerrilla organization.

SMIMFA: Sociedad Multidiciplinaria de Investigación Médica y Farmacológica Autoctona, the Medical-Pharmaceutical Research Society in Bolivia.

UMOPAR: Unidad Móvil de Patrullaje Rural, the name given to rural mobile patrol units in Bolivia and Peru.

UPPER HUALLAGA VALLEY: The main coca-growing area in Peru, encompassing parts of San Martín and Huanuco departments.

Index